P9-AGA-552

DATE DUE

DEMCO 38-296

REVIEWS IN ENGINEERING GEOLOGY
VOLUME XII

A PARADOX OF POWER:
VOICES OF WARNING AND REASON
IN THE GEOSCIENCES

Edited by

CHARLES W. WELBY
Department of Marine, Earth, and Atmospheric Sciences
North Carolina State University
Raleigh, North Carolina 27695-8208

and

MONICA E. GOWAN
GeoLogic Co.
P.O. Box 5237
Glacier, Washington 98224

Access to power must be confined to those who are not in love with it.
————Plato

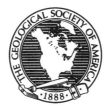

The Geological Society of America, Inc.
3300 Penrose Place, P.O. Box 9140
Boulder, Colorado 80301
1998

Riverside Community College
Library
4800 Magnolia Avenue
Riverside, CA 92506

TA 705 .P37 1998

A paradox of power

Copyright © 1998, The Geological Society of America, Inc. (GSA). All rights reserved. GSA grants permission to individual scientists to make unlimited photocopies of one or more items from this volume for noncommercial purposes advancing science or education, including classroom use. Permission is granted to individuals to make photocopies of any item in this volume for other noncommercial, nonprofit purposes provided that the appropriate fee ($0.25 per page) is paid directly to the Copyright Clearance Center, 27 Congress Street, Salem, Massachusetts 01970, phone (508) 744-3350 (include title and ISBN when paying). Written permission is required from GSA for all other forms of capture or reproduction of any item in the volume including, but not limited to, all types of electronic or digital scanning or other digital or manual transformation of articles or any portion thereof, such as abstracts, into computer-readable and/or transmittable form for personal or corporate use, either noncommercial or commercial, for-profit or otherwise. Send permission requests to GSA Copyrights.

Copyright is not claimed on any material prepared wholly by government employees within the scope of their employment.

The Reviews in Engineering Geology series was expanded in 1997 to include Engineering Geology Case Histories, 11 volumes of which were published by the Geological Society of America from 1957 to 1978 with ISBNs from 0-8137-4001-0 to 0-8137-4011-8. Beginning with Volume XI, Reviews in Engineering Geology may include both reviews and case histories, under the ISBN 0-8137-4111-4 and subsequent numbers.

Published by The Geological Society of America, Inc.
3300 Penrose Place, P.O. Box 9140, Boulder, Colorado 80301

Printed in U.S.A.

GSA Books Science Editor Abhijit Basu

Library of Congress Cataloging-in-Publication Data
A paradox of power : voices of warning and reason in the geosciences /
    edited by Charles W. Welby and Monica E. Gowan.
        p.   cm. -- (Reviews in engineering geology ; v. 12)
    Includes bibliographical references.
    ISBN 0-8137-4112-2
    1. Engineering geology.   2. Environmental health.   3. Health risk
assessment.   4. Environmental geology.   5. Environmental
geotechnology.   I. Welby, Charles W.   II. Gowan, Monica E.
III. Series.
TA705.R4 vol. 12
624.1'51 s   98-9275
[624.1'51] --DC21   CIP

10   9   8   7   6   5   4   3   2   1

Contents

Preface

Power (pou'er): 1. The ability or capacity to act or perform effectively. 2. . . .
3. Strength or force exerted or capable of being exerted; might. 4. The ability or official
capacity to exercise control; authority. (*American Heritage Dictionary*)
Enlightenment (en-lit' n-ment): The state of possessing knowledge and truth. (*American
Heritage Dictionary* synonyms for "knowledge")

This volume is about the power of geoscience in the context of environmental issues. Most North Americans consider themselves environmentalists on one level or another. Many seek environmental enlightenment; others wish to be perceived as environmentally enlightened. Yet there are a myriad of views on what constitutes "enlightenment." We live and work in a world of idealogical conflict over "true" environmental enlightenment where clashes between epistemological and theological belief systems can produce seemingly intractable situations. Often these conflicts are a struggle for power rather than insight.

Into this conflict steps the geoscientist. Because of our knowledge and professional judgment we are often asked by stakeholders to provide assistance for a magnanimous purpose: to sort out conflicts of fact and value; to protect public safety; to find resources; to help design or engineer solutions; or to provide scholarly answers. We are also asked to provide Machiavellian means to achieve certain ends. Whether the power struggle is social, economic, legal, or political, we are asked and sometimes expected to provide counsel that helps a client, agency, or organization "win" its wars. For either purpose the inescapable result is that stakeholders place us in a position where we can control or influence opinions and decisions.

Herein lies the paradox of geoscience knowledge. It puts us in a position of power, allowing us to use our knowledge as a tool or weapon. This power shoulders us with seemingly antithetical responsibilities to provide wise counsel in warning of potential risk or error yet to counter hysteria with discriminating thought or reason. Often we must meet these responsibilities with limited knowledge or conflicting evidence. This paradox challenges our ethics in our relationships with others, with the Earth, and with ourselves. It tests our steadfastness to truth, purpose, responsibility, and trust.

Out of this paradox and its concomitant challenges to ethics and soundness arose two theme sessions, Environmental Geology: The Voice of Warning and Environmental Geology: The Voice of Reason, which the Geological Society of America's Institute for Environmental Education (IEE) and the Committee on Geology and Public Policy sponsored at the 1992–1995 annual meetings. The sessions sought to focus on how geoscientists can meet this challenge by helping create an informed citizenry and by assisting decision-makers on environmental matters.

Many excellent presentations discussed new ways to express difficult concepts, to engage the public intellectually, to assess the viability of analytical methods, and to provide approaches to achieving conflict resolution. Some papers highlighted issues of data reliability and relevance and difficulties in determining causal relationships. Others clarified misconceptions of risk and offered philosophical perspectives on ethical, legal, pedagogical, social, economic, and political aspects of environmental issues. Thirteen of these papers have been selected for publication in this volume. They share an awareness that political realities can render the value of geoscience information moot if it does not provide the answers sought, yet they aspire to assist the citizen and decision-maker in asking the right questions. It is hoped that these papers provide insight on the application of geology to public policy issues and guidance for implementing effective approaches with personal integrity and scientific expertise. Perhaps they will also spawn valuable insight into the reader's own professional challenges and provoke a little philosophical musing on how the geoscience profession can best serve society.

The intent in developing the *Voices* sessions was to provide a forum for discussion on how geoscientists can be problem solvers in environmental conflicts. The sessions were guided by the belief that the best chance for creative solutions might lie in educating the public and decision-makers on *how to think* more than on *what to think* about environmental geoscience issues. Fred A. Donath, past executive director of IEE, supported the idea and saw it as complementary to IEE's goal of applying geology to the "wise use of Earth." David Gross, a former member of GSA's Committee on Geology and Public Policy, also believed in the idea and provided the support of the committee. Charles W. Welby and the Engineering Geology Division of GSA recognized the value of sharing a collection of papers in a publication. From this support of the *Voices* sessions came the current volume. It is my hope that you will find it valuable and a stepping stone to further discussion on the positive power of the science for which we share a passion.

Monica E. Gowan
November 1996

Introduction

In preparing this volume the editors have chosen papers to form chapters of the volume that examine the issues of public health and welfare from different aspects. We have placed the chapters into four major groupings to emphasize these aspects.

The first group addresses issues related to decision-making about land use and natural resources. The first two chapters provide a framework for decision-making—based in part on the variability of temporal and spatial scales in the geologic environment—that can be a tool for resolving environmental complexity. Gerhard calls for establishment of priorities and rejection of spurious issues through a matrix approach that analyzes environmental issues at the global through local level of interest. Pinet et al. apply a hierarchial classification to process-response elements of geomorphic systems to assist in assessing the impact of environmental effect. In the third chapter, Thorson et al. discuss how the public perception of environmental *wildness* may be incongruous with the true *naturalness* of wetlands in New England. Their emphasis is on the need to incorporate the geological perspective in the evolution of wetlands and in their attributed value.

Geology and health provide the context for several "voice of warning" discussions. Burns et al. illustrate a case history of public education about radon potential in Portland, Oregon, which empowered citizens to heighten their personal awareness of their relationship to environmental hazards. Jibson et al. document the first case of an outbreak of coccidioidomycosis (valley fever) being related unequivocally to an earthquake and attendant natural phenomena, opening a new area of concern in natural hazard preparation and response. Welby discusses the risk of ground-water contamination from application of biosolids to agricultural lands and the need for decision-makers to contemplate future possible uses of the land when considering biosolid land disposal. Levson et al. discuss concepts related to earthquake damage mitigation and the methodology by which regional potential hazards maps can be developed from existing information supplemented by additional geologic data. These maps can be used in land-use planning and for emergency planning purposes.

The next group of chapters illustrates ideas related to the "voice of reason" concept. They offer prudent alternatives to regulatory and engineering approaches in solving environmental problems. Reid and Carpenter note the facility with which asbestos-monitoring requirements can be waived based on the results of bedrock mapping. Keaton and Lowe discuss how a geological approach could have assessed more accurately and cost effectively debris-flow hazards in contrast to the engineering methods that incorrectly defined 100-year flood plains along the Wasatch Front.

Ethical and philosophical questions confronting geoscientists under the "paradox of power" are addressed in the fourth group of chapters. Cronin and Sverdrup set the stage for a discussion of ethics in the geosciences through their work to protect the public by proper fault identification in the Malibu Coast Fault Zone. Whether a fault is classed as active or is recognized as a "fossil fault" bears upon proper use of land and on property rights questions. Feld et al. note that in the Love Canal trial the search for truth varied in process and criteria, depending upon one's professional background and perspectives. Bjerstedt wrestles with the question of How much information is enough? in contemplating work at Yucca Mountain for a high-level radioactive waste disposal site. Boak and Dockery emphasize the need to access the validity of conflicting descriptions of reality when making long-term projections of geologic systems.

Although all the chapters discuss important issues in and by themselves, taken as a whole they provide a perspective of the relationship among geology, environmental questions about how humans use Earth's resources, and ethical questions about how best to integrate geologic knowledge into systems of human welfare and safety.

Acknowledgments

The editors acknowledge the assistance of a number of people who made this volume possible. First are those who encouraged the development of the GSA theme sessions between 1992 and 1995 in which the papers were first presented orally: Fred Donath and David Gross. Theme session co-chairs who guided the oral discussions included Calvin Alexander, William Berry, Scott Burns, Monica Gowan, Brett Leslie, Syed Hassan, Jeffrey Keaton, Mac Ross, and Charles Welby. Former chairs of the Engineering Geology Division, Jerome DeGraff, Rhea Graham, and Michael Hart, supported the development of the volume during their tenures.

Reviewers play an important role in the evaluation of papers for such a volume. Because of the variety of topics covered in the papers, the editors chose reviewers not only within the GSA family but among others who by reason of their professional responsibilities possessed knowledge and understanding that might make their review of particular value to the authors of the manuscripts. To these persons the editors and the authors are especially appreciative: Dyane Brown, Edward R. Burt III, John M. Dennison, Tom Drake, Dale Dusenbury, Duane A. Eversoll, David W. Folger, Richard M. Fry, G. David Garrett, Neil J. Gilbert, Charles H. Gardner, Monica E. Gowan, Bruce W. Hurley, Mark E. Landis, Matthew A. Mabey, Peter Malin, Christopher C. Mathewson, Malcolm Ross, William P. Scott, Henry M. Singletary, James E. Slosson, Edward F. Stoddard, and Gerald F. Wieczorek.

Finally, no volume can exist without the efforts and interest of the authors. To them the editors say, "Thank you" for the time and effort that each has spent on their respective manuscripts. The editors hope that we have set them in a context that makes them useful.

Geological Society of America
Reviews in Engineering Geology, Volume XII
1998

The dilemma of the geologist: Earth resources and environmental policy

Lee C. Gerhard

State Geologist and Director, Kansas Geological Survey, 1930 Constant Avenue, Campus West, Lawrence, Kansas 66047

ABSTRACT

American environmental policy has developed over the last 25 years under a preservation ethic, which is a dilemma for geologists who must explore for and develop earth resources for society. Geologists have a professional responsibility to provide the earth resources, upon which society absolutely depends, in a society that values unspoiled scenic vistas more than the earth resources they contain. Recent federal elections have amplified public debate over the appropriateness of current environmental laws and policy. Impacts of environmental preservation policies are seen in a decline in standard of living, in lack of consensus on priorities, and lack of science in risk management. In order to sustain society's needs for earth resources, we must reexamine our stance about environmental standards, and develop a holistic approach to balancing societal needs for resources with societal desires for a pleasant physical environment. Human health and safety should be our most important goals; recreation and esthetics are of lesser importance to most of the world's population.

THE PROBLEM

Environmental policy and law in the United States have been driven by a preservation ethic for more than 20 years but have come under increasing criticism in the last few years for perceived excesses detrimental to personal property, individual rights, and economic progress. Many of these issues are being fought out in the Congress and in court as this is written. Rhetoric on both sides is strong, but the media, which had favored environmental preservation, are now more equitably examining issues and effects (Ward, 1993).

In recent years grassroots organizations favoring individual rights, private property rights, and resource conservation have risen to challenge environmental preservation organizations in the legislative process. Legal challenges to environmental groups and assessment of litigation costs for frivolous complaints are now being instituted (The Anchorage Times, 1993). Questions about cost/benefit ratios and special interests now are routine, and there are frequent challenges to soft or poor science underlying popular issues. Zealots and their excesses have pulled the entire environmental movement and its hard-fought gains under scrutiny. Some of these gains have been unquestionably good for

the nation and all its people, but there is a backlash as fringe groups strive to press their agendas upon an increasingly perceptive and unwilling public. Congressional review of major environmental laws at any time may either improve the effectiveness of the legislation or simply change direction and focus of environmental law.

In consequence, it is absolutely necessary to reestablish the basic tenets of a national environmental policy that preserves an acceptable quality of life for all of American society in its equations of cost and benefit. National environmental policy must satisfy generally accepted norms for it to be successful, norms that include opportunities for citizens to be economically upwardly mobile, that create jobs for those who wish to work, that provide a realistically healthy life environment for all, and that provide a breadth of recreational opportunities accessible to all. Our national policies now conflict with these norms.

Further, our environmental policies must be science driven rather than agenda driven. Misleading science has no place in public policy. Science that is the basis of regulatory action must be separated from the regulatory actions themselves. Law that is contrary to science can not be tolerated if we are to keep public faith and support for sustaining the physical environment to

Gerhard, L. C., 1998, The dilemma of the geologist: Earth resources and environmental policy, *in* Welby, C. W., and Gowan, M. E., eds., A Paradox of Power: Voices of Warning and Reason in the Geosciences: Boulder, Colorado, Geological Society of America Reviews in Engineering Geology, v. XII.

which we aspire. We must confront inaccurate science, half-truths, and mistruths.

Geologists are the forefront of these issues because we are largely responsible for providing the earth resources upon which society is sustained, yet we find ourselves ever increasingly limited in where we can explore for and develop the energy and minerals the nation needs.

Five major areas of weakness are present in national environmental policy: (1) there is a lack of recognition of societal needs for earth resources to preserve the standard of living; (2) there are no established environmental priorities; (3) there is no consensus on environmental standards; (4) environmental policy is fractured by spurious issues, suffers from inflation of issue significance, and accepts direction by special interests; and (5) effective environmental action requires higher quality and more holistic science than now attained.

Let us examine some issues the American public must understand if we are to develop a rational and useful national policy. While I anticipate much debate about what is included in this conceptual base, it forms a nucleus about which to crystallize our debate.

LACK OF RECOGNITION OF SOCIETAL NEEDS FOR EARTH RESOURCES

The very fabric of society is rooted in earth resources, but there is no widespread public understanding of the relationship of standard of living, earth resource wealth, and costs of environmental policy. Earth resources are not accorded the significance in policy that they play in sustaining the economy and our social fabric. One reason for this lies in the divorcement of the American people from their earth resources: land, water, minerals, energy, agriculture, and forestry. Increasing urbanization has created a separation between resource use and understanding of resource origins. Little connection is made by "Aunt Sophie" between turning on her television set and mining coal; dressing in new man-made fiber clothing and drilling oil wells; or eating a bounteous meal and making fertilizers, products of those same oil wells. Many years ago we farm kids laughed at city kids who thought milk came from bottles in grocery stores. We did not correct then the problem of source and product divorcement, so now we reap conflict over resource access.

Why worry? I worry because the basis of American wealth that provides our standard of living is the monetary value of extracted American earth resources, plus the value added to these resources through manufacturing. The relationship can be expressed as:

$$S_{ol} = W/P$$

where S_{ol} = standard of living, W = national wealth, and P = population (Gerhard and Puderbaugh, 1993).

Limitation of national access to earth resources—be they water, timber, farmland, minerals or energy resources—assumes that the limitations will mean that fewer of the resources are used (Gerhard and Weeks, 1996). In fact, limitation of access and increased costs of value-adding simply substitute foreign earth resources for our own, and transfer American wealth elsewhere to pay for the substitution. Thus, the term "W" does not increase as much as it would if the access were unlimited. Population continues to grow, that of the United States growing from 125,000,000 to over 257,000,000 in my lifetime, from the mid-1930s to the present. The United States has managed to increase its wealth in proportion to its population growth until recently. The ratio is declining, and this reflects in a lessened rate of increase in standard of living. When coupled to the trade balance figures of the same years, there is an absolute decrease in standard of living indicated for the United States (Figs. 1, 2).

The obvious consequence of this change in standard of living growth is a reduced standard of living for the already financially disadvantaged of America. The effects of increased costs of resource access, environmental regulation, and importation fall most heavily on those least able to afford it; in effect, the environmental movement has become regressive. "Environmental racism" is a term frequently used in nonscientific literature to refer to siting of potentially environmentally hazardous or unsightly facilities in minority neighborhoods. Brimelow and Spencer (1992) argue that the early 1990s cost of environmental regulation by the Environmental Protection Agency (EPA), using EPA's own estimates of cost, was about $450 per person per year, with dramatic increases into this decade.

Our social fabric depends on continuation of our standard of living, despite arguments that the standard is too high. Too high for whom? Perhaps the financially advantaged will wish to voluntarily give up some of their toys, but an ever-increasing financially disadvantaged class who cannot find new jobs when displaced by the depressed economy, who have never found a stable job, and who live on taxpayer largesse have nothing left to give. I cannot address the unequal distribution of wealth in this paper, but it must be part of our environmental equation.

At this writing the national debate about balancing our federal budget rages. We cannot balance a budget without cutting social programs or increasing revenues. Current environmental regulations stifle economic progress and depress revenues, perhaps rightfully, but they are now viewed by many as part of a national problem.

ESTABLISHING ENVIRONMENTAL PRIORITIES

There is no prioritization of environmental issues in national policy today. Each group, each interest, devotes its energy, time, and resources to narrow and often counterproductive issues, without understanding the overall impact of the issue of the proposed solutions on the global setting. People think narrowly. Often the costs of mitigation are not proportionate to the problem, or larger problems are ignored in favor of popular sentiment for small-scale issues.

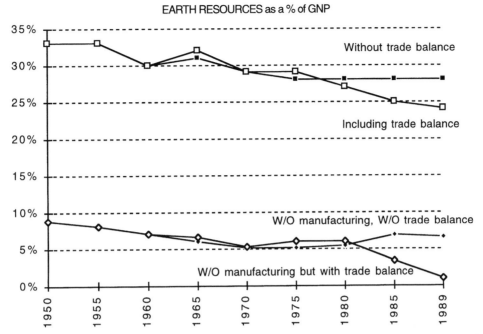

Figure 1. Percentage (%) of earth resources value in the gross national product (GNP). Upper curves of graph include "value-adding" manufacturing. Trade balance summed with curve as noted. Note that the percentage of earth resources in the GNP declined from 1950 to 1975, then stabilized, if trade balance is not included. However, when the balance of trade, largely controlled by the price of imported oil, is included, the percentage continues to drop. The lower curves reflect just the value of earth resources (agriculture, forestry, construction, fishing, and mining, including oil and gas extraction), without (w/o) the manufacturing value, divided by the GNP, without the trade balance, the curve shows a decline in percentage from 1950 to 1970, but increases slightly from 1980 to 1989. When the trade balance is included, the value drops precipitously from 1980 to 1989. All values are based on 1992 dollars. Data from post-1989 not available. Data from U.S. Bureau of Census (from Gerhard, 1996).

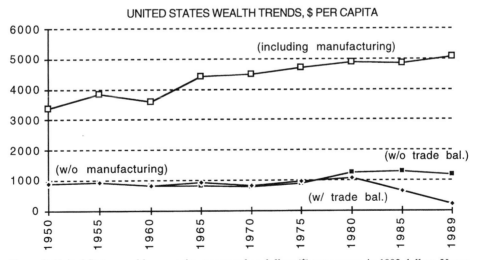

Figure 2. United States wealth per capita, expressed as dollars ($) per person, in 1992 dollars. Uppermost curve represents value of earth resources, including "value-added" manufacturing, which rises steadily in value per capita from 1950 to 1980. From 1980 to 1989 the rate of increase is very small. The lower curves present the earth resource wealth values per capita without (w/o) the "value-added" manufacturing. The upper curve does not include the trade balance (bal.), the lower curve does include the trade balance (w/ = with). Note the steep drop in wealth per capita from 1980 to 1989 as the increasing value of imported resources is summed into the total. Unequal distribution of wealth accounts for an apparent increasing standard of living of the wealthier portion of population, and the worsening plight of the financially disadvantaged. Data from U.S. Bureau of the Census (from Gerhard, 1996).

Scalar issues

In a previous paper (Gerhard, 1994), I outlined a base scaling of issues, ranging from microenvironmental issues to mega-issues, which I reiterate and amplify here.

Microenvironmental issues. Issues that are short term or in home are microenvironmental, such as disposal of household chemicals, lawn mulching, objections to sand and gravel extraction in the neighborhood, recycling of household wastes, and similar small-scale individual decisions. These are personal decisions, and although they impact the lives of others, their impact tends to be very local, and action agendas can be very personal.

Macroenvironmental issues. These issues are of larger temporal scale and cut across geographic boundaries. They include air pollution in large cities, single major aquifer contamination or dewatering, factory smokestack output, or single tributary stream basin issues. Frequently, like the preceding class, these are issues of NIMBY, "not in my backyard," but actions of no one person can realistically materially affect an issue.

Tackling these issues requires organizational action rather than personal action, but care must be exercised not to let parochial views override negative effects of actions on the community.

Mesoenvironmental issues. Regional in nature, these issues may have impact on very large numbers of people. The Mount Saint Helens volcanic eruption and the eruption of Mount Pinitubo in the Philippines are examples of natural phenomenon that fall into this category. Acid rain, when perceived as an issue, would have fallen into this category. Automobile efficiency and offshore drilling prohibitions are of similar scale in their potential long-term effects on standard of living. Population growth is at least this important. Pesticide regulation, predator control, insect control, and crop fertilization are all issues of this magnitude and have great impact on nearly all of society.

Great care must be exercised in the application of governmental power to insure that the issues solved are not symptoms, and that the solutions devised are real, necessary, and do not cause negative large scale–downstream effects. National government is responsible for exercising this concern and care, but must do so in an open and informed arena. The examination and treatment of environmental problems must be holistic.

Megaenvironmental issues. Global climate change, ozone concentrations, and biodiversity are the three most popular issues today in America, although the furor over ozone depletion seems to have waned. However, overpopulation, mass famine, soil erosion, desertification, and massive plague are much more pressing to the majority of the world. Mega-issues are of global scale.

Impacts on society

Once issues have been scaled in scope and size, they then can be scaled as to impact on society.

Human health and safety. There should be no argument that the highest priority for environmental action is about issues adversely affecting human health and safety, but the importance of an issue should reflect the geographic scale or number of individuals in need. For instance, global climate change, when it occurs, whether it is cooling or warming, would affect the entire global population. A spread of the *Ebola*-type virus could be a mega-issue of human health. Megaenvironmental issues affecting human health and safety are the most important issues of all.

Perturbations of natural systems. Earth systems suffer human interference poorly. Whether groins are installed to preserve one beach that in turn cause erosion farther along shore, or whether there is unwise construction on flood plains or in earthquake zones; much human suffering and death occurs when geologic systems are ignored. Thirty thousand deaths in a recent earthquake in India underscores the need to consider earth systems as one of the most significant environmental parameters affecting humans. The 1993 Midwestern United States floods also emphasize the problems of human interference in natural systems: artificial river control measures on rivers in the Midwest added significantly to flooding, and the unrestrained development of flood plains in these areas was responsible for preventable damage.

Societal interest issues. These issues are primarily conflicts between perceived environmental issues and property valuation. Facilities siting problems are at the root of most of these problems, although occurrence of pests, moderate air pollution, and other inconveniences resulting from human activity fall into this category. Frequently these issues are expressed as "NIMBY," (not in my backyard) issues. Many of these issues also reflect changing values and concepts of personal risk in society, such as using environmental laws and zoning to preclude mixing of incomes and social classes, establishment of social support facilities (such as halfway houses), and thoroughfares and bus routes in neighborhoods.

Esthetic issues. Many loudly contested environmental issues involving earth resources are simply esthetic issues: some people regard an oil well drilling location in the Rocky Mountains as an engineering marvel; others regard it as an invasion of pristinity. Mines and mining districts are variously regarded as environmental eyesores or as major historical artifacts of our heritage. For many of these issues perspective is individual and not based upon real long-term physical environmental effects. Haze in the national parks may be objectionable, but it has never been documented as a hazard. Many times arguments over esthetic issues pit region against region, or community against community, for some of the nastiest confrontations of all. Recreational interests have precipitated many confrontations, since many recreation issues benefit only the financially advantaged.

Graphic evaluation and prioritization. The scalar values for the environmental priorities versus the societal values can be cross-plotted to arrive at a generalized "significance factor" for each issue discussed, where ranking 1 = greatest long-term significance and 16 = least (Table 1).

This table provides a measurement for the importance of any issue. At a minimum, use of the table requires that each participant critically examine his or her stance, identify the perti-

TABLE 1. SCALE OF VALUES FOR EVALUATION OF ENVIRONMENTAL ISSUES

| | Societal Value | | | |
	(1) Health, Safety, of People	(2) Nat. Systems Perturbations	(3) Societal Interest	(4) Esthetics, Recreation
Scale Value				
(1) Mega-	1	2	3	4
(2) Meso-	2	4	6	8
(3) Macro-	3	6	9	12
(4) Micro-	4	8	12	16

nent aspects of his or her issue, and then argue for inclusion in a priority block.

By means of Table 1, earth scientists can focus on real resource and environment issues, while demonstrating to lay citizens the relative merit of other issues.

SUGGESTED OTHER ACTIONS

Building consensus on environmental standards

There are no consensus environmental standards. There is no national consensus about what our ultimate goals are. There can be no "pristinity," since it never existed. The biota and the earth have been changing for billions of years and will continue to change. Humans are part of the biota, their works and deeds are part of the equation with which we work, and wishful thinking and social engineering will not change that constraint. Therefore, we must agree on a set of standards to be attained. That agreement will not be by simple congressional vote or agency rule—it will have to be a consensus of the people. Why is this necessary? Simply, we are now enforcing environmental policy by ex post facto regulations and by constantly changing attainment standards. Our employers are never sure of their attainment goals, and the costs of constant change serve only to depress the economy and suppress capital development.

In order to build a national consensus on standards it is necessary to recognize that regional differences exist and adjust standards to these differences. For instance, the national 55 mile-per-hour speed limit instituted during the oil crisis of the 1970s was never truly enforceable in many states and resulted in the most massive civil disobedience since Prohibition. Laws that make little sense are rarely obeyed, and in Nevada and Montana, as examples, the speed limit law simply made lawbreakers out of average, law-abiding citizens. Yet, in the eastern states, the law made sense—there are many more passenger-miles driven in the populated east, distances are shorter, and traffic accidents more frequent. What was good for Massachusetts, however, was not useful for Nevada, where the opposite conditions exist. As one example of the current change in federal attitude, that law was repealed.

Similarly, methods of trash and garbage disposal in New

York City are not an individual option, and care must be exercised to insure that the mass of garbage and toxic chemicals disposed of in that teeming metropolis do not pollute the region; however, it is most difficult to argue reasonably that the trash and garbage of one remote Wyoming ranch should be subject to the same regulations as New York City. The costs of rural trash disposal under new federal law almost insures widespread passive disobedience. The town of Pretty Prairie, Kansas, faces the imposition of EPA fines and penalties for not having constructed a water purification plant to treat its town water, which the EPA contends violates the EPA nitrate standard. The cost of the plant would be about $600,000. The town has a property tax base of about $16,000 per year. There will be no locally funded water plant, no matter what EPA insists. Civil disobedience is the result of poor legislation and regulation.

Clearly, population density is a major controlling factor in environmental mitigation. The EPA has not established baselines including naturally occurring chemistry of water, air, and land. Acquisition of baseline information should be a first priority of the EPA. Then population density criteria should be developed to implement standards of "pristinity" that are truly appropriate to the various population densities.

Special interests and agendas

The environmental debate has been fraught with spurious issues, misinformation, and special interests. There is need to ask questions about issues, about motivation and group benefits (Heidelberg Appeal, 1992). There is need to weigh costs against accomplishment. There is need to analyze issues clearly and in language that all understand.

Our global environment is constrained first by its geology, second by its chemistry, and third by its biology. The role of natural earth systems in constraining the environment and controlling human effects is poorly understood except by geologists. Thirty thousand deaths in remote India from preventable earthquake damage is not a concern to most people, whereas the possibility of a few or perhaps tens of early deaths from natural radon is considered a major national issue. Floods annually kill and bankrupt people, but little is done to mitigate these controllable effects of natural events. We do not nationally recognize what level of natural risks we face.

Lack of geologic perpsective arises frequently. One of the great quasi-scientific mistruths is that we are "running out" of a resource (read oil, iron, copper, etc.). The geologic truth is that our resources are unlimited for all practical purposes. Most people do not understand that richness of resources controls price and value, and we simply run out of resources that we are willing or able to afford. During the oil embargo and consequent price rise, we conserved. Now, during the lowest prices in recent history, we use oil freely. Technology also provides resource alternatives when the marketplace demands them.

Possible global climate warming is another case in point. There is near hysteria about the catastrophic changes humankind is wreaking on global climate. Yet, we ignore that the only evidence for climate warming is increased CO_2 in the atmosphere. The climate has not yet changed. Greenland ice cores have provided striking information that makes our present CO_2 issue pale. The amplitude of earth climate variation documented in the Greenland ice core is great, but more important, the core documents two major human-interest issues. First, the last 8,000 years have been remarkably stable in climate, compared to all previous time. Human civilization has evolved in the last 8,000 years without regard to the natural climatic cycles of the past, but will almost certainly have to engineer society to survive the swings that will occur. The swings tend to occur with changes in atmospheric CO_2 concentrations, which also took place before civilization. Second, climate changes may not take centuries to evolve, they may take place in decades (Dansgaard et al., 1993; Mayewski, 1993).

John S. Perry recently wrote for the National Academy's Board on Global Change, "Yet each year will bring a new environmental crisis clamoring for redress in political councils—ozone depletion last year; climate this year; invasion of exotic species, ground water quality, chemical time bombs, tropospheric ozone, and so on in years to come" (Perry, 1992, p. 13, 14).

It is possible to advocate issues for personal or professional gain. There is much research money to be gained if your issue is perceived to be the "catastrophe of the year." Issues of "rangeland reform" and changes in the 1872 Mining Law are not about fees the federal government collects, but about recreation and esthetics; mines are not pretty when operating, and cattle are not native animals. Therefore all issues and any proposed solutions should be questioned, specifically targeting the beneficiaries of proposed policy. Some questions that need to be asked are:

1. Why is the policy, law, or action necessary? What are the costs, and what are the benefits?

2. Is "who benefits" identified, along with "who loses?" Do all citizens receive benefit from the action and is any group unfairly bearing the costs? Are the special interests identified?

3. Is the scale of action appropriate to the scale of effects?

4. Are the proposed changes scientifically sound or else scientifically innocuous? Will the action precipitate a worse problem? Is the risk being mitigated worth the risk being introduced?

5. Are anthropogenic effects carefully separated from natural effects?

Environmental action requires high quality and holistic science

Perhaps most important to us who work as scientists is the need for scientific integrity in the law and rule-making process. Legal language must be scientifically valid and arguments based more upon scientific fidelity of issues. The earth is a planet, a relatively solid body of minerals that happens to be enclosed in a thin envelope of fluids (oceans and atmosphere) in which we have evolved. That is our final constraint. It is incumbent upon us, geologists, to confront inadequate, dishonest, and poor environmental and resource science.

Science is not well-integrated in federal environmental law and regulations. Environmental law should be a statement of legislative principles and objectives. The implementing regulations are where objective science should play a very strong role, but where objective science is commonly sacrificed. For instance, the legal language of The Endangered Species Act contains a scientifically fraudulent definition of species that provides for the protection of subspecies, and does not provide standards for designation of therein defined species (subspecies) (The Endangered Species Act, P.L. 93-205 et seq.).

The Environmental Protection Agency sets standards for contamination that have become measurement-technology-based rather than based upon actual knowledge of human effects or human evolutionary tolerance. Where numeric standards are specified, they may lead to requirements that are not technically feasible. Where technology is specified rather than goals, market disruptions can occur. There is a clear need for objective science to support regulations and advise Congress about implications of proposed laws. There are two actions that the federal government can take to mitigate these problems.

The federal government should reorganize natural resources and environmental research to remove such research from the regulating agencies and into an independent agency focused on providing objective science. The National Aeronautics and Space Administration (NASA) is a suitable organizational structure model. Geologists should advise the federal government on needs and organization for natural resources and environmental research. A recent Hedberg Research Conference sponsored by the American Association of Petroleum Geologists Division of Environmental Geosciences recommended that the federal government should ensure that assessment of natural resources and environmental research is conducted by scientific, not regulatory agencies. Regulatory agencies should develop policy and regulations based on the objective research provided by a "natural resource and environmental science agency" (Gerhard et al., 1996).

Second, risk-based assessment and risk management must be the cornerstone of all public environmental policy. Much environmental regulation is based upon perceived risk and esthetic values. Human health and safety are of paramount concern, but risks are not well understood. Consequently, law and regulations may address issues of little consequence while omitting consideration of real issues. Much has been written about risk assessment in the human environment, and informal risk numbers are frequently used in television broadcasts and other media. The ultimate goal of science-based risk assessment is to prioritize the issues upon which public dollars and economic activity are expended. Choices include economic, human health, and intangible values, such as esthetics. Weighing risks among the options available and placing resources where we can save the greatest number of lives are obvious goals.

Geological responsibility. Finally, there is concern that the earth sciences are not playing an appropriate role in the public debate about natural resource access and production. Geologists and their professional societies have not met their public responsibilities to provide objective science to the legislative and regulatory process. Geology must be better represented in Washington to provide objective science to lawmakers and regulators. It is clear that those who propose new endangered species and other land withdrawals succeed unless objections are raised and appropriate science is presented to counter withdrawal arguments. Thus, agencies generally err on the conservative, correctable, side, and succumb to the "squeaky wheel" syndrome. The responsibility of the profession of geology is to provide the earth resources to society that society needs, even when society does not generally recognize its needs or the conflicts between its needs and desires.

SUMMARY

As a broadly educated geologist and natural scientist, I am most concerned with the issues revolving around the access to and extraction of earth resources, while cognizant of the broad chemical and biologic questions being raised. I am confused by rhetoric, rhetoric that decries the mere presence of humankind on earth while ignoring the explosive growth of global population and that is unwilling to address the population issue. I am confused by those who purport to investigate the scientific issues of environment, while choosing, against advice, to ignore the fundamental geological controls on global environment and biodiversity. I resent the regressive nature of current environmental policy that places a disproportionate share of environmental costs upon those least able to afford to pay.

The nation needs environmental leadership that can make positive advances, that can encompass all of its citizens, and be open to public scrutiny. We must strive to improve the process that develops our environmental policy. Our economy must be able to support the environmental costs, and provide for standard of living in addition to the environmental quality of life. We must develop policy that reflects a consensus of the people, and that encourages enthusiastic support and compliance. Setting standards, insisting upon high standards of ethics and truth, allowing for regional differences, and providing frameworks for evaluation of issues and results are crucial to long-term success. We have not yet reached these goals.

ACKNOWLEDGMENTS

The data used in this paper were in part extracted from a data base on environmental issues constructed by Bobette Puderbaugh, whose assistance and discussions have been invaluable to me.

REFERENCES CITED

The Anchorage Times, 1993, Fighting back: reprinted from The Anchorage Daily News by The Professional Geologist, v. 30, no. 12, p. 21.

Brimelow, P., and Spencer, L., 1992, You can't get there from here: Forbes Magazine, July 6, 1992, p. 59–64.

Dansgaard, W., and 11 others, 1993, Evidence for general instability of past climate from a 250-kyr ice-core record: Nature, v. 364, p. 218–220.

The Endangered Species Act (P.L. 93-205, approved December 28, 1973; as amended by P.L. 100-707, approved November 23, 1988) (16 U.S.C. §§1531–1543), §1532. (Definition of species includes: species is defined as subspecies . . . and population segments that interbreed when mature.)

Gerhard, L. C., 1994, Framing policies of resources and environment: Geotimes, v. 39, no. 5, p. 20–22.

Gerhard, L. C., 1996, Earth resources and our environment: resource and policy problems and solutions: Environmental Geosciences, v. 3, no. 2, p. 76–82.

Gerhard, L. C., and Puderbaugh, B., 1993, Earth resources and society: Kansas Geological Survey Open-File Report 93-10, 17 p.

Gerhard, L. C., and Weeks, W., 1996, Earth resources data: A basis for resource analysis and decision-making: Environmental Geosciences, v. 3, no. 2, p. 62–75.

Gerhard, L. C., Oglesby, C., and Rice, R., 1996, Rational science for rational policy: Environmental Geosciences, v. 3, no. 2, p. 57–61.

Heidelberg Appeal, 1992, Beware of false gods in Rio: The Professional Geologist, v. 30, no. 12, p. 15.

Mayewski, P. A., 1993, Greenland ice core "signal" characteristics: an expanded view of climate change: Journal of Geophysical Research, v. 98, no. D7, p. 12839–12847.

Perry, J. S., 1992, The United States global change research program: National Research Council, National Academy Press, 20 p.

Ward, B., 1993, The media turn skeptical: The Environmental Forum, v. 10, no. 4, p. 4.

Manuscript Accepted by the Society June 5, 1997

Printed in U.S.A.

Geological Society of America
Reviews in Engineering Geology, Volume XII
1998

Resolving environmental complexity: A geologic appraisal of process-response elements and scale as controls of shoreline erosion along southeastern Lake Ontario, New York

Paul R. Pinet and Charles E. McClennen
Department of Geology, Colgate University, Hamilton, New York 13346
Laura J. Moore
Earth Sciences Department, University of California at Santa Cruz, Santa Cruz, California 95064

ABSTRACT

Geomorphic systems are inherently complex and are the product of a unique integrative history of surface processes, making it difficult for engineers, scientists, and resource managers to regulate environmental change in order to attain a specific management goal. A powerful means for unpacking geomorphic complexity is hierarchical classification of the dominant process-response elements of a geomorphic system. We apply hierarchical analysis specifically to the evaluation of the probable environmental effects of erosion-abatement projects at drumlin bluffs along the southeastern shore of Lake Ontario, assessing their impact across a variety of spatial and temporal scales. Some of the conclusions about probable impacts of shore-stabilization structures on the Ontario lakeshore are not intuitive, but are logically derived from the systematic hierarchical analysis of the system's geomorphic complexity.

INTRODUCTION

Given that geomorphic systems, all of them, are inherently complicated, how does one engineer or manage environmental change? There are a variety of investigative strategies for understanding and evaluating change in geomorphic systems (Cooke and Doornkamp, 1990). One effective technique for unpacking environmental complexity is to examine geomorphic systems within an hierarchical framework, endeavoring to understand them in a variety of spatial and temporal spheres (Kennedy, 1977) that are relevant to the management problem at hand. Recognizing the multiplicity of spatial scales and time frames over which landscapes respond to and in turn influence the driving geomorphic forces is vital for effective decision making and planning (Leopold and Langbein, 1963). This assertion is particularly germane given that the contemporary documentation of geomorphic processes and responses is typically inadequate for elucidating the long-term evolutionary pathway of landscapes and their landforms (Church, 1980).

We report our research findings about the complex geomorphic character of the New York shore of Lake Ontario (Fig. 1) and their implications for understanding and managing environmental change. Our specific objectives in this paper are (1) to review briefly the many spatially and temporally based factors that produce complex causality in geomorphic systems, (2) to describe the technique of hierarchical analysis for understanding geomorphic change, and (3) to apply hierarchical analysis to managing bluff recession along the southeastern Lake Ontario shore.

THE NATURE OF ENVIRONMENTAL COMPLEXITY

The results of current studies, both theoretical and field-based, have deepened our understanding of the geomorphic behavior and history of landscapes and their associated sedimen-

Pinet, P. R., McClennen, C. E., and Moore, L. J., 1998, Resolving environmental complexity: A geologic appraisal of process-response elements and scale as controls of shoreline erosion along southeastern Lake Ontario, New York, *in* Welby, C. W., and Gowan, M. E., eds., A Paradox of Power: Voices of Warning and Reason in the Geosciences: Boulder, Colorado, Geological Society of America Reviews in Engineering Geology, v. XII.

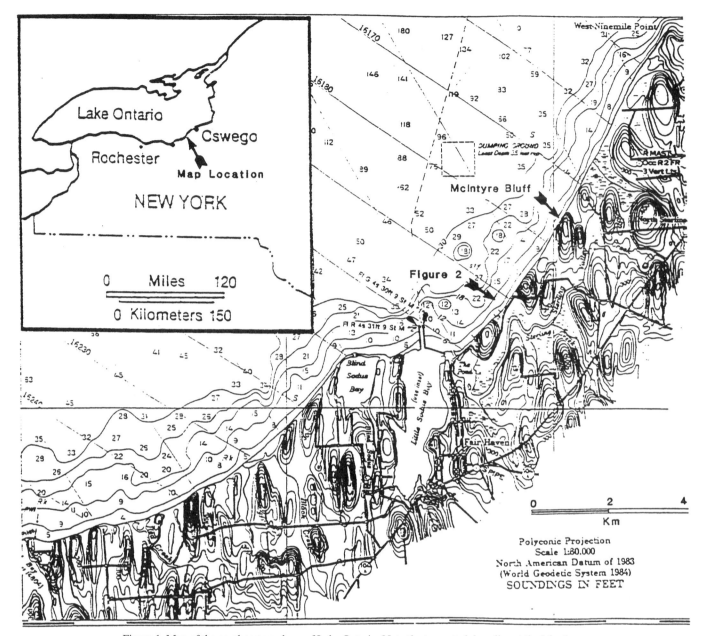

Figure 1. Map of the southeastern shore of Lake Ontario. Note the truncated drumlins at the lakeshore that supply sediment to a downdrift barrier located to the east of each bluff. The first arrow to the right of Little Sodus Bay indicates the beach that was measured to provide shore-recessional data (Fig. 2). The second arrow identifies McIntyre Bluff, where much of the field work on bluff development was completed.

tary deposits. Not only are the driving forces entangled across a variety of spatial and temporal domains, but also geological and biological responses to these stimuli are complex (Chorley, 1962; Swanson et al., 1988; Montgomery, 1989; Cooke and Doornkamp, 1990; Allen and Hoekstra, 1992; Burt, 1994). Each landform within a geomorphic landscape occupies a specific location and is the product of a unique integrative history of surface processes, which because of long relaxation times may not be in equilibrium with the present-day environmental conditions (Montgomery, 1989; Renwick, 1992). The geologic history of a landscape also affects the response of its landforms and sedimentary deposits to process stimuli, including their sensitivity to potential change (Brunsden and Thornes, 1979), and to crossing geomorphic thresholds (Schumm, 1973; Coates and Vitek, 1980). Additionally, fundamental chaotic behavior in geomorphic systems can arise in response to nonlinear interactions (Anderson, 1991; Phillips, 1992a, b, 1993). This mix of geologic processes acting on landforms imparts a singularity that renders short- and long-term predictions about explicit environmental change fraught with possible errors of judgment (Schumm, 1985; Hallet, 1990; Phillips, 1995) and, in the view of some researchers (Leopold and Langbein, 1963; Huggett, 1988), introduces fundamental indeterminacy in forecasting future change in a specific part of a geomorphic system.

To emphasize our point about the inherent complexity of geomorphic systems, consider Figure 2. It is a plot of the spatial variation of a beach, located 2 km downdrift (eastward) of Little Sodus Bay on Lake Ontario, New York (Fig. 1), relative to a fixed feature on land identified on aerial photographs. The data indicate unambiguously that this coastal sector is receding at close to 2 m/yr, a magnitude that is two to five times greater than that estimated for the mean short-term (0.8 m/yr) and mean long-term (0.4 m/yr) recessional rates for the southern shore of Lake Ontario (Drexhage and Calkin, 1981). What factor or combinations of factors have exacerbated erosion at this beach? Is the rapid retreat of the beach attributable to the installation of shore-stabilization structures that abound here (Brownlie and Calkin, 1981), or are the reasons intrinsic to the beach compartment itself, having more to do with its peculiar geographic location on the lakeshore, or perhaps with its internal geomorphic complexity or sediment composition (Phillips, 1993; Cooke and Doornkamp, 1990; Schumm, 1973)? Does the high rate of erosion reflect the accelerated removal of sediment from the compartment by longshore and offshore drift (output) or the diminishment of the beach's sediment supply (input), or both? Perhaps a geomorphic threshold was crossed or the beach's singular history and its internal dynamism (e.g., positive feedback loops) are creating higher than normal rates of coastal recession? Obviously, understanding the reasons for these changes is essential for implementing management procedures that can effectively ameliorate beach erosion at this site.

However, it does not end here. The intricacy of the analysis is compounded further by the fact that erosion tends not to proceed at a constant rate along the New York shore of Lake Ontario (Drexhage and Calkin, 1981; Brennan and Calkin, 1984; Frederick et al., 1991; Pinet et al., 1992). Rather, short periods of rapid shoreline retreat during unusually severe storms are separated by extended intervals of stability when the position of the shoreline remains fixed in place despite regular episodes of inclement weather, including large storm events (Pinet et al., 1992). In other words, short-term, intense erosional events cause rapid, local retreat of the southern Lake Ontario shoreline. These short-lived episodes interrupt temporally longer, less energetic processes that collectively produce a long-term trend characterized by a more gradual rate of coastal recession. In fact, the data of Figure 2 suggest a stepwise temporal retreat of this particular beach sector of Lake Ontario during the last 50 years.

What exact geomorphic role do short-lived, extreme events play in coastal evolution of Lake Ontario or, for that matter, in the geomorphic processes of any landscape (Wolman and Miller, 1960)? Are they more important at some spatial or temporal scale than the common, day-to-day, average processes? Obviously, successful management requires not only that the actual process-

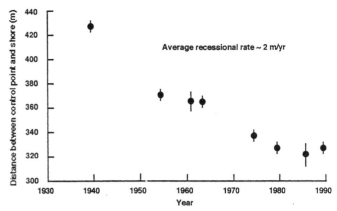

Figure 2. Based on analysis of aerial photographs, a beach located to the east of Little Sodus Bay, New York (Fig. 1), has receded during the past 50 years at a rate of 2 m/yr. Note the suggestion of "steps" in the retreat pattern; this indicates that the recessional rate has varied considerably over time.

response elements be identified, but also that the temporal nature of their coupling be understood, including the magnitude, frequency, and persistence of the driving forces (Schumm, 1985) and the relaxation time of the resultant landforms and deposits (Renwick, 1992). So, given the bewildering complexity of geomorphic systems, how does one study and manage environmental change, such as what is taking place along the coastline of Lake Ontario?

HIERARCHICAL ANALYSIS OF THE GEOMORPHIC COMPLEXITY OF THE ONTARIO LAKESHORE

Cooke and Doornkamp (1990) assess the difficulties of understanding geomorphic change and review possible approaches to its investigation. In our study we relied on the physical character of landforms and their associated deposits to deduce geomorphic process and change along the New York shore of Lake Ontario (Fig. 1). We modeled it as a complex, dynamic system of interdependent geomorphic elements that interact on vastly different time scales (Church, 1980; Lewin, 1980). This analytical procedure requires that the fundamental process-response elements of a geomorphic system be identified and distinguished from one another, including the relative magnitude and coherence of their interconnections across space and time (Kennedy, 1977; Huggett, 1988; Phillips, 1992b).

Hierarchical theory that focuses on scale allows the intricate process-response elements of natural systems to be unpacked formally and systematically, a technique of analysis that helps minimize confusion about the workings of complex systems (Anderson, 1991; Pinet, 1992; Allen and Hoekstra, 1992). For example, the geologic processes and geomorphic features (landforms and associated deposits) of a landscape (the geomorphic system) interact in different physical domains (Renwick, 1992). As such, the geomorphic elements of a landscape, like the Lake Ontario shoreline, can be ranked hierarchically (Table 1) as primary (operating or having an effect "everywhere" in the land-

TABLE 1. A MATRIX HIERARCHY

Time	Space			
	Primary	Secondary	Tertiary	Quaternay
Primary	Operating everywhere in landscape over thousands of years.	Operating regionally in landscape over thousands of years	Operating on a specific landform over thousands of years	Operating on a section of the landform over thousands of years
Secondary	Operating everywhere in landscape over tens to hundreds of years	Operating regionally in landscape over tens to hundreds of years	Operating on a specific landform over tens to hundreds of years	Operating on a section of the landform over tens to hundreds of years
Tertiary	Operating everywhere in landscape over years and months	Operating regionally in landscape over years and months	Operating on a specific landform over years and months	Operating on a section of landform over years and months
Quaternary	Operating everywhere in landscape over weeks and days	Operating regionally in landscape over weeks and days	Operating on a specific landform over weeks and days	Operating on a section of the landform over weeks and days

scape), secondary (operating or having an effect on a regional scale within the landscape), tertiary (operating or having an effect on a specific landform of the landscape), or quaternary (operating or having an effect on a portion of a landform).

The use of this hierarchical classification implies that a single landform of the shore, such as a particular coastal bluff, owes its geologic history, its present-day appearance, and its subsequent development to the dynamic interplay of tertiary, secondary, and primary processes acting on its preexisting morphology. Any section of that bluff—an incised gully, a slump scarp, or a talus slope—is influenced by the multiple impact of all of the aforementioned higher-order factors, *as well as by local quaternary processes*. This hierarchical approach to unpacking the complexity of environments indicates that a management plan, such as the regulation of water drainage in a particular gully of a coastal bluff, needs to address a complex assortment of process-response elements, including the site-specific quaternary determinants. Furthermore, because quaternary factors are specific to the local site, the carefully monitored responses of a similarly modified gully system elsewhere may not necessarily serve as an accurae predictor of the geomorphic response of the about-to-be-altered gully to the same set of environmental conditions, as is usually assumed by coastal researchers and land managers. Because landforms are unique in their location (space) and history (time), the extrapolation of a set of responses to environmental stimuli from one region to another without careful critical examination to the site-specific quaternary determinants can lead to gross errors of judgment (Huggett, 1988).

The application of hierarchical analysis to unraveling environmental complexity also serves to remind investigators and managers of the role of physical scale in understanding change in geomorphic systems (Kennedy, 1977). For example, an evalu-

ation of the probable environmental impact of management decisions on a physically large landscape is very different from assessing the complex response of one of its specific landforms to those same management procedures. The Lake Ontario shoreline is a landscape mosaic of bluffs, baymouth barriers, wetlands, and coastal bays (Fig. 1). The management assessment of a regional sector of this coast involves defining the collective influence of only secondary and primary geomorphic factors, because the environmental aspects of the landforms that are truly of tertiary and quaternary significance have little import on a regional scale. If they did, they would not be given a lower-order ranking. By extension, engineers, scientists, and resource managers assessing the probable impact of a proposed shore-stabilization structure at a specific site must consider the net effect of tertiary and quaternary factors that, although subsumed by the higher-order process elements, remain critical for understanding small-scale and short-term responses of the subsystem to being manipulated artificially.

Because the response and equilibrium states of landscapes are imbedded in time as well as in space (Lewin, 1980; Cooke and Doornkamp, 1990), the character of their process-response elements has an important temporal aspect that is scale dependent and, therefore, amenable also to hierarchical analysis. A time-hierarchical classification that seems appropriate for ordering geomorphic changes within the coastal landscape of Lake Ontario (Table 1) includes primary (operating or having an effect over geologically significant time spans $>10^3$ yrs), secondary (operating or having an effect over 10^1 to 10^2 yrs), tertiary (operating or having an effect over months and years), and quaternary (operating or having an effect over days and weeks).

A vital aspect of resolving environmental complexity is determination of the time framework that is compatible with the management goal. Is one managing an environment with a short-

(years), intermediate- (decades to centuries), or long-term (millennia) perspective in mind, or are the day-to-day changes crucial to the management scheme? A case in point is the marked difference between the short-term mean (0.8 m/yr) and long-term mean (0.4 m/yr) recessional rates for the southern Lake Ontario coastline (Brennan and Calkin, 1984). How exactly are the two recessional rates nested and integrated over different time frames? Is the proper decision for the long-term stewardship of a segment of the Lake Ontario shoreline to disregard intense, but short-lived erosional events (such as the collapse of a portion of a bluff, which has tremendous immediate impact locally), and to concentrate more on the regulation of environmental processes and responses over the long run? At the very least, configuring an environmental problem in a hierarchical time framework allows such questions to be raised, even if they cannot be answered precisely. This serves the useful purpose of alerting environmental scientist and managers about possible consequences of short-term (years to decades) engineering procedures on the long-term (centuries to millennia) resiliency or equilibrium state of the landforms being managed.

These aspects of the physical and temporal domains of the Lake Ontario shoreline are addressed in the remainder of the paper. However, before pondering the details of how to handle geomorphic complexity and change, we must review generally how the coastal bluffs of Lake Ontario evolve. The theoretical model presented below has been extensively field tested at nine Lake Ontario bluffs that are in various stages of geomorphic development (Moore et al., 1996).

BLUFF EVOLUTION ALONG THE SOUTHEASTERN LAKE ONTARIO SHORE

The southeastern shore of Lake Ontario (Fig. 1) consists of a series of coastal bluffs that are separated from one another by baymouth barriers. Composed of sand and gravel, the baymouth barriers isolate ponds, bays, and wetlands from the lake proper (Martin, 1901; Brennan and Calkin, 1984; Christensen et al., 1990). Ranging in height from 5 to 50 m above the lake level, the coastal bluffs slope lakeward at moderate-to-steep (> 45°) angles.

These coastal bluffs are erosion surfaces that have been cut across a series of north-south–trending Pleistocene drumlins by wave erosion and mass-wasting processes (Pincus, 1962; Brennan and Calkin, 1984; Pinet et al., 1992). The prevailing longshore currents flow eastward (Sutton et al., 1974) and the glacial till eroded from the drumlin bluffs supply downdrift beaches with sand and gravel (Pinet et al., 1992). As a first approximation, the southeastern shore of Lake Ontario can be modeled as a series of coastal compartments, each consisting of a morphological couplet—a drumlin bluff and a downdrift baymouth barrier (Pinet et al., 1993). Although these compartments seem to be closed on the short term (years to decades), whether or not significant amounts of sediment "leak" into adjoining compartments over the long term is not clear. However, we do know that sand and mud in

the nearshore is dispersed offshore by currents and ice rafting (McClennen et al., 1994 ; Mutch and McClennen, 1996).

All bluffs that we have examined along the southern edge of Lake Ontario are eroding and, judging from their morphology, this occurs in a variety of ways and at different rates (Martin, 1901; Pincus, 1962, 1964; Drexhage and Calkin, 1981; Brennan and Calkin, 1984). Some bluffs are eroding back in a planar fashion; others are gullied by a system of deep ravines with steep sides and head scarps, the most imposing example being the 50-m-high Chimney Bluff, located about 3 km northeast of Sodus Bay, New York (Fig. 1). In fact, there is a clear positive relationship between the height of a bluff and the degree of gullying (Fig. 3). The taller the bluff, the more deeply incised and larger the gullies tend to be; the lower the bluff, the more planar its surface tends to be (Covello et al., 1993).

According to field observations (Sunamura, 1977; Drexhage and Calkin, 1981; Frederick et al., 1991; Pinet et al., 1992; Covello et al., 1993; Yuengling et al., 1994), the volume of sediment supplied to the base of bluffs is most affected by their topographic height above the lake level and less on the till composition and internal structure of the drumlins. The large quantity of debris shed by high bluffs (> 20 m above the lake level) results in the formation of wide and thick colluvial fans at the mouths of gullies that build out onto the beach (Fig. 4). These fans consist of 1- to 4-m-thick sequences of superimposed mud-flow and water-laid deposits that may coalesce laterally with the fans of adjoining gullies and form a continuous terrace along the upper beach. The result is armoring of the cliff base and reduction in the frequency of wave notching of the bluff's toe. Without significant undercutting, the bluff's face tends not to collapse.

Persistent erosion by surface runoff and ground-water seepage excavates rills into the stable face of high bluffs. The rills widen and lengthen into deep, broad, steep-sided ravines

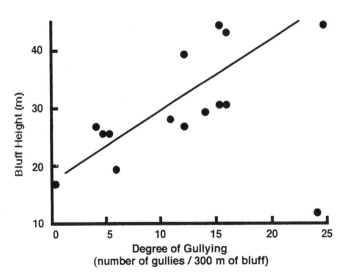

Figure 3. The degree of gullying along the southeastern Lake Ontario shoreline is strongly dependent on the height of the bluff above the lake level.

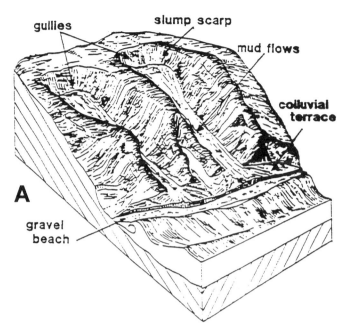

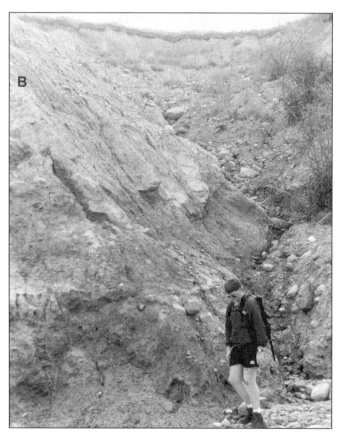

Figure 4. A, The gullied morphology associated with a high (>20 m) bluff; B, a view from the beach looking landward into a gully incised into McIntyre Bluff (Fig. 1).

(Yuengling et al., 1994) and eventually evolve into a classic gully-and-ridge morphology (Higgins et al., 1990). By contrast, the quantity of colluvium and beach deposits that collects at the base of low bluffs (< 10 m above the lake level) is modest because of the limited supply of debris from the cliff. This limited amount of debris allows frequent wave undercutting and destabilization of the bluff face, which are followed by slumping of the drumlin's till deposits. This ongoing process maintains a steep, planar cliff face (Fig. 5). In the case of small bluffs, gullying processes, so influential on the high bluffs, are overwhelmed by the high frequency of slump failures of the cliff face (Covello et al., 1993).

The above model describes the principal variations in the morphology of bluff faces as they exist at the moment along the southeastern shore of Lake Ontario. What about the temporal aspect of bluff evolution? Our field data indicate that bluffs undergo a regular style of geomorphic development that reflects the time-dependent interplay of drainage, sediment supply, slumping, and gullying. An elaboration of our model of bluff evolution follows.

A theoretical model of bluff evolution along the Lake Ontario shore

Wave-driven erosional retreat of drumlin hills produced a transgression of the southern edge of Lake Ontario during the Holocene. The initial scarp carved into each drumlin by waves was low. With continued erosion, the bluffs grew in height as the drumlins were cut back, attaining a maximum relief that was commensurate with the elevation of the topographic crest of each drumlin. Thereafter, the height of the bluffs diminished progressively as cliff erosion proceeded, until the glacial hills were totally removed. This relationship indicates that the height of the present-day coastal bluffs of the Ontario lakeshore will vary systematically in the future, as erosion bites deeper into the drumlin hills (Fig. 6).

The interplay of wave notching (which induces slumping and the formation of a planar cliff faces) and gullying (which produces irregular ravines that are deeply incised into the cliff faces) depends directly on sediment supply to the beach that is, in turn, controlled by cliff height. As a consequence, the Ontario lakeshore bluffs progress through a series of developmental stages—young, mature, old, and terminal (Figs. 6 and 7). Each stage is characterized by distinctive bluff morphologies that reflect time-dependent variations in the relative impact of wave notching and slumping on the one hand and gullying processes on the other (Table 2).

Young bluffs are dominated by frequent wave notching and slumping and therefore are low, steep, and planar (Moore et al., 1996). Rills tend to be small in size and ephemeral because they are eradicated by the regular collapse of slump masses from the steep cliff face. By contrast, mature bluffs are high and supply copious sediment to the beach, protecting the cliff base from wave attack and, hence, slumping. During the mature stage, erosion by channelized water cuts deeply into the drumlin hill and with time creates a vast, intricate gully system. Subsequently,

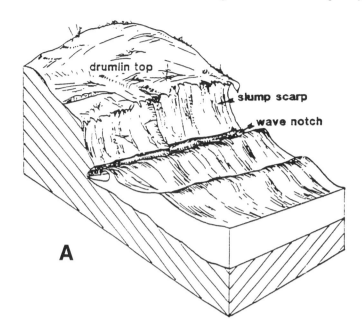

A

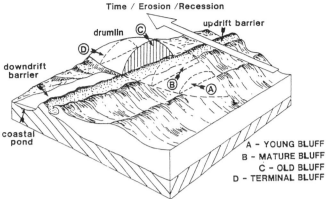

Figure 6. The progressive cutback of a drumlin causes the height of bluffs to vary over time, which results in a series of distinct morphological stages.

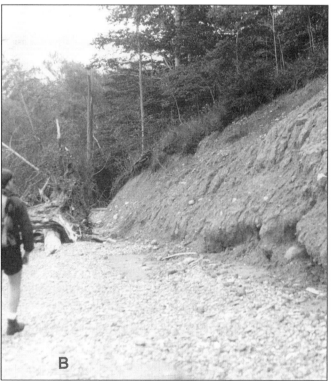

B

Figure 5. A, The slump-scarp morphology associated with a low (<10 m) bluff; B, a wave notch and slump face of a low bluff.

after about half of the drumlin hill has been eroded, the bluff enters the old stage of development. Gullies inherited from the mature stage become essentially inactive, because the dominant drainage of surface runoff and ground water is now directed landward, away from the bluff and its system of entrenched gullies (Fig. 8). Furthermore, as the old bluff is cut back, its height above

the lake level diminishes with time because of the convex shape of the drumlin's longitudinal crestline (Fig. 6). This reduces the supply of debris to the beach over time. The lack of toe protection allows wave notching and slumping to resume dominance of the bluff's morphological development. During the terminal stage of cliff evolution, the bluff is topographically low, the supply of sediment to the base is sparse, and wave notching and slumping rapidly eliminate the last vestige of the drumlin. Side-scan sonar records reveal the presence of boulder pavements on a nearshore wave-cut terrace of Lake Ontario that are interpreted as the trace of drumlins that have been completely beveled by coastal erosion (Mutch and McClennen, 1996).

Implications of bluff development model for coastal management

A crucial and unexpected aspect of our model that bears directly on management strategies is the specific response of both the base and top of the cliff to the erosive agents that dominate each stage of bluff evolution (Fig. 7). In the past, management personnel seem not to have discriminated between the recessional rates of the top and bottom surfaces of bluffs, assuming that the entire cliff face responds uniformly to erosional forces. Clearly, the top and base of bluffs retreat at a uniform rate during both the young and terminal stages of development, as a result of the commanding effects of wave notching and slumping that influence the entire vertical extent of planar cliff faces. However, in the case of bluffs in mature and old stages of development, the cliff's top and base are subjected to different erosional agents and thus behave independently of one another (Fig. 7). The top of a mature bluff is very irregular in plan view and retreats rapidly as a consequence of the headward erosion of its many gullies. Its cliff base, on the other hand, is stabilized by the deposition of ample quantities of colluvium that is swept out of the active gully mouths onto the beach. This material protects the cliff base from wave attack, and reduces its recessional rate. One consequence is a reduced average slope for the mature bluff (Table 2; Moore et

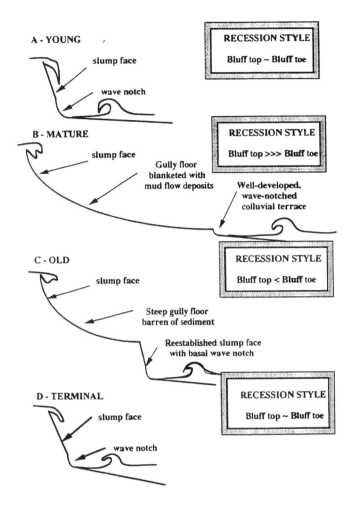

Figure 7. Idealized profiles of bluffs for each of the four developmental stages, showing their dominant morphologies and their recessional styles.

TABLE 2. BLUFF CHARACTERISTICS

Stage	Height (m)	Drumlin Eroded (%)	Slope (°)	Morphology	Geomorphic Processes
Young	<10	<25	65 – 90	Slump scarps	Wave notching and slumping
Mature	>10	25 – 50	30 – 90	Gullies and colluvial terrace	Gullying
Old	>10	50 – 75	30 – 90	Gullies and slump scarps	Wave notching and slumping
Terminal	<10	>75	65 – 90	Slump scarps	Wave notching and slumping

steps. These are to (1) classify the geomorphic factors of the coastal system into a space/time hierarchy, (2) examine generally how causality within the system varies with differing spatial and temporal scales, (3) define the management objectives and identify their appropriate spatial/temporal framework, (4) assess and evaluate the engineering proposals for reaching the specified managerial goal(s), and (5) anticipate the probable impact of ancillary environmental factors, such as the role of geomorphic thresholds. Below, we apply each step to a hypothetical erosion-control problem along the southeastern Lake Ontario shore.

Space/time hierarchy

The complexity of geomorphic systems can be examined hierarchically (Pinet and McClennen, 1995). Our studies indicate that the dynamic interplay between slumping and gullying determines the morphological character of drumlin bluffs that front the Ontario lakeside (Fig. 7). Domination of the system by slumping hinges on frequent wave notching of the cliff base and gullying on the channelized drainage of water across the cliff face during periods when wave attack of the cliff base is inhibited. Because this interaction operates on bluffs everywhere along the south shore of Lake Ontario, slumping and gullying have primary hierarchical status (Table 3). Secondary factors, those of regional import, involve: (i) bluff orientation and hence exposure to storm wave attack—west-facing shore segments receive the most wave energy, north-facing the least (Drexhage and Calkin, 1981); and (ii) the amount of bedrock frontage (Upper Ordovician Oswego Sandstone) along a stretch of the waterline, which like riprap can shield the cliff base from regular wave erosion. The critical tertiary determinant, which impacts individual drumlin bluffs, is the landform's present stage of evolutionary development (young,

al., 1996). Although similarly decoupled, the top of an old bluff retreats much more slowly than its base, a response that is opposite to that of a mature bluff. Headward erosion and deepening of the gullies in the old stage of bluff development are reduced, because surface runoff is directed down the landward-facing slope of the remaining half of the drumlin, leaving little water to drain through its gully system (Fig. 8). This yields a minimal supply of sediment to the bluff base, and without a significant supply of colluvium to armor its base, wave undercutting destabilizes the cliff face and induces slumping. Therefore, the bluff's top is relatively stable in contrast to its base, the latter receding relatively rapidly as storm waves cut it away and replace the moderate gully slopes with steeper slump scarps (Fig. 7).

ADDRESSING GEOMORPHOLOGICAL CHANGE FOR EFFECTIVE MANAGEMENT

Our procedure for analyzing the environmental consequences of bluff recession on Lake Ontario involves five basic

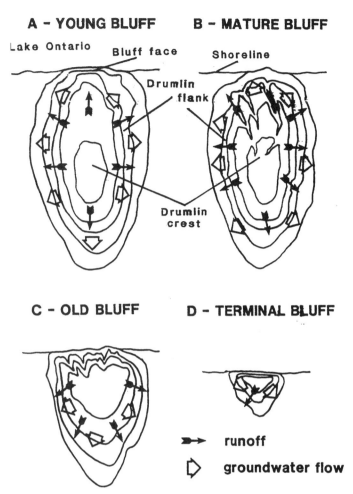

Figure 8. Theoretical drainage patterns of surface and subsurface water for the four bluff stages. Note that the gullies, which are active conduits of water and sediment during the mature stage, are inactive during the old stage because water drainage is directed landward away from the cliff face.

TABLE 3. HIERARCHICAL CLASSIFICATION OF GEOMORPHIC FACTORS

Level	Spatial Dimensions	Ontario Lakeshore Geomorphic Factors
Primary	Operating everywhere in the landscape	Slumping and gullying processes
Secondary	Operating regionally in the landscape	Bedrock frontage. Exposure to wave attack
Tertiary	Operating on a specific landform of the landscape	Stage of bluff development
Quaternary	Operating locally on a specific part of the landform	Till composition/stratigraphy. Geotechnical soil properties. Land development

mature, old, or terminal forms). The lowest-order factors relate to the local conditions and processes that act on parts of the cliffs; they include such factors as the composition and stratigraphy of the till deposits, the cliff material's geotechnical properties, extent and density of vegetative cover, local land development, and the presence of shore-stabilization structures.

Geomorphic causality across various spatial and temporal scales

The primary process elements of the bluff landscape of southeastern Lake Ontario—slumping and gullying—function everywhere in the system and, depending on the weather conditions, across all but the briefest time intervals (days and weeks). However, their relative effects at any site depend on the present-day evolutionary state of the cliff face; that is, whether it currently is in the young, mature, old, or terminal stage of development. The evolutionary state of any coastal bluff is easily established by consulting a topographic map, noting the extent of drumlin truncation (Table 2), and following with a field check, which is particularly needed if the map is dated. The bluff stage has an important bearing on the long-term assessment of geomorphic change because as the drumlin is cut back the cliff will pass from one evolutionary stage to another (Fig. 6) with a corresponding change in the relative interaction of the principal process elements (Table 2). For example, a bluff that is in the latest phase of the young stage—a state when the top and bottom of the planar cliff are coupled and retreating at similar rates (Fig. 7)—may suddenly enter the mature stage of development. The system then will be dominated by gullying processes, and the bluff crown will recede rapidly and irregularly relative to the now-stabilized cliff base. Also, rapid headward erosion will create steep headcuts and head scarps (Higgins et al., 1990). Thus, bluff evolution must be factored into any management scheme of the southern Ontario lakeshore.

Specific management goals

Specifying the management objectives clearly and in detail is critical to an overall environmental assessment of a natural system because it allows decision-makers to anticipate and perhaps compensate for possible environmental perturbations that seem to be associated with a particular space/time continuum of the system. Two questions must be addressed. If the goal is long term (centuries, millennia), then what will be the short-term (seasons, years, decades) consequences of the management scheme? Conversely, how will the cumulative environmental effects of short-term management strategies impact the long-term response of the geomorphic system?

Answers to these questions assure that researchers and planners examine management objectives across differing dimensions of space and time. Ignoring the space and time relationships increases the likelihood of mismanagement and failure to achieve the desired end. For example, is the intent to control bluff erosion from day-to-day or from year-to-year? Is the mandate to preserve the entire landscape (not merely a landform) over the long run (centuries, millennia), striving to mitigate the environmental repercussions of short-term human activity, such as land development or erosion abatement? Can managers impose an engineering solution to an acute, local erosion problem, such as the unusually rapid recession rate of the beach to the east of Little Sodus Bay (Fig. 2) and be reasonably assured that the long-term resiliency of another segment of the coastal system will not be compromised in some fundamental way? Or given the dynamics and interconnections of the various landform elements of a unified landscape, is it futile to expect a system to work "naturally" once humans intervene? How does one weigh environmental concerns with the needs and wants of people who legitimately desire (in a legal sense) to occupy and develop prime coastal real estate? Our point in raising these rhetorical queries is to underline the need for managers and policy makers to set priorities (local versus regional impacts; short-term versus long-term concerns; human needs versus environmental deterioration), so that the intended management goals are definable and articulated clearly to all concerned.

Evaluation of management strategies

By way of illustration, we evaluate the potential environmental aftermath of curtailing cliff erosion at a particular unprotected bluff on the southern Lake Ontario shore, a situation, let us say, that is gravely threatening the structural integrity of several expensive houses perched near the drumlin's hillcrest. We begin the analysis by addressing the specific management goal (step 3) in light of (i) the space/time hierarchical classification of the relevant geomorphological factors (step 1), and (ii) geomorphic causality for differing spatial and temporal dimensions of the geomorphic system (step 2). Because our charge as land-use planners is the amelioration of erosion of a particular drumlin bluff, we consider all of the geomorphic factors that operate at the tertiary, secondary, and primary hierarchical levels (Table 3). Quaternary environmental determinants have no special import for planning at the spatial scale of the project, because they operate locally on a section of the landform. Our bluff erosion model (Fig. 7) indicates that domination by one of the primary environmental agents—slumping versus gullying—depends directly on the drumlin's specific stage (young, mature, old, or terminal) of geomorphic development. Combining this information with the management goal—mitigation of bluff erosion—yields the results of Table 4. What follows is the systematic exploration of the plausible environmental impacts of the various land-change scenarios for different time frames.

If the bluff to be modified is in a young stage of development, our model indicates that the use of the time-honored, cost-effective engineering procedure of armoring the entire cliff base with riprap to eliminate wave notching and hence slumping will ultimately have dire consequences for the bluff face and the houses on the hilltop. The placement of riprap along the cliff's toe will in fact increase and not retard recession of the bluff's crown, if our model of bluff development is valid. This is a surprising deduction because it seemingly defies common sense and is clearly at odds with the experience of others who have used riprap elsewhere as a shore-protection measure. However, reducing cliff attack by storm waves should induce an ill-timed, overhasty shift of the young bluff to a mature stage of development, in which water runoff and ground-water seepage, rather than wave notching and slumping, dominate the system (Fig. 7). With time, this water drainage will excavate furrows into the cliff face, leading to the entrenchment of channels and their eventual enlargement into an extensive, branching gully network. As such, the top of the bluff will be decoupled from its

TABLE 4. ENVIRONMENTAL IMPACT ASSESSMENT

Bluff Stage	Engineering Strategy	Rationale	Probable Impact
Young	Any attempt to protect the bluff's base must also include control of water drainage and vegetation of slopes	Must prevent the initiation of gullying	Minimal impact downdrift because of small sediment supply from bluff
Mature	Redirect water drainage, control ground-water seepage, and vegetate slopes; no protection of bluff base is needed	Must stabilize the bluff crown	Minimal impact downdrift provided bluff base is not armored
Old	Riprap to protect base of bluffs; nourishment of downdrift barrier	Bluff top is stable because gullies are inactive	Major impact downdrift requiring beach nourishment
Terminal	Reprap to protect bluff's base	Prevent wave notching and slumping	Minimal impact because downdrift barrier is in a naturally starved state due to limited sediment supply

base (Fig. 7), and the recessional rate of the upper bluff surface will *increase dramatically* as headward erosion cuts deeply and rapidly into the drumlin hill, threatening the perched houses much more so than before the "solution" to the problem. In effect, the proposed course of action—the emplacement of riprap—will aggravate rather than mitigate the erosion problem for property owners.

What can be done in lieu of this? In order to reduce wave notching and cliff collapse and not cause the system to change over to the mature stage of bluff development, engineers may decide to do the following (Table 4): construct a revetment with backfill and proper drainage outlets; reduce the steepness of the cliff slope by grading; control surface runoff and ground-water drainage; and stabilize the sediment of the bluff face by promoting the dense growth of native (ideally) vegetation. Obviously, these engineering projects are high-priced items, and their cost will have to be weighed against the value of the threatened property. Also, there is an additional consequence of erosion abatement of the bluff—the elimination of the single most important source of sand, gravel, and cobbles to the beach and to the downdrift baymouth barrier. With a reduced supply of sediment, the downdrift barrier will be sediment-starved and thus erode, becoming increasingly susceptible to overwash by storm waves with time. However, because the drumlin bluff–baymouth barrier is a geomorphic couplet, the human-induced environmental impact likely will be confined to the immediate region of the coastal compartment and, at least in the short run (decades?), not adversely affect the sediment budget of shore segments outside of the compartment.

Erosion abatement at a mature bluff is straightforward in theory but difficult in practice. Gully development controls the morphology of a bluff in a mature stage of development (Fig. 7 and Table 2). The top of the drumlin cliff is irregular in plan view with headcuts and ridge shoulders that slope steeply into the main channel of the gully. Headward and lateral erosion are rapid because gullies are active conduits that funnel water and sediment debris to the bluff's base. These thick deposits of colluvium protect the bluff from wave notching and stabilize its base. Because flowing water is the dominant erosional agent, surface runoff and ground-water seepage and sapping of headscarps have to be controlled to lessen the deepening and lengthening of the gullies. In this case, armoring the base with riprap is clearly of little use for erosion abatement because the problem is with the crown and not the foot of the cliff. Rather, engineers must redirect the natural surface runoff by diverting water away from the gully system. Also, driveways and paved roads that are directing water to the bluff need to be redesigned to that same end. Control of ground-water flow at a bluff is problematical. At the very least, improper septic systems and leaky swimming pools can be remedied, and the excessive watering of lawns can be curtailed. In seepage-induced gullies, measures to stabilize the headslope and to stem ground-water outflow need to be implemented in order to retard cliff sapping and headward erosion. Finally, as sideslopes, headslopes, and channels of active

gullies are typically unvegetated, their sediment is susceptible to mass transport processes (slides, slumps, and mud slurries) and to entrainment by flowing water. Hence, efforts at promoting the growth of a lush carpet of turf with a dense root system can effectively bind and thereby stabilize the sediment of sideslopes and headscarps.

The drawback to all of these engineering measures is that the cliff base is denied its natural input of sediment debris from the gullies (Table 4). As such, waves will erode the older colluvial fan deposits that form at the gully mouths, and eventually reexpose the bluff's base to wave notching and slumping. However, once water drainage through the gullies is controlled, downdrift barriers will be denied their natural supply of sediment. After removal of the colluvium by wave erosion, the situation will be rectified naturally, as waves attack the glacial till of the cliff base (provided that it has not been protected artificially) and longshore drift resupplies the downdrift barrier with coarse sediment.

The erosion of bluffs in old and terminal stages of development is easily and economically addressed (Table 4). The placement of riprap along the cliff's base will eliminate wave notching in both cases. Gullying processes in the old stage of bluff evolution are of no consequence, because these gullies are inactive, according to our model, and receive no significant surface and subsurface drainage of water (Fig. 8). Because no significant water drainage is directed toward these cliff faces, controlling erosion of bluffs in a terminal stage of development is straightforward—the use of riprap. The main environmental drawback to armoring the cliff base with riprap for both old and terminal bluffs is the interruption of a sediment supply to their downdrift barriers (Table 4). These barriers, however, are already sediment starved due to the limited supply of sediment from their updrift bluffs. Reducing the input of sand and gravel to these barriers will increase beach erosion, and lead to overwash processes and the subsequent landward migration of the barrier into the adjoining bay, pond, or wetland. Nourishment of the beach fronting the barrier with gravel and cobbles should help counter this effect.

Because the sediment yield varies directly with the stage of bluff development, the flux of sediment across inlets that are cut into downdrift barriers will fluctuate over time as well. Maximum dredging of channel inlets and mouths will be required when bluffs are in a mature stage of geomorphic development, a time when gullies are large and active, and sediment supply to the downdrift part of the compartment is high. This obviously has clear implications for harbor and marina maintenance.

Anticipated natural and human-induced ancillary effects on the landscape/landform

Rates of erosion averaged over a long time (e.g., Fig. 2) are of limited use for dealing with short-term development of a specific portion of a landscape. A landform, for example, may be poised at a geomorphic threshold, a metastable condition under which a land feature can undergo a significant, abrupt transformation in its morphological state *without an obvious change in the external conditions* (Patton and Schumm, 1975). This metastable state, if unforeseen, is disastrous for making precise predictions of impending environmental changes due to land-control measures. In the case of the Lake Ontario shore, specific bluffs or even parts of a single bluff may be in the waning phase of the young developmental stage, a state when slumping predominates and the crown and foot of the cliff are coupled and receding at comparable rates (Fig. 7). Such ungullied slopes are extremely unstable and may cross the geomorphic threshold independent of the environmental controls. Suddenly and for no obvious reason the system crosses to the mature stage of bluff evolution and the tempo and character of the geomorphic changes of the bluff shift abruptly. With the crossover intense and rapid gullying, rather than slumping, controls the cliff face's morphology (Table 2); this will result in the erosional retreat of the bluff's crest and colluvial deposition at its base. The upper surface of the bluff retreats at an alarming rate as headward erosion of nascent gullies cut deeply into the drumlin hill, while at the same time colluvial deposition widens the beach.

Precise predictions of the timing of such events are impossible to make (Patton and Schumm, 1975). In fact, bluffs elsewhere on the lakeshore that are similarly poised at geomorphic thresholds likely will respond differently or not at all to the same external conditions. However, if threshold conditions for a bluff or a particular slope of a bluff are recognized, then managers and engineers at the very least can proceed with caution, always anticipating the possiblity of impending and rapid geomorphic change. Furthermore, it may be possible to assess whether the management procedures may contribute to or even precipitate the sudden crossing of a geomorphic threshold by some part of a landform.

CONCLUSIONS

As noted above, geomorphic systems are complex, because landscapes are the product of a variety of driving forces that interrelate in different ways and to different degrees across different time frames (Cooke and Doornkamp, 1990). An understanding of this environmental complexity by environmental engineers, scientists, and managers is fundamental for the successful implementation of erosion-abatement projects and of land-use practices that reduce the likelihood of negative environmental impacts, howsoever defined. As demonstrated for the Ontario lakeshore, hierarchical analysis is a powerful technique for fostering clear-sighted understanding of geomorphic complexity and for making sound decisions for effective landscape management.

REFERENCES CITED

Allen, T. F. H., and Hoekstra, T. W., 1992, Toward a unified ecology: New York, Columbia University Press, 384 p.

Anderson, D. W., 1991, Long-term research—A pedological approach, *in* Risser, P. G., ed., Long-term ecological research: An international perspective: New York, John Wiley and Sons, p. 115–134.

Brennan, S. F., and Calkin, P. E., 1984, Analysis of bluff erosion along the southern coastline of Lake Ontario, New York: Albany, New York, New York-Sea Grant Institute, 74 p.

Brownlie, W. R., and Calkin, P. E., 1981, Effects of jetties, Sodas Bay, New York: Great Lakes Coastal Geology: Albany, New York, New York Sea Grant Institute, 27 p.

Brunsden, D., and Thornes, J. B., 1979, Landscape sensitivity and change: Transactions of the Institute of British Geographers, v. 4, p. 463–484.

Burt, T. P., 1994, Long-term study of the natural environment—perceptive science or mindless monitoring?: Progress in Physical Geography, v. 18, p. 475–496.

Chorley, R. J., 1962, Geomorphology and general systems theory: U.S. Geological Survey Professional Paper 500-B, p. B1–B10.

Christensen, S., McClennen, C. E., and Pinet, P. R., 1990, Coastal erosion: Southeastern Lake Ontario shore: Geological Society of America Abstracts with Programs, v. 22, p. 7.

Church, M., 1980, Records of recent geomorphological events, *in* Cullingford, R. A., Davidson, D. A., and Lewin, J., eds., Timescales in geomorphology: New York, John Wiley & Sons, p. 13–29.

Coates, D. R., and Vitek, J. D., editors, 1980, Thresholds in geomorphology: London, Allen & Unwin, 498 p.

Cooke, R. U., and Doornkamp, J. C., 1990, Geomorphology in environmental management, Oxford, Clarendon Press, 410 p.

Covello, D. M., Knotts, K. A., Pinet, P. R., and McClennen, C. E., 1993, Erosional dynamics and morphological analysis along the southeastern Lake Ontario shoreline: Geological Society of America Abstracts with Programs, v. 25, p. 10.

Drexhage, T. F., and Calkin, P. E., 1981, Historic bluff recession along the Lake Ontario coast, New York: Albany, New York, New York Sea Grant Institute, Great Lakes Coastal Research Series, 123 p.

Frederick, B., McClennen, C. E., and Pinet, P. R., 1991, Quantification of differential erosion patterns on a drumlin bluff along the coast of southeastern Lake Ontario: Geological Society of America Abstracts with Programs, v. 23, p. 31.

Hallet, B., 1990, Spatial self-organization in geomorphology: From periodic bedforms and patterned ground to scale-invariant topography: Earth-Science Review, v. 29, p. 57–75.

Higgins, C. G., Hill, B. R., and Lehre, A. K., 1990, Gully development, *in* Higgins, C. G., and Coates, D. R., eds., Groundwater geomorphology: Geological Society of America Special Paper 252, p. 139–155.

Huggett, R. J., 1988, Dissipative systems: Implications for geomorphology: Earth Surface Processes and Landforms, v. 13, p. 45–49.

Kennedy, B. A., 1977, A question of scale?: Progress in Physical Geography, v. 1, p. 154–157.

Leopold, L. B., and Langbein, W. B., 1963, Association and indeterminacy in geomorphology, *in* Albritton, C. C., ed., The fabric of geology: Reading, Addison-Wesley, p. 184–192.

Lewin, J., 1980, Available and appropriate timescales in geomorphology, *in* Cullingford, R. A., Davidson, D. A., and Lewin, J., eds., Timescales in geomorphology: New York, John Wiley & Sons, p. 3–10.

Martin, J. O., 1901, The Ontario coast between Fairhaven and Sodus Bay: American Geologist, v. 27, p. 331–334.

McClennen, C. E., Schaefer, R. A., and Pinet, P. R., 1994, Nearshore-ice complex and preliminary assessment of sediment transport of southeastern Lake Ontario: Geological Society of America Abstracts and Programs, v. 26, p. A178.

Montgomery, K., 1989, Concepts of equilibrium and evolution in geomorphology: The model of branch systems: Progress in Physical Geography, v. 13, p. 47–66.

Moore, C. F., Pinet, P. R., and McClennen, C. E., 1996, A field test of a bluff erosion model for the southeastern shoreline of Lake Ontario: Geological Society of America Abstracts with Programs, Northeastern Section, v. 28, p. 84.

Mutch, A., and McClennen, C. E., 1996, Side-scan sonar images of contemporary sediment transport and lag deposits on a coastal erosion terrace along the southeastern shore of Lake Ontario: Geological Society of America Abstracts with Programs, Northeastern Section, v. 28, p. 86.

Patton, P. C., and Schumm, S. A., 1975, Gully erosion, northwestern Colorado: A threshold phenomenon: Geology, v. 3, p. 88–90.

Phillips, J. D., 1992a, Qualitative chaos in geomorphic systems, with an example from wetland response to sea level rise: The Journal of Geology, v. 100, p. 365–374.

Phillips, J. D., 1992b, Nonlinear dynamical systems in geomorphology: revolution or evolution?: Geomorphology, v. 5, p. 219–229.

Phillips, J. D., 1993, Instability and chaos in hillslope evolution: American Journal of Science, v. 293, p. 25–48.

Phillips, J. D., 1995, Self-organization and landscape evolution: Progress in Physical Geography, v. 19, p. 309–321.

Pincus, H. J., 1962, Recession of Great Lakes shorelines, *in* Pincus, H. J., ed., Great Lakes basin: Baltimore, American Association for the Advancement of Science Publication 71, p. 123–137.

Pincus, H. J., 1964, Retreat of lakeshore bluffs: Journal of the American Society of Civil Engineers, v. 90, p. 115–134.

Pinet, P. R., 1992, Unpacking complexity in the analysis of environmental and geological problems: Geological Society of Amererica Abstracts with Programs, v. 23, p. 243.

Pinet, P. R., and McClennen, C. E., 1995, Mitigation of coastal bluff erosion: Moving beyond the simple and obvious: Geological Society of America Abstracts with Programs, v. 27, p. A234.

Pinet, P. R., McClennen, C. E., and Frederick, B. C., 1992, Sedimentation-erosion patterns along the southeastern shoreline of Lake Ontario, *in*

April, R. H., ed., New York State Geological Association Field Trip Guide Book: Hamilton, New York, Colgate University, Department of Geology, p. 155–169.

Pinet, P. R., McClennen, C. E., and Moore, L. J., 1993, Coastal compartments of the southeastern shoreline of Lake Ontario: Geological Society of America Abstracts with Programs, v. 25, p. A368.

Renwick, W. H., 1992, Equilibrium, disequilibrium, and nonequilibrium landforms in the landscape: Geomorphology, v. 5, p. 265–276.

Schumm, S. A., 1985, Explanation and extrapolation in geomorphology: Seven reasons for geologic uncertainty: Transactions of the Japanese Geophysical Union, v. 6, p. 1–18.

Schumm, W. H., 1973, Geomorphic thresholds and complex response of drainage systems, *in* Morisawa, M. E., ed., Fluvial geomorphology: Binghamton, New York, State University of New York, p. 299–310.

Sunamura, T., 1977, A relationship between wave-induced cliff erosion and erosive force of waves: Journal of Geology, v. 85, p. 613–618.

Sutton, R. G., Lewis, T. L., and Woodrow, D. L., 1974, Sand dispersal in eastern and southern Lake Ontario: Journal of Sedimentary Petrology, v. 44, p. 705–715.

Swanson, F. J., Kratz, T. K., Caine, N., and Woodmansee, R. G., 1988, Landform effects on ecosystem patterns: BioScience, v. 38, p. 92–98.

Wolman, M. G., and Miller, J. P., 1960, Magnitude and frequency of forces in geomorphic processes: Journal of Geology, v. 68, p. 54–74.

Yuengling, K. R., Pinet, P. R., and McClennen, C. E., 1994, Lake Ontario bluff morphologies explained by a drumlin erosion cycle: Geological Society of Amererica Abstracts with Programs, v. 26, p. 82.

MANUSCRIPT ACCEPTED BY THE SOCIETY JUNE 5, 1997

Printed in U.S.A.

Geological Society of America
Reviews in Engineering Geology, Volume XII
1998

Colonial impacts to wetlands in Lebanon, Connecticut

Robert M. Thorson
Department of Geology and Geophysics and Department of Anthropology, University of Connecticut, Storrs, Connecticut 06269-2045
Andrew G. Harris and Sandra L. Harris*
Department of Geology and Geophysics, University of Connecticut, Storrs, Connecticut 06269-2045
Robert Gradie III
Department of Anthropology, University of Connecticut, Storrs, Connecticut 06269-2176
M. W. Lefor
Department of Geography, University of Connecticut, Storrs, Connecticut 06269-2148

ABSTRACT

The expansion and contraction of the agricultural economy in Lebanon, Connecticut, a seventeenth century New England colonial village, was associated first with conversion of "wilderness" to a pastoral landscape, and later with nearly whole-scale reforestation. Freshwater wetlands throughout the area were strongly impacted by this discrete pulse of landscape disturbance, but the response of each wetland to local and upstream land use was site specific. The individualistic nature of wetland responses can be understood only by treating the drainage basin as a linked physical system that integrates geomorphic processes in a downstream direction.

Our study is based on the historical geography of 61 wetlands within a very small watershed (Susquetonscut Brook; 14 km²), on the stratigraphy of 18 widely distributed sites (as interpreted from conventional geomorphic, lithologic, radiocarbon, and pollen techniques), and on numerical modeling of historic flood discharges. Our results indicate that (1) presettlement wetlands were strongly impacted either directly or indirectly by English land-use practices; (2) the hydrogeologic setting of each wetland was responsible for either mitigating or amplifying these impacts at downstream sites; (3) the pulse of disturbance from the colonial period (1695–1787) continues to govern the modern sediment budget, flood regime, and riparian habitat of wetlands and watercourses throughout the area; (4) wetland impacts from Native American populations were not significant enough to be detected by our study; and (5) although many swamps were drained by the colonists, these wetland losses were more than offset by the amount of wetlands created.

*Present address: U.S. Geological Survey, Water Resources Division, Marlboro, Massachusetts 01752.

Thorson, R. M., Harris, A. G., Harris, S. L., Gradie, R., III, and Lefor, M. W., 1998, Colonial impacts to wetlands in Lebanon, Connecticut, *in* Welby, C. W., and Gowan, M. E., eds., A Paradox of Power: Voices of Warning and Reason in the Geosciences: Boulder, Colorado, Geological Society of America Reviews in Engineering Geology, v. XII.

INTRODUCTION

Widespread public support for wetlands protection derives from the general perception that wetlands are ancient, pristine, stable ecosystems of high intrinsic value. This is clearly not the case for many freshwater wetlands in the glaciated uplands of southern New England, a setting that was dramatically impacted by a wave of European agricultural technology that passed over the landscape like a storm beginning in the late seventeenth century and culminating shortly after the American Revolution. A tangible, quantifiable record of serious wetland impacts resulting from this ecological transition (or catastrophe) lies within the sediments of swamps and floodplains throughout this reforested region.

Wetland regulation is arguably the most contentious environmental issue in the United States with respect to the conflict between public and private property rights (National Research Council, NRC; 1995). Hence, the identification and delineation of wetland ecosystems must follow explicitly standardized legal procedures. Specifically, the recent NRC guidelines for wetland regulation (1) make no provision for the *origin* of wetlands, (2) require the identification of sites that have been *recently altered* by anthropogenic or natural events, and (3) allow wetlands on *agricultural* lands to be treated differently. These guidelines make sense when the alterations are very recent and are self-evident. But when wetland impacts have been naturally mitigated for centuries, and when abandoned, but reforested, agricultural land is not considered, the convenient assumptions underlying the regulatory process break down.

The investigation of historically impacted wetlands also has scientific merit because it provides a framework for evaluating landscape response to disturbance within the context of human ecology (Naveh and Leiberman, 1990; Worster, 1990; Chase, 1995). Most hydrogeologists who investigate wetlands understand that the impacts at any site were influenced by the integrated effects of all upstream sites, and that linkages between sites, however obscure, influence the differentiation of natural changes from anthropogenic ones. This watershed-scale perspective, however, is seldom applied in routine wetland investigations, especially in other disciplines, owing to the complexity of the issues involved (Phillips, 1992).

Our investigation lessens the problems of a watershed-scale approach by (1) focusing on a high concentration of wetlands in a very small area, (2) selecting a reforested agricultural area in which historic settlement occurred as a discrete pulse, and (3) selecting a watershed in a physiographic setting that would amplify, rather than attenuate, flood response in a downstream direction. Our study area is a small (14 km²) watershed at the headwaters of Susquetonscut Brook in the highlands of east-central Connecticut (Fig. 1). During the middle of the eighteenth century, the entire watershed was agricultural land within the colonial town of Lebanon, a small geographic area adjacent to, and governed by, a municipal Town Center (Fig. 1). Lebanon's land-use history, which begins in 1692 (Figs. 2–4), documents the agricultural conversion of the upland soils, the regulation of

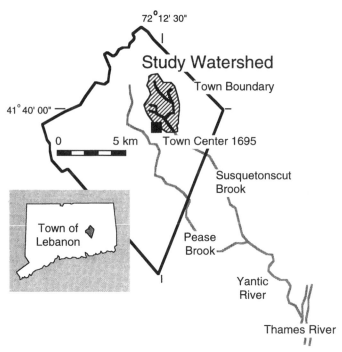

Figure 1. Location of study watershed area (hachured) within the headwaters of Susquetonscut Brook, in the town of Lebanon. Watershed is enlarged as Figures 2, 3, 5, and 9.

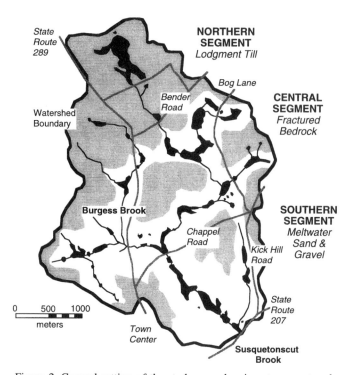

Figure 2. General setting of the study area showing stream network, roads, physiographic sections, and localities mentioned in the text. Boundaries between physiographic segments trend northeast-southwest parallel to the strike of the bedrock. Wetlands examined in this study (black) are shown. Areas above 122 m (400 ft) elevation are shaded. Dominant aquifers are listed for each segment.

streamflow for hydropower, the use of floodplains for grazing, deliberate wetland drainage, mining of wetlands for bog iron, the local extinction of beaver, and the construction of roads and bridges. The watershed had a variety of wetlands present at the time of settlement that attracted use as drained cropland and water-supply reservoirs. The outlet of Susquetonscut Brook was tightly constricted by artificial fill associated with a highway bridge built before 1720; this facilitated our treatment of the watershed as a closed physical system with a low sediment delivery ratio. Our results are broadly applicable because the rural-suburban character of the town and its large percentage of second-growth (or third-growth) forest are typical for southern New England.

This review is a case study addressing the physical evidence for hitherto unrecognized human impacts on the riparian wetlands in Susquetonscut Brook. We began with a field traverse of the stream network to identify, locate, and describe human influences on the channels and adjacent slopes. Next, we used aerial photographs to map all wetlands within the watershed and to classify them according to land-use history, rather than by traditional methods. Our main objective, however, was to reconstruct the recent development of the wetland system at the watershed scale by using sedimentary evidence from cores and natural exposures, and by hydrologic modeling of former conditions.

Our results demonstrate that (1) hidden human impacts to the wetland system were pervasive and ubiquitous, (2) stratigraphic evidence for the predicted effects of land-use changes is indeed present, and (3) that modern conditions continue to be influenced by the colonial deforestation that began more than three centuries ago. There is nothing "pristine" left in the scenic rural wetlands of Lebanon.

BACKGROUND

The sedimentary record

The ecological transformations that swept New England during the seventeenth and eighteenth centuries were recognized in their time (Deane, 1790) but were infrequently documented and are poorly understood, especially in quantitative terms. Ecological impacts on the presettlement flora, fauna, and indigenous peoples are known reasonably well because these were subjects of scientific interest to colonial writers. Anecdotal descriptions of transient changes in soils and hydrology are also available because these phenomena were vital to the agricultural economy (Cronon, 1983). But historic documents are inadequate to assess the "naturalness" of our present landscape in areas where historic structures (farmsteads, enclosures, dams for water supply) are not readily apparent (Thorson and Harris, 1991). At what scale of resolution (Urban et al., 1987) is the landscape the same, or different, from precolonial times?

The invasive nature of colonial agricultural technology, its broad geographic application, and its intensification through time ensured that permanent changes in the soils and streams of south-

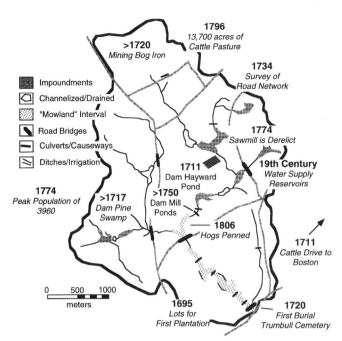

Figure 3. Map showing location of anthropogenic changes to the drainage network. Evidence from primary historic accounts (tax, deed, etc.) in boldface and listed by date; > symbol indicates structure in place before the date shown. Evidence from ground reconnaissance shown symbolically. Impoundments (dark gray) are located in central section where gradients are high. "Channelized" indicates rerouting of the main channel. Stone concentrations interpreted as former causeways are particularly abundant along the main stem.

ern New England occurred before original conditions could be adequately documented. The limited depth of prehistoric archaeological sites on slopes above wetlands, the dearth of presettlement soils (Hill et al., 1980), and the ubiquitous gridwork of stone walls demonstrates that upland soils were pervasively disturbed. Strata from wetlands, however, can be reliable indicators of land-use changes because they are sites of net deposition, and therefore act as recorders of changes in the flux of nutrients, sedimentary particles, and pollen grains (Bormann et al., 1974; Carter, 1986; Phillips, 1989). Thus, presettlement conditions at the landscape scale, the baseline from which environmental "alteration" must be measured, require field investigations of sedimentary strata within small freshwater wetlands.

Previous studies of wetland impact in New England have relied on a range of techniques. Pollen records confirm the known changes in watershed vegetation associated with land clearing, agricultural use, and abandonment to pasture and forest cover (Brugam, 1978; Kelso and Beaudry, 1987) and demonstrate that Native American populations had little impact on vegetation beyond the larger estuaries and floodplains (McAndrews, 1988). Engineering studies indicate that sediment transport at the Atlantic scale (Meade, 1982) was relatively insensitive to deforestation. The elevated sedimentation rates in New England lakes during historic time (Webb and Webb, 1988) tell us almost nothing about landscape change at the scale of farms, villages, and

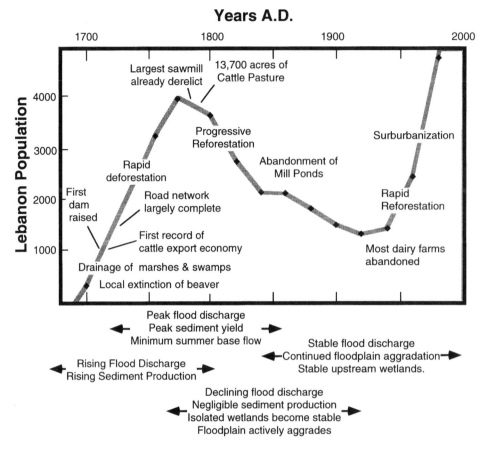

Figure 4. Graph illustrates changes in population of Lebanon from official census data (Milne, 1986). Specific historic events (lines) and general land use activities are superimposed on the population curve. Blocks of text beneath graph describe general hydrogeologic response to human activities, with arrows indicating general time range of response.

towns. The poor correlation between modern agricultural activities and sediment yield of larger New England streams (Gordon, 1979; Toney, 1987) belies the dramatic relationship between these variables in smaller drainages.

Our conclusion that small headwater wetlands in southern New England are the most (rather than the least) impacted by human disturbance is counterintuitive to the general perception that these remote wetland areas largely escaped the imprint of human hands (Adamus, 1983). Ironically, strict regulations are now mandated in the same watersheds that were once mined for ore, clear-cut of forest, mired by livestock, and dammed for hydropower. But unlike the obvious global effects of mining and agriculture in more arid landscapes (Hooke, 1994; Turner, 1990) the best record of equivalent landscape changes in New England lies buried beneath our protected wetlands.

The study area

Susquetonscut Brook is one of two major tributaries that meet to form the Yantic River near Norwich in southeastern Connecticut, a drainage network created by differential erosion of high-grade metamorphic rocks during Tertiary time (Denny, 1982). Our study area constitutes the northernmost 14 km² of the Susquetonscut Brook drainage (Fig. 2), centered on 41°40'00" N; 72°12'30"W. The watershed is approximately 5 km long, 4 km wide, and lies about 8 km south of the nearest city, Willimantic, Connecticut. The western third of our study area is drained by Burgess Brook; the eastern two-thirds by an unnamed stream. These tributaries merge just north of Chappel Road to form a single channel, here referred to as the main stem. Surface soils are sandy loams and stony sandy loams classified as dystrochrepts and udorthents (Cunningham and Ciolkosz, 1984), which reflect moderate to weak horizonification under acidic postglacial conditions. A discontinuous mantle of loamy topsoil above the till created by late-glacial eolian deposition (Thorson and Schile, 1995) and Holocene biomantle production (Johnson, 1990) is responsible for most of the suspended sediment transported to the streams.

The watershed consists of three physiographic segments,

each covering about one-third of the area and each containing highlands above 122 m elevation (400 ft). In the *Northern Segment*, elevations reach approximately 152 m (500 ft) and are underlain by sandy glacial till of low permeability with moderate local relief (Clebnik, 1980). A perched water table often occurs in shallow depressions. Local summits are glacially streamlined hills with broad, till-covered summits, and were ideal sites for upland colonial agriculture. In the *Central Segment*, watershed relief reaches a maximum; streams occupy bouldery ravines at about 90–100 m deep as they cross through a belt of resistant rock, and hill summits project above 182 m (600 ft) elevation. Ground water availability is dominated by flow within fractured rock. In the *Southern Segment*, a well-developed modern flood-plain lies terraced below a broad, gravely valley fill deposited by meltwater deltas and streams during glacier recession about 17,000 years ago. The most transmissive aquifers occur within these glacial sedimentary basins, insuring persistent wetness throughout the year. These meltwater deposits are, in turn, flanked by till-covered drumlinoid slopes rising to 134 m (440 ft) elevation, which recharge the stratified drift aquifer.

Vegetation in the study area is classified as the Appalachian Oak Forest Section of the Eastern Deciduous Forest (Bailey, 1978), and consists of areas reforested after abandonment of farms. Dominant trees include oak, maple, hickory, ash, hemlock, and white pine; chestnut was prominent prior to the outbreak of chestnut blight in the early twentieth century. The modern climate is temperate, with a mean precipitation of about 1,200 mm distributed evenly throughout the year (Ruffner, 1985), although the year-to-year variability of rainfall is high. Proximity to the Atlantic Ocean moderates extreme variations in temperature and is responsible for high-intensity precipitation events associated with strong frontal activity and hurricanes. Major hurricane floods occurred in 1927, 1938, and 1955, with storm precipitation exceeding 125 mm in a three-day period (Patton, 1988). The water budget is dominated by infiltration and evapotranspiration during the winter and summer months, respectively (Thomas et al., 1967).

The regional pollen stratigraphy and climatic modeling experiments (Webb et al., 1993) demonstrate that peak postglacial warmth was delayed until sometime between 9,000 and 6,000 B.P., owing to the persistent effects of the Laurentide Ice Sheet. Slightly cooler and moister conditions characterized the last several millennia (Davis, 1983). Historic climate records begin in 1742 (Landsburg, 1967). In the most general terms, average conditions for the period 1780–1840 were colder, drier, and more variable than present; the period 1840–1890 was colder, wetter, and more variable than present; and the period 1890–1990 has shown a broad trend towards warmer, drier, and more stable conditions.

Land-use history

The abundance of Native American names and the presence of late Woodland and contact-period artifacts indicate that the town of Lebanon was occupied by Mohegan peoples before being "transferred" to a collective of colonists in 1692. The town was named by John Fitch, who, noting the majestic cedars within local swamps, compared the area to that of the Holy Land (Milne, 1986). Ironically, what is now the village green (listed on the National Register of Historic Places), was once a perched swamp, the draining of which may have been the first serious impact to a local wetland. Another early historical impact took place at the largest wetland in the study area, which was mined for bog iron between the late 1720s and early 1730s.

The narrow, original house lots dating to 1695 fronted on the town common and extended eastward, downslope across the floodplain of Susquetonscut Brook, between Chappel Road and Route 207 (Figs. 2 and 3). The pattern of stone walls, collapsed bridge abutments, and ditches runs perpendicular to the brook and indicates that individual landowners each maintained his own causeway across the marsh. An early deed describes "mowlands" in the floodplain of Susquetonscut Brook, suggesting that at least part of the floodplain was being used (and artificially drained) at this time. Government surveys indicate that the present network of roads and villages was established before 1734.

The population of Lebanon grew from about 350 inhabitants at the time of settlement to a premodern peak of nearly 3,960 inhabitants (including 116 slaves) in 1774 (Fig. 4). Colonial population growth was fueled by an export agricultural economy that accelerated in the decades before and during the American Revolution. For example, cattle drives to Boston occurred as early as 1711, and the tax list for 1796 describes 13,700 acres as cattle pasture, nearly all of which has since been reforested. Evidence for early and intense deforestation is found in a 1774 deed referring to the largest saw mill in the area as "old" (generally meaning derelict). A second deed in 1806 indicates the commercial penning of hogs, which implies that forest clearing may have been essentially complete. After its peak, the population of Lebanon declined steadily throughout the nineteenth and early twentieth centuries, rising again only after the automobile provided convenient access to nearby cities.

The widespread occurrence of mills, reservoirs, and irrigation ditches demonstrates the degree to which water was regulated in the basin during colonial times. Specific historical descriptions are available for six of the eight artificial impoundments in the basin. Associated with these ponds were at least six industrial enterprises, including a grinding shop, a grist mill, a saw mill, a cider press, a distillery, and a shop of undetermined function. The historic accounts of these structures and reconnaissance archaeological investigations indicate that industrial development of the Brook reached its peak between 1775 and 1825. Additionally, cattle watering would have required many artificial ponds in this rocky and generally well-drained hill country.

The earliest evidence for the deliberate management of water is a 1711 deed for Hayward Pond, which was impounded by a "nine-foot" stone-faced earthen dam to power a grist mill that operated through the end of the nineteenth century. Pine Swamp (Fig. 3) was impounded by 1717. Two dams were raised near the head of the steep ravine between Hayward Pond and Chanski Basin sometime before 1750 (Sawmill Pond, Fig. 3). Two other nineteenth-century dams (Manning Pond and Unnamed Dam) are located directly above Hayward Pond, and probably were used to regulate streamflow to it as part of an integrated water-management scheme. Two more dams, both located below Hayward Pond, were discovered in field surveys.

Irrigation ditches and structures are also sporadically mentioned in written accounts, and were observed during our reconnaissance. The upper dam along the main stem and the dam above Hayward Pond have been reinforced and continue to function as unregulated stock ponds. Most of the other dams are partly collapsed, but still retain ponds.

CRONON'S HYPOTHESIS

William Cronon (1983, p. 122–124; Table 1) summarized historical accounts from the eighteenth and nineteenth centuries regarding how colonial land-use practices impacted the hydrologic regimes in New England. Based on his analysis, the earliest hydrologic changes in colonial Lebanon would have been associated with the local extinction of beavers (*Castor canadensis*), whose persistent presence in southern New England for the past 12,000 years (Kaye, 1962) was an important component of the fluvial system (Naiman and Johnson, 1988). Breaching of beaver dams, which may have been abandoned as early as 1640, would have released sediment from storage, and their dams could no longer have attenuated flood peaks.

Historical accounts also indicate that removal of the forest canopy in Susquetonscut Brook would have increased both the frequency and magnitude of floods, and would have greatly elevated the flux of suspended sediment from the upland landscape. Enhanced flooding would have been a direct consequence of many factors, chief among them being the decreased permeability associated with the deeply frozen and compacted soils of cultivated and pastured areas, and with the enhanced rate of spring snowmelt in exposed areas. The effect of deforestation on the ground-water budget of wetlands in Susquetonscut Brook, however, would have been case-specific. In some cases, the reduced infiltration responsible for enhanced flooding would have caused a reduction in ground-water recharge, leading to greater drying of soils and the loss of wetlands. Elsewhere, decreased evapotranspiration losses resulting from deforestation led to greater aquifer recharge and higher base-flow discharge to wetlands.

These historically based accounts of change are consistent with the results of modern empirical studies based on deforestation experiments (Hornbeck et al., 1970), flood discharge (U.S. Army Corps of Engineers, 1981) and water budget (Miller and Focazzio, 1988) models, regression analyses of watershed response to known changes (Pickup, 1988), case studies of wetland impacts (O'Brien, 1977), and by stratigraphic records (Jacobsen and Coleman, 1986).

The consistency between historical and empirical approaches suggests that the hydrologic impacts of the colonial land-use changes on wetlands in Susquetonscut Brook can be considered as a single broad hypothesis. Specific predictions from Cronon's hypothesis include the following.

1. Land clearing, grazing, and cultivation would have

TABLE 1. EXPECTED HYDROLOGIC IMPACTS OF COLONIAL LAND USE CHANGES*

Purpose	Specific Action	Local Impacts	Downstream Discharge			Sediment Load		Relative Importance
			Total Runoff	Base Flow	Peak Flood	Direct	Indirect	
Transportation	Roads, trails	Drainage occlusion	+	−	+/−	−	+	Low
Hydropower	Mills, dams, sluiceways	Reservoir storage. Local rise in water table	+	+	−	−	−	High
Drainage	Ditching, channelization	Local sediment production. Peat decomposition	0	−	+	+	+	Low
Food Production	Tillage, pasture	Sediment production. Decreased infiltration. Ground freezing	+	−	+	+++	+	Medium
Property Division	Stone walls/fencing	Drainage occlusion. Sediment retention	+	−	+/−	−	−	Low
Forestry/Clearing	Clearing	Sediment mobilization. Limited infiltration	+	+	++	++	+	Very high
Trapping	Beaver extinction	Sediment source from abandoned dams	−	−	−	++	+/−	Medium

*Qualitative relative estimate for the significance of selected impacts on selected parameters. Major increase = +++; moderate increase = ++; slight increase = +, decrease = −, or no effect = 0.

increased both total discharge and base flow, owing to increased runoff from bare soils and decreased evapotranspiration from denuded watersheds, respectively.

2. Sediment transport would have increased due to erosion of exposed upland soils, and to enlargement of channel banks in response to increased flood flows.

3. The subsequent construction of mill dams during the late eighteenth and early nineteenth century would have attenuated and desynchronized peak flood flows by mass storage in reservoirs, and simultaneously increased the permanent storage of sediment in reservoirs and ponds.

4. Expansion of the transportation network (roads, cartways, causeways, and trails) and the construction of fences and stone walls would have created site-specific occlusions of the drainage network, leading to enhanced retention of sediment on the upstream sides, causing wetter conditions, the enhanced growth of obligate hydrophytes, and additional retention of sediment.

5. Ditching and channelization of streams would have contributed to the release of sediments from storage through the effects of increased stream power, and through the aerobic decomposition of organic soils in situ by bacterial respiration.

These specific predictions can be tested by comparing them with the actual changes at wetland sites as reconstructed from stratigraphic records in a range of hydrogeologic settings.

METHODS

Mapping and classification

To map the wetlands in the watershed we used aerial photographic stereo pairs from the spring of 1986 at an approximate contact scale of 1:12,000. By simultaneously examining wetland boundaries from the National Wetlands Inventory of the Willimantic Quadrangle (Metzler and Tiner, 1992) and the aerial photographs, we developed an operational definition of a wetland for mapping purposes (a flat landform where the photographic tone contrasted strongly with the adjacent terrain and where prolonged wetness was consistent with geomorphic setting and field observations). Our population of wetlands (n = 61) is based strictly on the interpretation and field checking of the aerial photographs against the ground distribution of hydric soils (Tiner and Veneman, 1989), and includes all sites that were large enough to map at a scale of 1:12,000. We included all sites linked by the drainage network but excluded recently excavated farm ponds on the upland. Although the lower floodplain of Susquetonscut Brook is continuous along the main channel, we subdivided it into four sedimentary basins (wetlands) between constrictions, all of which were partly human in origin (Fig. 5; Tables 2–4). The spatial density of wetlands examined (4.4 per km²) was sufficient to characterize the watershed qualitatively, and is representative of terrain throughout eastern Connecticut.

The classification system used by the National Wetland Inventory (Cowardin et al., 1979) was inappropriate because

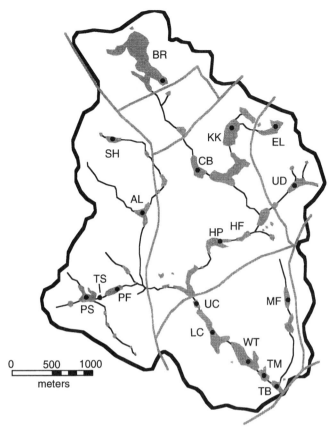

Figure 5. Map showing wetlands investigated in this study. Full names for abbreviations and wetland characteristics are given in Table 3. Large black dots show locations of natural exposure, sediment cores, or transects of cores for stratigraphic interpretation that are summarized in this report (additional details are given in Thorson, 1992).

every wetland in our study area belonged to the same subclass (Broad-leaved Scrub-shrub Palustrine Wetlands; Fig. 4). A classification based on surficial geology (Clebnik, 1980) and soils type (U.S. Soil Conservation Service, 1983) failed because the mapped units were independent of wetland stratigraphy. A hydrological classification of wetlands (Gosselink and Turner, 1978) required surface-water data that was unavailable. The most consistent and meaningful classification that we could devise was based on apparent land use (Table 2).

We obtained quantitative data for each wetland and its upstream watershed (Table 3) in order to examine the relationship between wetland response to geomorphic setting. Data on wetland elevation and stream gradient were obtained from the U.S. Geological Survey topographic map of the Willimantic Quadrangle (7.5' series scale 1:24,000). Parameters associated with the geomorphic setting of each wetland including wetland area, the length of stream channel draining directly into the wetland without an intervening wetland, and the number of known occlusions upstream of a wetland were obtained from aerial photographs.

TABLE 2. LAND-USE CLASSIFICATION OF WETLANDS*

Category	Subtype	Operational Definition	Number	Percent
Intentionally Created	Dams	Marshes, swamps, and remnants of open water impounded by unmaintained stone-faced and earth-fill dams	8	13
Intentionally Created	Ponds	Ponds upstream from artificial constriction; generally stock ponds	18	30
Intentionally Created	Quarries	Marsh and open-water within active or abandoned quarries as of March 22, 1986. Does not include small excavations and swimming pools in residential areas	5	8
Unintentionally Created	Occlusion	Swamps upstream of historic structure such as abandoned roads, walls, and cattle fords	20	33
Apparently "Natural" Wetlands	Constriction	Wetland upstream from constriction for which no evidence of a historic structure is present	7	11
Apparently "Natural" Wetlands	Other	Meets operational definition of wetland but none of the criteria above	3	5
Total			61	100

*Field-checked from 1986 aerial photographs at 1:12,000 scale.

Field reconnaissance and sampling

To examine the wetlands mapped from aerial photographs, we walked approximately half of the length of the stream network. We paid particular attention to intentional changes in the drainage network such as channelization and causeway construction, and to the structure, storage capacity, and spillway mechanisms of all historic impoundments.

To investigate the more subtle historic impacts on our population of 61 wetlands, we selected a sample of 18 sites for field study (Fig. 5; Table 4). We did not follow an objective, statistical sampling strategy. Instead, we chose sites based on the constraints of road access, permission to work on private property, and the presence of a thick sedimentary record, while simultaneously attempting to balance the broadest geographic distribution and variety in hydrogeologic settings. Although our sample (n = 18) was qualitatively selected and is biased toward sites with a thick sedimentary record, we believe that it is broadly representative of all large (> 1 ha) wetlands in the watershed. Almost all of the wetlands investigated were unnamed; thus we gave each an informal local name and a two-letter code (Table 4).

Field investigation

Field mapping of sites was based on soil morphology. Sedimentary records were obtained from natural exposures, centrally located cores in small wetlands, or traverses of multiple cores across larger wetlands. We selected sites from natural exposures (n = 5) as representative of streambanks in the vicinity. In most of the wetlands, we used a stainless steel probe to determine the depth to the underlying glacial substrate, and thus, the overall configuration of the wetland sediments. For areas underlain by more than a meter of sediment we used a 5-cm-diameter device to extract short cores in order to examine near-surface variability in composition. At sites where the near-surface deposits were similar over a broad area (n = 13), we estimated where the sediments would be thickest, and extracted a single piston core to the maximum depth of penetration. Routine procedures for measurement and for estimating sediment compaction were used. In wetlands having substantial variability in subsurface stratigraphy (n = 5), we used a transect of two or more cores taken from a surveyed baseline. Unit thickness was measured to the nearest centimeter, although variations in the height of the ground surface and in compaction errors introduce an uncertainty of several centimeters into all measurements. All cores were field wrapped in plastic, aluminum foil, and PVC pipe for transport. We attempted to obtain a core from two of the larger wetlands (Hayward Pond, Sawmill Pond), but could not extract the near-surface sediments because of their high water content.

Laboratory procedures

Qualitative observations on sedimentary texture, grain size and shape, compaction, bulk density, organic content, and degree of decomposition (indicated by the proportion and selective preservation of plant fibers and the color and texture of the matrix) were made for each lithologic unit following conventional procedures (Aaby, 1986). Measured data include moist Munsell color, the size of large particles, bed thickness, bed orientation, and the location of intrastratal lenses. Organic content was measured using loss on ignition. Munsell colors were recorded but are reported here without numerical coding. Pollen samples were taken above and below all lithological contacts and at regular intervals within thick units, usually at 10-cm intervals. Samples were extracted, prepared, counted, and plotted using the procedures outlined by Faegri and Iversen (1975). At least 200 grains were counted for each sample. Macrofossils were identified using standard taxonomic keys and a reference collection.

We obtained chronological control from 10 radiocarbon dates, 34 biostratigraphic horizons, and 15 instances where the historic disturbance horizon could be identified. Although the wave of colonial settlement in the watershed was diachronic (1695–1774), we assign a uniform age of 250 yrs. B.P. to the set-

TABLE 3. FIELD AND MAP DATA FOR SAMPLE OF WETLANDS IN STUDY AREA*

Identification Code	Local Name	Data Source	Number of Stratigraphic Sections	Selected Parameters Wetland Elevation (m)	Selected Parameters Wetland Area (ha)	Selected Parameters Upstream Gradient (m/km)
AL	Alice's Swamp	Core	1	105	3	62
BR	Bender Road	Core	1	160	12	26
CB	Chanski's Basin	Bank	2	114	3	25
UC	Chapel Hill, Upper	Bank	2	79	8	20
LC	Chapel Hill, Lower	Transect	5	78	8	20
EL	Ellis Pond	Core	1	114	3	109
HF	Hayward Floodplain	Bank	1	na	1	na
HP	Hayward Pond	Test core	0	na	2	na
KK	Kalmon Kurcnik's	Core	1	114	7	199
MF	Manning Floodplain	Transect	2	102	2	78
PS	Pine Swamp	Core	1	99	3	62
PF	Pogmore Floodplain	Transect	2	96	1	101
TS	Typha Swamp	Core	1	98	0	119
SH	Sweet Hill	Core	1	168	1	37
TB	Trumbull Bridge	Core	1	75	7	16
TM	Trumbull Marsh	Core	1	76	7	17
UD	Unnamed Dam	Core	1	111	3	132
WT	Wet Transit	Transect	3	76	7	17

*Map data from U.S.G.S. Willimantic Quadrangle, scale 1:24,000.

tlement horizon for the purposes of rate calculations. Radiocarbon samples consisted of hand-picked wood obtained from wet-sieved peat, and were obtained above or below lithological core breaks. All dates were given standard counts following routine laboratory pretreatment procedures, and are reported in radiocarbon years before present (1950) based on a half life of 5,568 years. Biostratigraphic dates were assigned through comparison of pollen diagrams for each wetland with the well-established regional pollen stratigraphy (Deevey, 1939; Davis, 1969; Gadreau and Webb, 1985) and are supported by the available radiocarbon and macrofossil evidence. The arbitrary error assigned to each presettlement biostratigraphic date ($\pm$ 500 yr) includes both our vertical sampling resolution and the chronological error inherent in the regional pollen record; this error is not included in estimated rates for sediment accumulation.

Stratigraphic interpretations

Biostratigraphic dates follow the zonation and dates of Davis (1969) and Gaudreu and Webb (1985; Fig. 6). The most easily recognized biostratigraphic horizon is the pine/oak transition (Zone B/C-1 boundary) dating to approximately 8,500 [14]C B.P. Next in order of prominence is the C3a–C3b zone boundary, which marks the arrival of the Europeans (Brugam, 1978) and is consistently expressed as an increase in ragweed and grass pollen and a decrease in tree pollen. An abrupt first occurrence of chestnut pollen to a level of about 10 % of the total pollen count marks the local arrival of chestnut at about 2,000 B.P. The chestnut rise coincides with an increase in the abundance of

hickory pollen (5,000 B.P.) in most cores from Susquetonscut Brook, indicating a negligible background sedimentation rate during this interval. The transition between a spruce-fir assemblage and the pine-dominated assemblage in our cores is correlated with the Zone A–Zone B pollen zone boundary at about 10,000 B.P. We assign a date of 12,000 B.P. to the transition between a sedge/herb/heath pollen assemblage to one dominated by spruce (Zone T–Zone A).

We interpreted wetland prehistory based largely on first-order, macroscopic, sedimentary evidence (Fig. 7). Bedded strata consisting largely of inorganic grains indicate slackwater sedimentation from turbid streams, generally under lacustrine conditions. Aquatic (limnic) peats are fine grained, detrital, and frequently contain the seeds of aquatic taxa. Matted (interwoven) fibrous peats with a dominance of cryptogam and monocot tissue and a dearth of wood often coincide with times of high mineral sedimentation, and indicate accumulation in unforested marshes. Variations in the ratio between organic and inorganic content is a function of the availability of sediment from the upstream watershed.

Peat accumulation in swamps is indicated by autochthonous humified peats with abundant wood, especially in situ roots. Thoroughly decomposed horizons (Saprists) with a high mineral content in woody peat sequences indicate net decomposition of peat, an interpretation often supported by a hiatus in bracketing dates. Topstratum (overbank) sedimentation is indicated by bioturbated mineral horizons occasionally interbedded with peaty lenses. Coarse-grained topstratum deposits often exhibit cross-stratification, basal scouring, and load structures, indicating rapid

TABLE 4. QUALITATIVE DESCRIPTION OF WETLANDS IN STUDY WATERSHED*

Wetland Code	New London County Soil Map[†]	National Wetlands Inventory[§]	Surficial Geology[**]	Land-Use Subtype[‡]	Stratigraphic/ Hydrogeologic Setting[‡]
AL	Adrian Muck	P-SS-1	Stratified drift	Other	Tributary confluence
BR	Ridgebury e.f.s.l.	P-SS-1	Till	Occulsion	Artifical occlusion
CB	Adrian Muck	P-SS-1	Stratified drift	Occlusion	Drained
UC	Rippowam	P-SS-1	Stratified drift	Constriction	Main flood plain
LC	Rippowam f.s.l.	P-SS-1	Stratified drift	Occlusion	Main flood plain
EL	Adrian Muck	P-SS-1	Bedrock	Occlusion	Bedrock basin
HF	Ridgebury e.f.s.l.	P-SS-1	Stratified drift	Occlusion	Drained
HP	Ridgebury e.f.s.l.	P-SS-1	Stratified drift	Dam	Upland stream
KK	Ridgebury e.f.s.l.	P-SS-1	Bedrock	Occlusion	Artifical occlusion
MF	Ridgebury e.f.s.l.	P-SS-1	Till	Occlusion	Upland stream
PS	Ridgebury e.f.s.l.	P-SS-1	Stratified drift	Occlusion	Tributary confluence
PF	Ridgebury e.f.s.l.	P-SS-1	Bedrock	Dam	Bedrock basin
TS	Canton vsfsl	P-SS-1	Stratified drift	Dam	Upland stream
SH	Rippowam f.s.l.	P-SS-1	Till	Occlusion	Upland stream
TB	Rippowam f.s.l.	P-SS-1	Stratified drift	Occlusion	Main flood plain
TM	Carlise Muck	P-SS-1	Stratified drift	Occlusion	Main flood plain
UD	Carlise Muck	P-SS-1	Till	Dam	Bedrock basin
WT	Rippowam f.s.l.	P-SS-1	Stratified drift	Occlusion	Main flood plain

*Soil texture abbreviations are: e.f.s.l. = extremely stony fine sandy loam; f.s.l. = fine sandy loam; P-SS-1 = subclass Palustrine shrub-Scrub broadleaved.
[†]Soil Conservation Service, 1983.
[§]Cowardin et al., 1979.
[**]Clebnik, 1980.
[‡]This report.

deposition by current traction on a soft floodplain surface. Immature floodplain soils (Aquents) are recognized by their blocky structure, incipient mottling, root casts, and surface relief. The specific identification of plant macrofossils, diatom frustules, and pollen also aided in identification of these environments.

Flood discharge modeling

Quantitative estimates for how deforestation and dam impoundment affected peak flood discharge were obtained using HEC-1, a widely used flood discharge model developed by the U.S. Army Corps of Engineers (1981; Table 5). For the purposes of this report, we modeled the peak flood discharge at the Lower Chapel Road wetland that would have been produced by a storm with a one-year recurrence interval from unfrozen soil. To implement the model, we divided the 14 km^2 watershed into 26 sub-basins, each of which yielded runoff, based on soil properties and average slope (Harris, 1993). Discharges from each subbasin were then summed and routed in a downstream direction at a rate controlled by the hydraulic configuration of the channel in each reach (roughness, size, gradient, etc.).

We directly calibrated the model to Susquetonscut Brook for a series of storms using weather data from USGS stations, map data for present land use and reservoir geometry, and field measurements of storm discharge and lag time from a gauging station installed near the Lower Chappel Road wetland. We calibrated the model by iteratively changing the land-use input parameters

until they yielded the observed storm discharges. We then inverted the model to retrodict peak discharge, total discharge, and ground-water recharge for two separate historic land-use scenarios. Our presettlement scenario assumes no reservoirs and complete forest cover; it does not take into account the effect of beavers, which have been reintroduced into the watershed, the effects of which are already included in model calibration. Our "developed" scenarios are based on unpublished data from nearby Worcester County, Massachussetts (John Larkin, Research Director, Sturbridge Village, Inc., written communication, 1993), which suggests that two thirds (67%) of the terrain was "improved" (10% tillage and 57% pasture) with the remaining third (33%) being woodlot, outcrop, and other uses. We could not model active human management of stormflows, hence the impoundments modulate flood discharges based solely on their preabandonment shapes and spillway cross sections.

RESULTS

Deliberate channel alterations

The only site-specific, historically documented changes in the stream network within Susquetonscut Brook are short reaches of the channel that have been submerged by extant water-supply reservoirs (Hayward Pond, Sawmill Pond, Pine Swamp, Unnamed Dam). During our field studies, however, we discovered that deliberate changes to the stream network are nearly

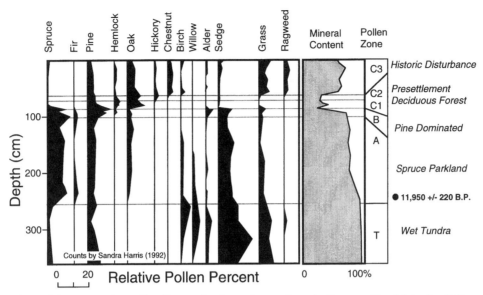

Figure 6. Representative pollen diagram for the study area from the Pogmore Floodplain site. Pollen abundance (black), mineral content (shaded), and pollen zonation (Davis, 1969) are given. Approximate boundary dates for biostratigraphic zones are T/A = 12,000; A/B = 10,000; B/C1 = 8,500; C2/C3 = 250 B.P. Core stratigraphy is given in Figure 7.

ubiquitous and have taken many forms. Most modifications appear subtle in the field, owing to secondary growth of forest, burial beneath alluvium, and turbation by tree blowdowns; in many cases, attributing human cause to channel change was based solely on anomalously large boulders or channel widths.

We did not do an archaeological inventory of these deliberate modifications but noted them when discovered (Fig. 3). Among the many changes that we observed were (1) draining of the main stem by ditching and diking of the meadows between the Kalmon Kurcnik and Ellis wetlands, (2) straightening of the stream by channelization (excavation and bank-armoring) of the main stem in the Hayward Floodplain wetland, and of the tributary to the south of Pine Swamp, (3) excavation of irrigation channels below Sawmill Pond, (4) drainage of Alice's Swamp and Pine Swamp by deepening of the channel, (5) drainage of riparian meadows by ditches parallel to the Lower Chappel road wetland, and (6) a variety of anomalous stone concentrations across the channel, which can be easily mistaken for bouldery, natural riffles in many cases.

The channel-crossing stone concentrations are particularly abundant, occur in a variety of forms, and are clearly artificial. Where they occur in ravines between reservoirs (Sawmill Pond, Hayward Pond) and mills we interpret them as check dams (designed to reduce peak stream power during floods). Where two or more of the stones remain fitted together along the channel margin (Trumbull Bridge, Trumbull Marsh, Lower Chappel Road, Hayward Pond, Bender Road), we interpreted them as abutments for wooden bridges; where unfitted we interpret them as crude fords (or foundations for private wooden bridges) when the stones were simply heaped into the channel. When the stones extended into swamps, rather than channels, we interpreted them as primitive causeways for livestock.

Every wetland that we examined had a stone concentration of one form or another at its constricted outlet that could be, but often probably is not, of human origin. Proving such an assertion is complicated by the construction activities of beavers, which have recently been re-introduced and which have incorporated stone slabs up to 10 kg into their dams.

Flood retrodictions

Results from HEC-1 modeling indicate that peak discharges (mean annual flood) during the time of maximum colonial development were twice as high as the undisturbed, base-line scenario (Table 5), despite the mitigating influence of the reservoirs and check dams. Most of the increase results from enhanced overland flow on deforested, compacted soils. Modern flows are actually lower than those of the undisturbed condition, owing to the continued presence of abandoned dams, which attenuate peak flows through the effect of reservoir storage. First-order infiltration to the ground-water table (assumed to be the reciprocal of storm runoff) would have been substantially lower during colonial times, suggesting that upland streams would probably have been drier at peak agricultural expansion, more than two centuries ago. This interpretation is supported by the increased development of local ponds during the nineteenth century.

Watershed-scale effects

We used conventional regression and correlation techniques to investigate the quantitative relationships between wetland and watershed characteristics (Table 3; wetland elevation, wetland area, stream gradient, watershed area) but were unable to find any meaningful correlations. Apparently, the distribution and

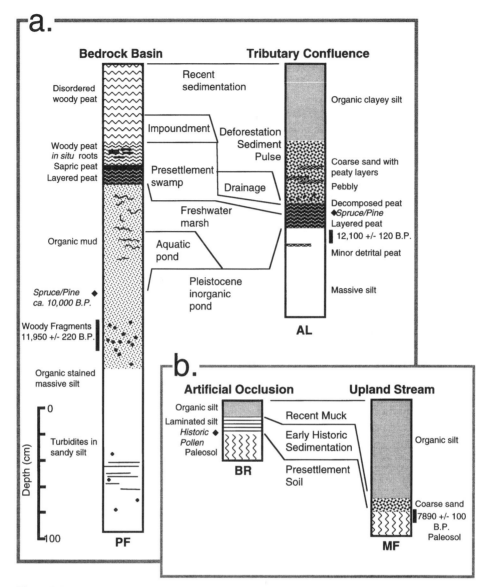

Figure 7. Measured stratigraphic sections of type wetlands for four hydrogeologic settings as discussed in text. Descriptions, radiocarbon dates (solid bar), and pollen dates (diamond) are listed on outside of columns. Interpretations and correlation lines are presented between columns. a, Longer, more continuous records of Pogmore Floodplain (PF; on left) and Alice's Swamp (AL; on right); b, Shorter, simpler records of Bender Road (BR; on left) and Manning Floodplain (MF; on right).

configuration of wetlands in Susquetonscut Brook are not governed by simple hydrologic, topographic, or hypsometric relationships. Instead, wetland characteristics represent site-specific, individualistic responses to local geology and anthropogenic impact.

The only wetland characteristics found to be highly correlated were those obtained from the stratigraphic analysis described below. Our results demonstrate that the flux of mineral sediment to wetlands was initially high prior to about 8,000 B.P., but diminished to negligible rates prior to European settlement. Since settlement, the average sedimentation rate increased several orders of magnitude at almost all sites (Fig. 8). Geologic age is thus associ-

ated with sedimentation rate, regardless of hydrogeologic setting. The modern wetlands of Susquetonscut Brook are overloaded with sediment.

Our land-use classification of wetlands provides an additional semiquantitative measure of landscape change (Table 2). Eighty-four percent of the wetlands in the study area watershed of Susquetonscut Brook appear to have been modified by human action, and more than half were either created or deliberately changed in some way prior to the federal management of wetlands. The largest single land-use category of wetlands appears to be wetlands inadvertently created upstream from drainage occlusions.

TABLE 5. PREDICTED STREAM DISCHARGES FROM CALIBRATED MODEL (HEC-1)*

| Scenario | Land Use | | | Rainfall | Peak Flood | | Storm Runoff | |
	Forest (%)	Improved (%)	Reservoirs (n)	(mm)	(m³/sec)	(% modern)	(mm)	(% modern)
Before 1692	100	0	0	69	7	118	14	74
Maximum Development 1754–1825	33	67	6	69	12	211	30	158
Modern, 1930–1996	78	22	6	69	6	100	19	100

*Based on 1-year storm recurrence. Improved land is 10% tillage, 57% pasture for developed scenario, 3% tillage, 19% pasture for modern scenario.

Wetland stratigraphy

The stratigraphy of 18 wetlands in Susquetonscut Brook is known with enough detail (Thorson, 1992) so that we can establish the geologic origin of each and document how colonial land use altered the environment from its presettlement condition (Figs. 7, 8). Each wetland responded to human impact in an individualistic manner. However, qualitative similarities in the pattern of stratigraphic change were clearly related to the hydrogeologic setting in which the wetland was located. Such similarities provided a basis for classifying each of the 18 wetlands studied into one of six categories. In turn, this permitted us to restrict the need for detailed description to only six sites (Appendix 1). Stratigraphic records for the remaining 12 wetlands are summarized as Table 6 and Figures 7 and 9. Our taxonomic approach underscores the importance of hydrogeologic setting in controlling wetland impact and provides a conceptual framework for integrating effects in a downstream direction.

Upland streams. These wetlands (Manning Floodplain, Sweet Hill) occur as expanded reaches of small, ephemeral streams at high elevations near the edges of the watershed and always occur immediately above constrictions. The till-covered slopes above these wetlands are sites of net erosion and are locally devoid of Holocene topsoil. The stratigraphy of these wetlands is dominated by an abrupt pulse of traction-deposited agricultural sediment (bedload sand and fine gravel) that overlies a well-defined presettlement horizon. Presettlement deposits in these settings are largely absent, and are instead represented by incipient poorly drained soils, now preserved beneath the bioturbated historic valley fills.

Entrapment of sediment from disturbed agricultural soils at drainage occlusions created the upland stream wetlands. The steep gradients and poorly drained soils of their watersheds, together with the potential for their use as pasture, is consistent with the sedimentary evidence.

Bedrock basins. Pogmore Floodplain, Ellis, and Unnamed Dam are examples of the bedrock basin wetlands that occur near the headwaters of the drainage network within the rugged, central physiographic segment. They lie within an east-west–trending belt of near-surface, heavily fractured bedrock where the stony meltout till is highly permeable and where the local relief exceeds 100 m. Each wetland parallels a prominent fracture zone in the local bedrock and is a zone of ground-water discharge from the fractured bedrock aquifer. Additionally, each wetland has a narrow outlet.

The bedrock basin wetlands have been sites of net organic deposition for all of postglacial time, and the sediments are dominated by limnic and marsh peats containing negligible watershed-derived (allogenic) mineral sediment. Prior to settlement, all of these sites were wooded swamps characterized by conditions of slow peat accumulation. Historic impacts to the three basins were similar, and are dominated by an abrupt rise in the water table to ponded conditions accompanied by strong siltation from topsoil erosion in their small steep watersheds. The abrupt rise in the water table at all sites is clearly shown by the drowning of woody peats, and was almost certainly caused by the raising of small dams at their outlets. The observation that these wetlands contained, but were not overwhelmed by, topsoil loss is consistent

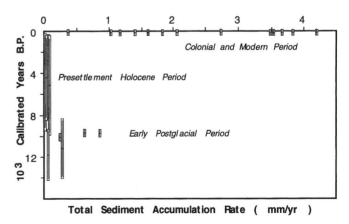

Figure 8. Plot showing changes in average sedimentation rate through time in wetlands from Susquetonscut Brook. All estimates are based on the compaction-corrected thickness between intervals dated by biostratigraphy and radiocarbon. All rates are subject to large uncertainties.

TABLE 6. SUMMARY OF HISTORIC CHANGES BASED ON STRATIGRAPHIC RECORDS*

		Depositional Environment at Different Times		
Code	Wetland Basin Locality	Presettlement Condition	Early Historic Changes	Recent Trends
UC	Upper Chappel Road	Unknown	Channel erosion. Pulse of coarse TSS followed by organic TSS	Reduced deposition of coarse TSS
TB	Trumbull Bridge	Unknown	Channel erosion? Bridge occludes drainage. Marsh deposits	Reduced deposition of coarse TSS
LC	Lower Chappel Road	Marshy flood plain. Slow peat accumulation	Pulse of coarse TSS followed by organic TSS	Second pulse of coarse TSS
WT	Wet Transit	Marshy flood plain. Hiatus in Holocene peat accumulation	Pulse of coarse TSS. Deliberate ditching. Soil?	Reduced deposition of coarse TSS
TM	Trumbull Marsh	Marsh; Hiatus in Holocene peat	Pulse of coarse TSS. Deliberate ditching. Soil?	Second pulse of coarse TSS
PS	Pine Swamp	Stable wooded swamp	Deliberate drainage. Impounded to aquatic pond. Siltation	Collapse of dam. Reverted to wooded swamp
AL	Alice's Wetland	Stable wooded swamp	Deliberate drainage. Strong pulse of coarse TSS	Continued TSS, but finer grained and at reduced rates
TS	Typha Swamp	Stable wooded swamp	Impounded to aquatic pond. Siltation	Siltation
EL	Ellis Wetland	Peat accumulation in wooded swamp	Impounded to aquatic pond. Limited siltation	No change
PF	Pogmore Floodplain	Peat accumulation in wooded swamp	Impounded to aquatic pond. Strong siltation	Reduced siltation. Collapse of dam, reverted to wooded swamp
UD	Unnamed Dam	Peat accumulation in shallow aquatic pond	Siltation. Impounded to deeper aquatic pond. Limited siltation	Reduced siltation
MF	Manning Floodplain	Seasonally wet bottomland. Incipient soil development	Strong pulse of coarse TSS	Continued TSS, but finer grained and at reduced rates
SH	Sweet Hill	Seasonally wet bottomland. Incipient soil development	Impounded to inorganic pond. Rapidly filled with slopewash	Unknown. Deliberate drainage?
BR	Bender Road	Seasonally wet slope. Incipient soil development	Occluded to shallow inorganic pond. Slopewash deposition	Reverted to wooded swamp
KK	Kalmon Kursnik's	Unknown	Occluded to shallow muddy pond. Siltation?	Deliberate drainage to wooded swamp
CB	Chanski's Basin	Forested levee of stream in basin	Strong pulse of coarse TSS	Continued TSS, but finer grained and at reduced rates
HF	Hayward Floodplain	Sinuous sand/gravel channel	Channelization to single straight channel	Well-drained soil above ditch
HP	Hayward Pond	Stream channel?	Impounded to aquatic pond. Strong siltation	Reduced siltation

*Event history is based on field stratigraphy of each site, independent of written records. TSS is an abbreviation for topstratum sedimentation. All events are listed in relative sequence.

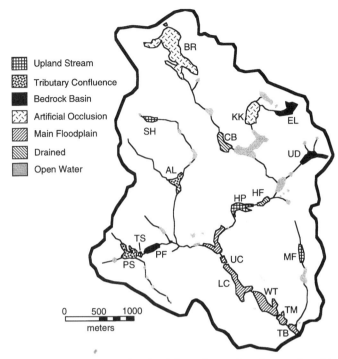

Figure 9. Classification of wetlands in study area based on stratigraphic response to colonial impact, which was governed by the hydrogeologic setting (boxes) at individual sites. Areas above 122 m (400 ft) are shaded. Refer to text for explanation. Full names for abbreviations and wetland characteristics are given in Table 3.

with the poor agricultural potential of the stony soils in their watersheds and the resistance of these soils to erosion. There seems to have been no attempt to drain or ditch these wetlands because their bedrock outlets were impossible to excavate with available technology and because the steep hydraulic gradients and high fracture permeability around their edges created numerous springs.

Tributary confluences. Located at the confluences of first-order tributaries, these wetlands (Pine Swamp, *Typha* Swamp, Alice's Swamp) occur where perennial stream flow often reaches its upstream limit in response to decreased channel gradient and increased catchment area. Such sites are often small sedimentary basins underlain by fine-grained glaciolacustrine sediment capable of supporting a perched water table. The stratigraphy of these settings consists of a pulse of bioturbated alluvium containing historic pollen overlying a thin, degraded, oxidized peat dominated by pollen of tundra and boreal taxa, in one case radiocarbon-dated to over 12,000 B.P. In two of the swamps (Pine Swamp, *Typha* Swamp), the unconformity between the Pleistocene peat and historic alluvium was buried by younger aquatic peats caused by subsequent impoundment.

The decomposition of the peat and absence of Holocene sediments beneath a thick historic fill almost certainly indicates the intentional drainage of presettlement swamps for colonial tillage and hayfields. Impoundment of these sites would have led to the preservation of woody peats, as was the case for the

deposits of bedrock basins. Our interpretation is supported by the proximity of the basins to the early road network, by the flat expanse of land that would have become available upon drainage, and to the anomalous channel geometry (steep banks) of the outlet streams. The sequence of initial drainage followed by later impoundment is also consistent with the early historic priority for meadows and mowlands followed by a later priority associated with stock watering and hydropower development (Gradie and Poirier, 1991).

Main floodplains. The riparian wetlands of the main floodplains (Upper Chappel Road, Lower Chappel Road, Trumbull Bridge, Wet Transit, Trumbull Marsh) are restricted to the perennial main stem of Susquetonscut Brook below Hayward Pond. Like wetlands at upland confluences, these sites are underlain by glacial meltwater sediment, but it is much more coarsely grained, and forms part of an abandoned system of kame terraces paralleling the valley wall. Ground-water recharge from the flanking till slopes discharges along the edge of the modern floodplain by seepages from these productive aquifers.

In all cases, the stratigraphy of these sites is dominated by vertically accreted mineral sediments associated with frequent overbank flows. Presettlement conditions at these sites are typified by a thin horizon of humified marshy peat lying above early postglacial alluvium and Holocene topstratum sediments. Reconnaissance observations of the main stem between Chappel Road and Route 207 (notably the absence of a modern organic topsoil and the presence of levees along the stream bank) indicate the net vertical accretion of topstratum sediments along much of the modern floodplain. This accretion appears to be particularly rapid at the Lower Chappel Road wetland, where the gravely channel bed is locally aggraded, where levees are most prominent, and where basal radiocarbon dates postdate nuclear testing. Rates of vertical accretion appear much slower between Chappel Road and Hayward Pond.

Evidence for a pause in topstratum accumulation associated with agricultural activity followed later by renewed topstratum accumulation is present at most sites (Fig. 10). The antiquity of the radiocarbon date for the humified presettlement peat lying immediately beneath the historic topstratum sediments suggests that the site was drained prior to its burial by mineral sediment derived from upstream reaches.

Artificial occlusions. Occlusion of the stream immediately downstream from the site formed these wetlands (Bender Road and Kurcnik's), which are of postsettlement age. The pulse of pond sedimentation at the Bender Road wetland—laminated silts of historic age grading into organic muck—indicates that topsoil erosion from disturbed soils coincided with wetland creation: presettlement conditions at this site were a poorly drained forested soil at the base of a slope. The same stratigraphic sequence is preserved in Kurcnik's wetland, but the historic age of the occlusion could not be confirmed because our cores did not penetrate to presettlement sediments. Evidence for historic ditching and artificial fill is especially prominent along the northeastern margin of this wetland.

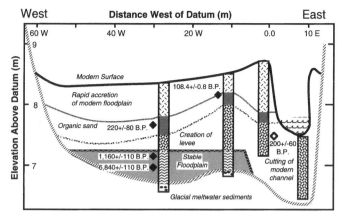

Figure 10. Cross-section across the main stem below Chappel Road (LC wetland) based on ground observations and four cores. Interpretations shown by correlation lines. Height and shape of the presettlement flood-plain shown by shaded area. Radiocarbon dates from Thorson (1992) and Harris (1993).

DISCUSSION

Most wetland investigations attempt to examine human impacts in either time or space. We have attempted to integrate both approaches by focusing on a very small watershed and by drawing conclusions from qualitative wetland histories. Although we have demonstrated that human impacts to the wetlands in Susquetonscut Brook were pervasive and that wetland response was governed by hydrogeologic setting, the dates at which most of the events occurred, the rates at which wetlands responded, and the specific mechanisms responsible for wetland interaction remain elusive. In this context, the value of our review lies not so much with its scientific rigor but in its research strategy.

The pace of landscape change prior to disturbance by European land-use practices was negligible in human terms. The rate of sediment influx for the preceding 8,000 years, even in the most efficient of sediment traps, was not measurably higher than the influx of airborne dust from the continental interior. An explanation for the limited transfer of sediment within the watershed under "natural" conditions is not well understood, but the persistence of beavers, the negligible impact of indigenous inhabitants, and the insensitivity of the forest to broad changes in climate, wildfires, pathology, and severe storms are probably important.

With the arrival of the colonists, however, came a rapidly applied, large-scale, drastic alteration of land use, cultivation practices, water management, and animal husbandry, collectively the most disruptive landscape event since the melting of the Pleistocene glaciers 17,000 years earlier. The abandonment of farms throughout the study area did not bring the wetlands back to their presettlement conditions because the modern flood regime and mechanisms of sediment transfer remain permanently altered by previous soil erosion and by the construction of a now-derelict water management infrastructure, most of which is now overlooked.

More specifically, the nature of historic impacts to wetlands depended principally on their hydrogeologic settings. In streams

near the headwaters of the watershed, especially below till-covered slopes, sediment mobilized by erosion of deforested slopes was trapped in the first available tributary confluence or occluded site, where it buried the former valley bottom. Colonial impacts at these sites were immediate, long lasting, and typical of the responses of headwater streams to agricultural conversion elsewhere in the eastern United States (Costa 1975; Trimble, 1981). Most of this sediment, which entered the system as a single pulse during the eighteenth century, remains stored high in the watershed, where it is now being intermittently entrained and mobilized down-valley.

In lowland swamps underlain by permeable sand and gravel aquifers, a similar pulse of agriculturally produced sediment took place *after* an interval of peat decomposition. Because the regional water table has likely risen slightly within the last few thousand years (Webb et al., 1993; Thorson and Webb, 1991), this decomposition probably resulted from deliberate drainage of swamps prior to denudation of the upstream watersheds. This geological interpretation is consistent with eighteenth century advice for draining swamps (Eliot, 1760), and with our observations of drainage ditches. Peat decomposition also may have been accentuated by the diminished ground-water recharge associated with deforested slopes. The absence of decomposition horizons in bedrock-rimmed basins probably results from the prohibitive cost of drainage.

The broad sediment-covered floodplain of Susquetonscut Brook is essentially a modern landform. Its present instability—rapid topstratum deposition, strong bank erosion, and thalweg aggradation—are governed by changes set in motion three centuries ago. In the constricted reaches just south of Chappel Road (Upper Chappel Road), the presettlement channel was first enlarged by lateral bank erosion, and later infilled by gravelly lateral bars. In expanded reaches to the south (Fig. 10), coarse-grained overbank strata deposited by floods with no prehistoric counterparts underlie more than a meter of historic alluvium. Ironically, overbank sedimentation is so fast that it precludes pedogenesis and peat accumulation, even though much of the watershed has been reforested for more than a century. The thickness (110–130 cm) and shape of topstratum deposits along the main stem are similar to those reported for postsettlement alluvium elsewhere in the unglaciated eastern United States (Knox, 1977; Trimble, 1970; Jacobson and Coleman, 1986; Scully and Arnold, 1981). The observed changes in channels size are consistent with disturbed rivers at a variety of scales (Kesel et al., 1992).

The disproportionately large floods of the historic period noted along the Connecticut (Jahns, 1947) and Housatonic (Patton, 1988) Rivers have been attributed to the enhanced runoff of deforested landscapes. This effect appears to have been accentuated in the smaller drainage of Susquetonscut Brook and is consistent with the results of our HEC-1 runoff models. The width of the channel along the main stem has remained nearly constant in many areas (as indicated by the pattern of stone walls, bridge abutments, inset terraces, and large second-growth trees), and significant downcutting has not occurred (bouldery channel lag horizons are common). Thus, the historic accumulation of leveed topstratum deposits probably represents both the need to pass larger storm discharges (either a higher mean annual flood or modal dominant discharge) and the availability of loamy sand from bank erosion of upland sites.

The very low sediment delivery ratio from the watershed and the continuous existence of a reservoir in Hayward Pond (since 1711) indicates that the sediment responsible for aggradation of the main stem came from channel erosion between Hayward Pond and Chapel Hill Road. This interpretation is supported by field observations from this reach. Topstratum deposits above historic soils are proportionately thinner (20–40 cm); the channel has a more rectangular cross section; and the frequency of unstable banks is higher. Additional sediment is being contributed from Burgess Brook because the modern channel is now downcut below a gravely terrace of historic age. Despite the clear evidence that sediment mobility was enhanced during the historic period, most of the sediment produced by colonial disturbance remains in upstream storage, and the total yield of agricultural sediments to the Yantic and Shetucket Rivers has been relatively small. Channel erosion is the main source of sediment. Point-source management of sediment "pollution" at upland sites seems to have little influence at downstream sites.

Historic documents indicate that peak rates of deforestation occurred early (ca. 1720–1754), prior to the intensive period of water regulation that peaked between 1775 and 1825. These relations suggest that an early phase of enhanced flooding caused by deforestation should have been followed by a period when peak discharges along the main stem were reduced by intentional water management. Abandonment and partial destruction of the hydropower infrastructure would then be followed by a return to the preimpoundement, deforested, flood regime.

The organic and agriculturally modified central part of the topstratum sequence may represent a time of reduced flood discharges associated with the period of intensive water management. This change may have been superimposed upon a reduction in mineral sediment production caused by abandonment of farms, as suggested by the reduced siltation rates in upland cores, and by deforestation experiments (Boormann et al., 1974). However, any anthropogenic changes would have been superimposed on natural climatic variation. Alternatively, a decrease in critical stream power during channel-forming floods may have led to aggradation of the bed, which in turn, may have forced an increase in the rate of topstratum sedimentation.

The trend toward increased wetness during the transition from base-line to historic conditions in Lebanon is consistent with the historic accounts, suggesting that lowland areas became wetter while the adjacent terrain simultaneously became drier (Marsh, 1869). These effects would have been amplified by the generally colder conditions of the eighteenth century. Thus, the unwanted growth of wetlands at occlusions would have occurred simultaneously with the increasing need to create artificial reservoirs for hydropower regulation (Gradie and Poirier, 1991), irrigation, and stock watering. At the same time, the increase in wetland cover caused by impoundments, occlusions, and sediment erosion would have increased runoff-generating area during storms, and contributed to the observed increase in bankfull discharge. Finally, we cannot rule out the possibility that peak flood discharges during historic time were associated with the catastrophic failure of earthen dams now completely collapsed or were associated with exceptionally severe storms that went unrecorded.

The landscape position, land-use history, and stratigraphy of the Susquetonscut wetlands lead us to a view of past changes that are in conflict with frequently assumed notions of landscape stability and orderly progress to a land-cover end point (Egler, 1977). Glaciation, as a land-reshaping pulse, led to a period of dynamic instability during which the soils and streams readjusted for thousands of years, then stabilized. The subsequent pulse of landscape instability caused by European settlement mimicked that of the late-glacial recovery period, a pulse from the which the physical landscape is still recovering. Meaningful regulation of contemporary wetlands in Susquetonscut Brook must therefore be predicated on viewing these environmental "resources" as evolving representatives of a changing landscape, not on viewing them as ancient, pristine ecosystems.

CONCLUSION

Stratigraphic and geomorphic evidence can be used to document historic human impacts to wetlands in Lebanon, Connecticut. A variety of wetlands were present prior to colonial settlement, but they were fewer in number, smaller in area, much more stable, and less encumbered with sediment than those we vigilantly try to protect today. Modern riparian wetlands on the floodplain of Susquetonscut Brook are still adjusting to a pulse of change initiated more than three centuries ago.

ACKNOWLEDGMENTS

Funding for this research was provided by grants from the Joint Highway Research Advisory Council of the Connecticut State Department of Transportation. The research design was an outgrowth of a fellowship by the senior author at Yale University under the sponsorship of William Cronon. Sabbatical support for the senior author from Dartmouth College, under the sponsorship of Robert Brackenridge, is greatly appreciated. Lucinda McWeeny (Yale University) contributed macrofossil identifications. Able field assistance was provided by Wayne Bugden, Brain MacInnich, and Ryan Paquet. Access to private property was freely given by dozens of Lebanon residents, most of whom also contributed bits of local landscape history.

APPENDIX 1. DETAILED STRATIGRAPHY OF WETLAND LOCALITIES USED AS TYPE EXAMPLES FOR DIFFERENT HYDROGEOLOGIC SETTINGS

Hydrogeologic Setting: Bedrock Basin
Example Wetland: Pogmore Floodplain (PF)
Site Description: The modern stream meanders through a swampy forested bottomland below Pleistocene terrace scarps. At the wetland

coring site the channel has negligible gradient and occupies a channel no more than 2-m-wide cut into organic strata. Fifty meters down valley, however, it flows rapidly over stony artificial fill interpreted here as the collapsed remnants of an unreported earthen dam.

Stratigraphy: Prior to about 12,000 B.P., the site was undergoing rapid sedimentation within a watershed dominated by tundra vegetation (Figs. 6 and 7). The transition to boreal forested conditions at a depth of about 2.5 m is indicated by the arrival of spruce in both the pollen and macrofossil records. Evidence for a mosaic of habitats at this time is indicated by the presence of horsetail, violet, water lily, and pond weed in the macrofossils.

An upward decrease in the concentration and continuity of mineral strata, and an increase in the abundance of hydrophytic local pollen indicate that the Pogmore Floodplain wetland changed from a sediment-laden boreal marsh to a stable organic pond as the watershed became progressively mantled and stabilized with coniferous forest. The spread of pine forest shown in the pollen records (Zone B; ca. 11,000–8,500 B.P.) marks an abrupt transition from a silty boreal marsh to a wooded swamp. A highly decomposed (sapric peat) layer, dating from between 8,500 ^{14}C B.P. and the arrival of hickory pollen about 5,000 B.P., represents peat decomposition under intermittently aerated (drier) conditions during peak warmth of the mid-Holocene (Webb et al., 1993). Strata above the residual layer (also in situ layered woody peats) indicate the return to slow peat accumulation under wetter conditions of the last few thousand years.

The top unit, a highly turbated sediment-rich organic muck, abruptly overlies decomposed woody peat. The sharp lithologic transition coincides with the settlement pollen horizon, which is clearly marked by the increase in ragweed, grass, and chestnut pollen, but not with the lower limits of rootlets, mottling, or evidence for water-table fluctuation. Hence, the abrupt lithologic transition represents a sedimentary event, rather than a change in bulk density associated with auto-compaction (George, 1975). The base of the postsettlement unit occurs just above a concentrated zone of light-colored fibrous tissue that intrudes the youngest presettlement peats, and which we interpret as the in situ roots and rhizomes of woody vegetation that are dead, but not completely decomposed. Collectively, these features indicate that the postsettlement stratum was caused by an abrupt transition to ponded conditions at a time of strong siltation. This interpretation is supported by the presence of the collapsed primitive dam downstream and with historic evidence for water use at upstream sites.

Hydrogeologic Setting: Upland stream
Example Wetland: Manning Floodplain (MF)
Site Description: The core was extracted about 20 m west of a small intermittent stream channel, and upstream from a forest-covered stony occlusion of unknown origin. Based on multiple test cores that exhibited an eastward-thickening stratum of recent mineral sediment, the coring site was located near the distal margin of a broad levee of loamy overbank sand. Prolonged seasonal inundation of the coring site during spring flooding is indicated by the absence of a surface soil.

Stratigraphy: The bulk of our sediment core (80 cm) contains a thoroughly bioturbated black mineral silt with a characteristic postsettlement pollen spectrum. This amorphous silt grades downward to a coarse, granule-bearing sand with an erosional basal contact.

This fining-upward sequence of historic sediment overlies a black fine sandy loam containing oxidized mottles, root casts, decomposed wood fragments, and a characteristic pedogenic crumb structure. These features are collectively interpreted as the A horizon of an incipient paleosol (aquent), the development of which was inhibited by poor drainage. A bulk radiocarbon date for the horizon of 7,890 ± 100 B.P. confirms the antiquity and stability of this small floodplain prior to settlement.

Hydrogeologic Setting: Tributary confluence
Example Wetland: Alice's Swamp
Site Description: The site is a small, flat lowland at the confluence of two unnamed tributaries of Burgess Brook, upstream of a bedrock ravine. The core from Alice's Swamp was taken about 40 m north of the tributary confluence, midway between the bordering streams. It is dominated by a thick sequence of modern alluvium.

Stratigraphy: The radiocarbon date of 12,100 ± 120 B.P. was obtained on detrital twigs within silty lacustrine strata at depth of 1.3 m, indicating that the wetland is the site of a sediment-filled Pleistocene pond. A strongly humified, herbaceous peat just above the radiocarbon sample consists almost entirely of monocot tissue, is devoid of mineral sediment coarser than silt, and contains a pollen spectrum dominated by spruce, pine, and sedges predating the arrival of deciduous forest. This unit indicates that the pond was replaced by a small freshwater marsh as sediment influx from the watershed diminished.

Lying with sharp unconformity above the freshwater marsh deposits is a graded sequence of coarse mineral detritus nearly 50 cm thick of postsettlement age. The unit is pebbly near its base, but grades upward into an interbedded sequence containing lenses of sandy silt, detrital organic fragments, and organic horizons, all of which contain a historic pollen assemblage. The uppermost 50 cm of this sequence is dominated by sandy silt, and extends upward to the modern surface of the swamp, which is periodically inundated by storm flow.

The abrupt and sustained reversal from conditions of a slackwater, freshwater marsh to conditions of rapid mineral sedimentation resulted from deforestation and erosion of upland soils during the colonial period, followed by sediment transport to the site by strong flood flows. The absence of wood and deciduous pollen within the youngest presettlement peat and its strongly humified character suggest that Alice's Swamp was a site of net peat decomposition prior to the influx of historic sediment. The aeration and decomposition of this decomposed, peaty soil is likely to have resulted from deliberate drainage of the swamp.

Hydrogeologic Setting: Main floodplain
Example Wetland: Lower Chappel Road (LC)
Site Description: This site spans the full width of the floodplain of Susquetonscut Brook near the upstream end of an expanded reach below Chappel Road. The stratigraphy was investigated by excavations along the stream bank supplemented by four cores taken in a transect perpendicular to the main channel (Fig. 10).

Stratigraphy: At the base of each core are current-bedded fluvial deposits associated with channel bed and bar deposition overlain by mineral overbank strata; this unit of inorganic strata was deposited during late glacial downcutting of the former glaciofluvial plain.

Overlying these late glacial deposits is a relatively uniform mantle of Holocene floodplain sediments dominated by interbedded silt and reddish brown herbaceous peats containing detrital wood fragments, discrete interbeds of medium sand, and no postsettlement pollen. Radiocarbon dates from near the top of this sequence at Lower Chappel Road are late Holocene in age (1,160 ± 110 to 220 ± 80 B.P.), whereas a similar sample from Trumbull Marsh, just downstream, yielded a mid-Holocene date of 6,480 ± 110 B.P. The limited thickness of sediment accumulation, the presettlement ages, and the composition of floodplain strata indicate that the long-term Holocene history of Susquetonscut Brook was characterized by negligible sediment transport in a marshy, seasonally inundated floodplain only rarely affected by severe floods.

Overlying the Holocene floodplain is a thick sequence of mineral-rich sediments deposited by overbank flows containing both coarse sand as well as detrital wood dating at 200 ± 60 B.P. Although highly variable from site to site, this topstratum sequence at Lower Chappel Road consists of an early coarse-grained phase followed by a finer grained, bioturbated interval. This organic deposit is devoid of sand horizons, and contains exotic pebbles, incipient soil structure, and rootlet mottling, all features suggestive of an agricultural soil. Above the organic interval the third topstratum unit, coarser grained, extends upward to the modern surface and is still undergoing rapid deposition. A radiocarbon date of 108.4 ± 0.8 B.P. from the base of this deposit indicates the modern alluvium postdates nuclear weapons testing in the mid-twentieth century.

Hydrogeologic Setting: Artificial occlusion
Example Wetland: Bender Road (BR)
Site Description: This site has the largest area and highest elevation of any wetland in the watershed. It is a contiguous swamp consisting of many coalesced perched basins above the upland till. At its southern limit, it drains southward across an eighteenth century road through a collapsed nineteenth-century stone culvert.
Stratigraphy: The saturated, bioturbated muck beneath much of the surface of the swamp near its southern limit overlies an unoxidized laminated sandy silt of lacustrine origin that contains historic pollen. These historic lacustrine deposits lie sharply above an incipient paleosol similar to that at the Manning Floodplain wetland. These relationships indicate that the southern part of this large wetland was converted to a localized pond when southerly drainage from the basin was impeded by road construction.

Hydrogeologic Setting: Drained wetlands
Example Wetland: Hayward Floodplain (HF)
Site Description: This broad terrace above a channelized stream has a distinct distal edge where it impinges on the flanking valley.
Stratigraphy: The surface is overlain by a thick, organic-rich loamy soil. It formerly was a stream floodplain, but no longer receives sediments owing to its elevated position above the channelized stream, and perhaps to upstream impoundments.

REFERENCES CITED

Aaby, B., 1986, Palaeoecological studies of mires, *in* Berglund, B. E., ed., Handbook of Holocene palaeoecology and palaeohydrology: New York, John Wiley & Sons, p. 145–164.

Adamus, P. R., 1983, A method for wetland functional assessment, Vol. I. Critical review and evaluation concepts: Washington, D.C., U.S. Department of Transportation Federal Highway Administration, FHWA IP-82-23, 176 p.

Bailey, R. G., 1978, Ecoregions of the United States: Ogden, Utah, U.S. Forest Service Intermountain Region, 77 p.

Boorman, F. H., Likens, G. E., Siccama, T. G., Pierce, R. S., and Eaton, J. S., 1974, The export of nutrients and recovery of stable conditions following deforestation at Hubbard Brook: Ecological Monographs, v. 44, p. 255–277.

Brugam, R. B., 1978, Human disturbance and the historical development of Linsley Pond: Ecology, v. 59, p. 19–36.

Carter, V., 1986, An overview of the hydrologic concerns related to wetlands in the United States: Canadian Journal of Botany, v. 64, p. 364–374.

Chase, A., 1995, In a dark wood: The fight over forests and the tyranny of ecology: New York, Houghton-Mifflin Company, 535 p.

Clebnik, S. M., 1980, The surficial geology of the Willimantic Quadrangle: State Geological and Natural History Survey of Connecticut, Quadrangle Report No. 39, scale 1:24,000.

Costa, J. E., 1975, Effects of agriculture on erosion and sedimentation in the Piedmont Province, Maryland: Geological Society of America Bulletin, v. 86, p. 1281–1286.

Cowardin, L. M., Carter, V., Golet, F. C., and LaRoe, E. T., 1979, Classification of wetlands and deepwater habitats of the United States: U.S. Fish and Wildlife Service, FWS/OBS-79/31, 131 p.

Cronon, W., 1983, Changes in the land; Indians, colonists, and the ecology of New England: New York, Hill and Wang, 241 p.

Cunningham, R. L., and Ciolkosz, C., 1984, Soils of the northeastern United States: Pennsylvania State University Agricultural Experiment Station Bulletin 848, 47 p.

Davis, M. B., 1969, Climate changes in southern Connecticut recorded by pollen deposition at Rogers Lake: Ecology, v. 50, p. 409–422.

Davis, M. B., 1983, Holocene vegetational history of the eastern United States, *in* Wright, H. E., Jr., ed., Late Quaternary environments of the United States, Volume 2, The Holocene: Minneapolis, University of Minnesota Press, p. 166–181.

Deane, S., 1790, The New England farmer or georgical dictionary: Worcester, Isiah Thomas.

Deevey, E. S., 1939, Studies on Connecticut lake sediments I, A postglacial climatic chronology for New England: American Journal of Science, v. 237, p. 691–724.

Denny, C. S., 1982, Geomorphology of New England: U.S. Geological Survey Professional Paper 1208, 18 p.

Egler, F. E., 1977, The nature of vegetation: Its management and mis-management: Norfolk, Connecticut, Aton Forest, 527 p.

Eliot, J., 1934, Essays on field husbandry in New England and other papers *in* Carmen, H.J. and Tugwell, R.G., eds.: New York Columbia University Press, 261 p.

Faegri, K., and Iversen, S., 1975, Textbook of pollen analysis: New York, Hafner Press, 137 p.

Gaudreau, D. C., and Webb, T., III, 1985, Late Quaternary pollen stratigraphy and isochrone maps for the northeastern United States, *in* Bryant, V. M., Jr., and Holloway, R. G., eds., Pollen records of late Quaternary North American sediments: Tulsa, Oklahoma, American Association of Stratigraphic Palynologists Foundation, p. 247–280.

George, J. E., 1975. Anomalous transmission of water through certain peats—a discussion: Journal of Hydrology, v. 27, p. 359–361.

Gordon, R. B., 1979, Denudation rate of central New England determined from estuarine sedimentation: American Journal of Science, v. 279, p. 632–642.

Gosselink, J. G., and Turner, R. E., 1978, The role of hydrology in freshwater wetland ecosystems, *in* Good, R. E., Whigham, D. F., Simpson, R. L. and Jackson, C.G., eds., Freshwater wetlands, ecological processes and management potential: New York, Academic Press, p. 63–78.

Gradie, R. R., III, and Poirier, D. A., 1991, Small-scale hydropower development; archaeological and historical perspectives from Connecticut: Industrial Archaeology, v. 17, p. 47–66.

Harris, A. G., 1993, Recent human disturbance at Susquetonscut Brook, Connecticut: Final Report to the Nature Conservancy, Connecticut Chapter.

Hill, D. E., Sautter, E. H., and Gonick, W. N., 1980, Soils of Connecticut: New Haven, Connecticut Agricultural Experiment Station Bulletin 787, 36 p.

Hooke, R. LeB., 1994, On the efficacy of humans as geomorphic agents: GSA Today, v. 4, p. 217–225.

Hornbeck, J. W., Pierce, R. S., and Federer, C. A., 1970, Streamflow changes after forest clearing in New England: Water Resources Research, v. 6, p. 1124–1132.

Jacobson, R. B., and Coleman, D. J., 1986, Stratigraphy and recent evolution of Maryland Piedmont floodplains: American Journal of Science, v. 286, p. 617–637.

Jahns, R. H., 1947, Geologic features of the Connecticut Valley, Massachusetts, as related to recent floods: U.S. Geological Survey Water Supply Paper 996, 158 p.

Johnson, D. L., 1990, Biomantle evolution and the redistribution of earth materials and artifacts: Soil Science, v. 149, p. 84–102.

Kaye, C. A., 1962, Early postglacial beavers in southeastern New England: Science, v. 138, p. 906–907.

Kelso, G. K., and Beaudry, M. C., 1987, Pollen analysis and urban land use; The environs of Scottow's Dock in 17th, 18th, and early 19th century Boston: Historical Archaeology, v. 24, p. 61–81.

Kesel, R. H., Yodis, E. G., and McCraw, D. J., 1992, An approximation of the sediment budget of the lower Mississippi River prior to major human modification: Earth Surface Processes and Landforms, v. 17, p. 711–722.

Knox, J. C., 1977, Human impacts on Wisconsin stream channels: Annals of the Association of American Geographers, v. 67, p. 323–342.

Landsberg, H. E., 1967, Two centuries of New England climate: Weatherwise, April 1967, p. 52–57.

Marsh, G. P., 1869, On man and nature, or physical geography as modified by human action: New York, Scribner, 527 p.

McAndrews, J. H., 1988, Human disturbance of North American forests and grasslands; the fossil pollen record, *in* Huntley, B., and Webb, T., III, eds., Vegetation history: Dordrecht, Netherlands, Kluwer Academic Publishers, p. 673–697.

Meade, R. H., 1982, Sources, sinks, and storage of river sediment in the Atlantic drainage of the United States: Journal of Geology, v. 90, p. 235–252.

Metzler, K. J., and Tiner, R. W., 1992, Wetlands of Connecticut: Connecticut Department of Environmental Protection Report of Investigations No. 13, 113 p.

Miller, D. R., Focazzio, M. J., Dickinson, M. A., and Archey, W. E., 1988, A user's guide to model for estimating the hydrological effects of land use changes: Storrs, Connecticut, U.S. Dept. Agriculture Cooperative Extension Service, University of Connecticut, University of Massachusetts, 28p.

Milne, G. M., 1986, Lebanon, three centuries in a Connecticut hilltop town: Canaan, New Hampshire., Phoenix Publishing, 287p.

Naiman, R. J., and Johnston, C. A., 1988, Alteration of North American streams by beaver: Bioscience, v. 38, p. 753–762.

Natural Research Council, 1995, Wetlands characteristics and boundaries: Committee on characterization of wetlands: Washington, D.C., National Academy Press, p. 13.

Naveh, Z., and Lieberman, A. S., 1990, Landscape ecology; theory and application, student edition: New York, Springer-Verlag, 356 p.

O'Brien, A. L., 1977, Hydrology of two small wetland basins in eastern Massachussetts: Water Resources Bulletin, v. 13, p. 325–342.

Patton, P. C., 1988, Geomorphic response of streams to floods in the glaciated terrain of southern New England, *in* Baker, V. R., Kochel, R. C., and Patton, P. C., eds., Flood geomorphology: New York, John Wiley & Sons, p. 261–277.

Phillips, J. D., 1989, Fluvial sediment storage in wetlands: Water Resources Bulletin, v. 25, p. 867–873.

Phillips, J. D., 1992, Nonlinear dynamical systems in geomorphology: revolution or evolution?: Geomorphology, v. 5, p. 219–229.

Pickup, G., 1988, Hydrology and sediment models, *in* Anderson, M. G., ed., Modeling geomorphological systems: New York, John Wiley & Sons, p. 153–215.

Ruffner, J. A., 1985, Climate of Connecticut, *in* Climate of the states, Volume I, Alabama–New Mexico: Detroit, Michigan, Gale Research Company, p. 165–176.

Scully, R. W., and Arnold, R. W., 1981, Holocene alluvial stratigraphy in the upper Susquehanna River basin, New York: Quaternary Research, v. 15, p. 327–344.

Thomas, M. P., Bednar, G. A., Thomas, C. E., Jr., and Wilson, W. E., 1967, Water resources inventory of Connecticut, Part 2, Shetucket River basin: Connecticut Water Resources Bulletin No. 11, 96 p.

Thorson, R. M., 1992, Remaking the wetlands in Lebanon, Connecticut, Final Report, Project 89–3: University of Connecticut Joint Highway Research Advisory Council Report JHR 92–215, 157 p.

Thorson, R. M., and Harris, S. L., 1991, How "Natural" are inland wetlands? An example from the Trail Wood Audubon Sanctuary in Connecticut, U.S.A.: Environmental Management, v. 15, p. 675–687.

Thorson, R. M., and Schile C. A., 1995, Deglacial eolian regimes in New England: Geological Society of America Bulletin, v. 107, p. 751–761.

Thorson, R. M., and Webb, R. S., 1991, Postglacial history of a cedar swamp in southeastern Connecticut: Journal of Paleolimnology, v. 6, p. 17–35.

Tiner, R. W., Jr., and Veneman, P. L. M., 1989, Hydric soils of New England: Amherst, Massachusetts, University of Massachusetts Cooperative Extension Revised Bulletin C-183R, 27 p.

Toney, J. D., 1987, Historical sediment storage and pollen stratigraphy in the Connecticut River estuary [M.A. thesis]: Middletown, Connecticut, Wesleyan University, 168 p.

Trimble, S. W., 1970, The Alcovy River swamps: The result of culturally accelerated sedimentation: Bulletin of the Georgia Academy of Science, v. 28, p. 131–141.

Trimble, S. W., 1981, Changes in sediment storage in the Coon Creek basin, driftless area, Wisconsin, 1853–1975: Science, v. 214, p. 181–183.

Turner, B. L., Clark, W. C., Kates, R. W., Richards, J. F., Mathews, J. T., and Meyer, W. B., eds., 1990, The Earth as transformed by human action: Cambridge, U.K., Cambridge University Press, 713 p.

Urban, D. L., O'Neill, R. V., and Shugart, H. H., Jr., 1987, Landscape ecology: Bioscience, v. 37, p. 119–127.

U.S. Army Corps of Engineers, 1981, HEC-1, a flood runoff model: U.S. Army Corps of Engineers, Technical release. Davis, California, Hydraulic Engineer Center.

U.S. Soil Conservation Service, 1983, Soil Survey of New London County, Connecticut: U.S. Dept. Agriculture Soil Survey Report, 154 p.

Webb, R. S., and Webb, T., III, 1988, Rates of sediment accumulation in pollen cores from small lakes and mires of eastern North America: Quaternary Research, v. 30, p. 284–297.

Webb, T., III, Bartlein, P. J., Harrison, S. P., and Anderson, K. H., 1993, Vegetation, lake levels, and climate in eastern North America for the past 18,000 years, *in* Wright, H. E., Jr., Kutzbach, J. E., Webb, T., III, Ruddiman, W. F., Street-Perrott, F. A., and Bartlein, P. J., eds., Global climates since the last glacial maximum: Minneapolis, Minnesota, University of Minnesota Press, p. 415–467.

Worster, D., 1990, Transformations of the earth; Toward an agroecological perspective in history: Journal of American History, v. 76, p. 1087–1106.

MANUSCRIPT ACCEPTED BY THE SOCIETY JUNE 5, 1997

Printed in U.S.A.

Geological Society of America
Reviews in Engineering Geology, Volume XII
1998

Presentation of radon potential maps to the public: A case history for Portland, Oregon

Scott F. Burns and Stuart G. Ashbaugh
Department of Geology, Portland State University, Portland, Oregon 97207-0751
Ray Paris and George Toombs
Radiation Protection Services Section, Oregon Health Division, 800 N.E. Oregon Street, Portland, Oregon 97232-2162

ABSTRACT

Most of Oregon has been mapped as having low radon potential. Overall, elevated levels of indoor radon are found in only 4% of Oregon homes compared to 8% of homes nationally. Most maps show Portland, Oregon's largest city, as having low to moderate potential for indoor radon. Using data collected by the Oregon Health Division's Radiation Protection Services Section, we found Portland to have elevated radon values in 22% of homes. A radon potential map has been produced for 39 zip code regions of Portland based on the rank sums of maximum radon values, average indoor radon values, and the percentage of homes with radon values >4 pCi/l. Eight zip codes have high, 15 moderate, and 16 low radon potential. The maps were constructed by taking the indoor radon values from 1,135 homes, categorizing the data in terms of radon values, and plotting the points geographically by zip codes. Trends became obvious when geologic maps were compared to the areas of radon potential. Most of the high potential sites lie on highly permeable Missoula flood sediments. The data and map of radon potential were presented to the public through television and radio interviews and newspaper articles in June of 1994. The public, already familiar with the zip codes, could understand how to use the map. People in high to moderate categories were strongly encouraged to test their homes. A telephone number was given to receive free information on radon testing and mitigation.

INTRODUCTION

Radon is a naturally occurring, odorless, tasteless, radioactive gas produced mainly as one of the decay products of the uranium decay series. It comes from rocks, soil, and ground water. It has a short half life of 3.82 days in the uranium series, but it is present long enough to create a health hazard to humans (Nero, 1988). Until 1984 exposure to elevated radon and its decay products resulted in primarily pulmonary diseases that were viewed as isolated cases among miners working with mining residuals enriched in uranium in pitchblende mines (Miller, 1990). This viewpoint changed in 1984 after the discovery of elevated indoor radon levels in the Reading Prong region of eastern Pennsylvania. As a result, widespread public and scientific interest over radon-related health issues has been generated (Hopke, 1987).

Radon and radon decay progeny (primarily polonium and bismuth) are considered to be the principal components of natural radiation exposure to the general population (Nero et al., 1990). Radon is a health hazard, primarily as a cause of lung cancer (Otton, 1992). It is estimated that for the general population the average lifetime risk of lung cancer caused from exposure to radon and radon decay progeny is at 0.4%, or approximately 20,000 cases of lung cancer annually within the U.S. population (Nero et al., 1990). This means that one in every seven lung can-

Burns, S. F., Ashbaugh, S. G., Paris, R., and Toombs, G., 1998, Presentation of radon potential maps to the public: A case history for Portland, Oregon, *in* Welby, C. W., and Gowan, M. E., eds., A Paradox of Power: Voices of Warning and Reason in the Geosciences: Boulder, Colorado, Geological Society of America Reviews in Engineering Geology, v. XII.

cer deaths in the United States could result from radon. It has also been suggested that radon is a causative factor in inducing myeloid leukemia, melanoma cancer of the kidney, and some childhood cancers (Henshaw et al., 1990).

In 1984 the Environmental Protection Agency (EPA) established its radon division to study the health effects of indoor radon. In 1988 the Oregon Health Division initiated the Oregon Radon Project, and in 1991 the Portland State researchers joined the study to try to relate the indoor radon values to the geology of the region. "Broad brush" evaluations of the radon potential from bedrock geology, aeromagnetic studies, and soil radionuclides led to earlier radon maps that have placed Portland in the low to moderate potential zone (Ashbaugh, 1996; Duval et al., 1989; EPA, 1993). Yet, when actual indoor radon values were collected, some parts of Portland had very high values.

Radon radioactivity is commonly measured in picocuries/liter (pCi/l). One pCi is equal to the decay of about two radioactive atoms per minute (Otton, 1992). Outdoor air ranges from less than 0.1 pCi/l to about 30 pCi/l but averages about 0.2 pCi/l (Otton, 1992). Indoor radon ranges from less than 1 pCi/l to about 3,000 pCi/l, but it averages between 1 and 2 pCi/l (Otton, 1992).

The EPA has chosen a level of 4 pCi/l as the action level for radon. It is recommended that occupants of houses containing levels greater than this amount of radon take action to reduce the radon levels. This action level is only an estimate of a concentration target to which indoor levels should be reduced. Living in an environment with an indoor radon level of 4 pCi/l is equivalent to receiving a radiation dosage one would receive from having 200 chest x-rays in a year (EPA, 1986b). This action level has been questioned, and some believe that it might be too low (Stone, 1993).

On a national scale, one in every 12 homes is reported to have elevated levels of radon above the action level (Keller, 1996). In Oregon an extensive study by the Bonneville Power Administration (1993) of over 15,000 homes showed that only one in every 25 homes had elevated levels of radon. Our study of 1,135 homes in the Portland area revealed elevated indoor radon levels in one in every five homes, a value that is more than twice the national average and over five times the Oregon average.

Indoor radon values are controlled by the following factors: bedrock under a house, soil porosity and permeability, construction of the house, ground-water levels, and the presence of faults (Otton, 1992). The concentration of uranium in the bedrock controls the radon potential. Most rocks contain low amounts of uranium (about 3 parts per million; ppm) so they are low generators of radon, but rocks such as granite, light-colored volcanic rocks, dark shales, sedimentary rocks containing phosphates, and metamorphic rocks derived from these rocks generally contain as much as 100 parts per million of uranium and are good generators of radon (Otton, 1992). Uranium ores can contain several thousand parts per million uranium. Soils with high porosity and permeability allow movement of the radon gas from a radon-generating bedrock or sediment to a house. High ground-water levels retard the movement of radon (Otton, 1992). Older foundations in homes have more cracks and therefore are more susceptible to radon movement (Otton, 1992).

The high incidence rate of radon in Portland homes led to this project. The following discussion summarizes how these Portland area radon data were mapped to discern geological and geographical trends, were summarized for easy interpretation by the general public, and were presented to the public through the media for rational adaptation to mitigation.

STUDY AREA: THE PORTLAND METROPOLITAN AREA

The study area encompasses approximately 3,300 sq km that includes the City of Portland, Oregon, and its surrounding communities (Fig. 1). The population is approximately 1.9 million people. There are approximately 60 postal zip codes in the study area. Portland and its suburbs lie in the Willamette Valley of northwest Oregon, a north-south–trending synclinal trough of Columbia River basalt that is filled with sediments (Orr et al., 1992). To the east lie the Cascade Mountains and to the west lies the Coast Range. The area is centered at 45° north latitude and 123° west longitude.

The Portland and Tualatin basins, which have been interpreted to be pull-apart basins formed by right-lateral strike slip and dip slip faults as part of the regional tectonic setting (Beeson et al., 1989), underlie the area. Separating the Portland and Tualatin basins are the Tualatin Mountains, a northwest-southeast–trending highland composed dominantly of Miocene Columbia River basalt and Pleistocene Boring lava (Beeson et al., 1989, 1991).

The geology of the Portland area is mainly volcanic rocks with sediments (Beeson et al., 1989, 1991; Madin, 1990; Fig. 1). The bedrock of each of the basins is Miocene Columbia River basalt (Tcr), and the basins are filled with Pliocene to Pleistocene age sediments of the Troutdale Formation (QTs) and the fine-grained Sandy River Mudstone (Tsr) to a maximum depth of 500 m (Fig. 1). Much of the basin is overlain by late Pleistocene fine-(Qff) and coarse-grained (Qfc) catastrophic flood deposits from Glacial Lake Missoula. Older Eocene basalt outcrops in the middle of the study area are called the Waverly basalts (Twh). The late Pliocene–Quaternary age Boring basalt (Qtb) outcrops on both sides of the Portland basin. Holocene alluvium (Qal) and alluvium and fill (Qaf) are both found along the Willamette and Columbia Rivers. Elevations above 90 m in the Portland area are often covered with loess of varying thickness.

Indoor radon potential for the Portland area has been previously interpreted as being low. A study based on radiation values taken from an airplane put the area into the low to middle range of "low" potential (Duval et al., 1989). The EPA's map of radon potential for the United States has classified Portland in Zone 2 or "moderate" potential (EPA, 1993). Ashbaugh (1996) completed a regional study of northwest Oregon using soil radionuclides to determine radon potential. All of northwest Oregon is in the low potential classification with 70% being in the upper low class and 30% in the lower low class.

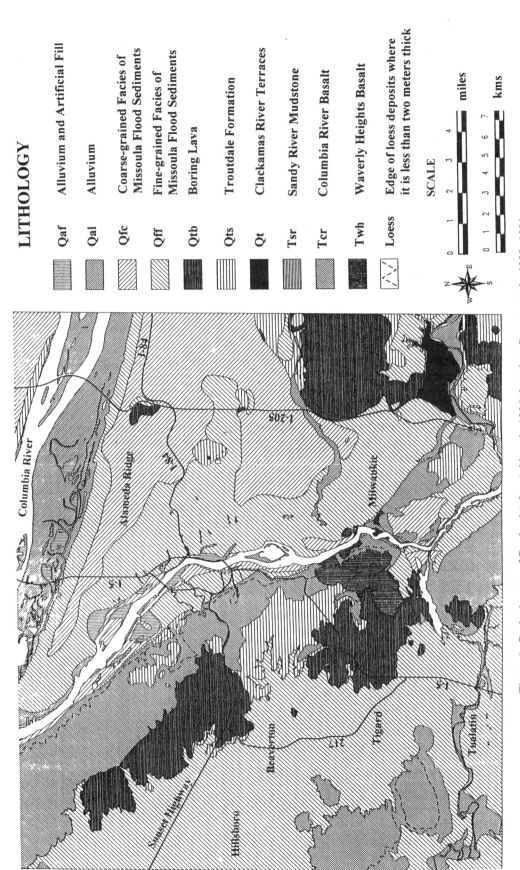

Figure 1. Geologic map of Portland (after Ashbaugh, 1996; based on Beeson et al., 1989, 1991; Madin, 1990).

METHODS

Sampling of indoor radon data

Indoor radon values were collected in the late 1980s and early 1990s by the Oregon Health Division using alpha-track detectors that were left in the homes for at least three months. These devices record etchings left behind by the energy released during the alpha decay of radon or its decay progeny. The canisters had to be placed in the living area to be used in the data set; therefore crawl space values were not included. We believe that the data set is conservative because it contains values from many places in homes, not just basements.

Mapping of the indoor radon data

In order to preserve the anonymity of the homes used in the study, only zip codes were recorded for the location of the radon values. Four maps representing different compilations of the raw data were produced. We mapped three radon values for each zip code. First, we included the maximum value recorded for the zip code for it represents the maximum potential for that area. Second, we calculated the average radon value for each zip code. This number is a better evaluation of radon potential than the maximum value because one "hot spot" will not necessarily give a high average, although if the data set is small, one high or low value could raise or lower the average disproportionately. Third, we calculated the percentage of homes with indoor values greater than 4 pCi/l, the EPA action level guideline. We believed the percentage value to be the best measure of radon potential because one high or low value in a small data set cannot skew the results. We divided the values into three groupings of high, moderate, and low and mapped them on individual maps.

Maximum values of indoor radon. We divided the maximum radon values for each zip code into three categories: high potential (>10 pCi/l), moderate potential (4 to 9.9 pCi/l), and low potential (<4 pCi/l). The rationale for the breaks was based on distributions and the standard EPA action level of 4 pCi/l. We felt that if no maximum value was more than 4 then it would be low potential. Many regions had values between 4 and 10 pCi/l, but few zip codes had values greater than 10.

Average indoor radon values. We divided the average indoor radon values for each zip code into three categories: high potential (>4 pCi/l), moderate potential (2–4 pCi/l), and low potential (<2 pCi/l). These categories follow the indoor radon classes designated by EPA.

Percentage of homes with radon >4 pCi/l. We divided the percentage of homes with values above 4 pCi/l into three categories: high potential is >35% of the homes, moderate is 16–35%, and low potential is <16%. Our boundaries are arbitrary and are narrower compared to some similar categories used by the U.S. Geological Survey in a similar study of Montgomery and Prince Georges Counties, Maryland, and Fairfax County, Virginia, where their boundaries were 33% and 50% (Otton et al., 1988).

Overall radon potential map based on rank sums. We wanted to have one overall indoor radon potential map that combined all of the above maps. We calculated the rank sum for each zip code and listed it at the right side of Table 1. For each map the high category is given a value of 3, moderate 2, and low the value of 1. For the map on percentage of homes with values over 4 pCi/l, if the value was zero percent having indoor values over 4 pCi/l, we gave 0 as the rank sum value. A total for each zip code was calculated with 9 being the highest (a high rating on each map) and 2 being the lowest (low values on two maps and a zero percentage on Fig. 2). The overall high potential for this map was assigned to zip codes with rank sums of 8 or 9; moderate potential for rank sums of 5, 6, or 7; and low potential for rank sums of 2, 3, or 4.

Presentation of radon potential maps to the public

A very important decision that we made was to work with the Portland State University and Oregon Health Division public relations staff who are experienced in working with the press. These staffs provided invaluable guidance on how best to get the information to the public.

First, they took our attempt at a press release and fashioned it into something that could be used by the media. They did put the news release out a few days early and put a "news embargo" on it (i.e., not be released until a specific date). This early release was a mistake because two radio stations started running the story early and "scooped" the rest of the media. We recommend providing the news release on the day of the press conferences.

Instead of having one press conference where all of the media come to hear the information once, our media people scheduled personal interviews with each television station and radio station and newspaper. This was a lot more work for us, but the stories got more air time coverage because each reporter had his or her own story. We scheduled the newspapers the day before the television and radio people so the print media people could also break the news at the same time as the others.

For the press conferences we prepared packets of information on radon, a brief summary of the report with one radon potential map (Fig. 3), one data sheet (Table 1), and a few pieces of trivia for soundbites. We also supplied an 800 number (1-800-SOS-RADON) that the public could call for a packet of information on radon and lists of local companies who supply test kits and mitigation.

RESULTS

Radon maps

The maximum indoor radon values map has the greatest number of high potential regions of all of the maps (Fig. 4). There are 25% of the zip codes in the high potential class, 42% in the moderate, and 33% in the low potential class. The high potential areas are mainly along the Alameda Ridge in north Portland (zip codes: 97211, 97212, 97213, 97217, 97218, 97220, and 97230).

TABLE 1. INDOOR RADON VALUES FOR PORTLAND, OREGON

Place in Oregon	ZIP Code	Records	Picocuries/liter Max.	Avg.	%>4	Rank Sum	Potential
Beaverton	97005	28	3.6	1.3	0	2	Low
NW Beaverton	97006	19	3.7	1.2	0	2	Low
Aloha	97007	23	15.4	2.8	13	6	Moderate
Gresham	97030	24	7.7	2.9	17	6	Moderate
Lake Oswego	97034	40	8.4	2.4	23	6	Moderate
Lake Oswego	97035	23	8.3	1.6	9	4	Low
Oregon City	97045	14	6.4	2.8	14	5	Moderate
Troutdale	97060	12	3.4	1.5	0	2	Low
Tualatin	97062	16	11.7	2.3	19	7	Moderate
West Linn	97068	19	25.5	4.6	26	8	High
S. Gresham	97080	16	2.4	1.2	0	2	Low
S. Hillsboro	97123	11	20.9	4.4	18	8	High
N. Hillsboro	97124	10	4.6	1.4	10	4	Low
Sherwood	97140	10	4.8	2.6	20	6	Moderate
Portland	97201	36	4.9	1.4	6	4	Low
Portland	97202	37	7.5	3.1	22	6	Moderate
Portland	97203	52	9.6	2.5	21	6	Moderate
Portland	97206	12	13.8	3.6	25	7	Moderate
Portland	97210	29	5.0	1.6	3	4	Low
N. Portland	97211	41	35.5	4.8	44	9	High
N. Portland	97212	84	18.4	4.4	40	9	High
N. Portland	97213	71	20.5	5.2	52	9	High
N. Portland	97214	17	6.3	2.2	18	6	Moderate
N. Portland	97215	27	3.7	2.0	0	3	Low
Portland	97216	10	2.6	1.7	0	2	Low
N. Portland	97217	17	10.2	4.3	44	9	High
N. Portland	97218	23	14.3	4.7	48	9	High
Portland	97219	48	6.1	1.3	8	4	Low
N. Portland	97220	32	33.9	6.6	47	9	High
Portland	97221	36	7.0	1.7	8	4	Low
Portland	97222	16	7.2	2.2	19	6	Moderate
Tigard	97223	36	8.3	1.7	6	4	Low
Tigard	97224	24	3.8	1.5	0	2	Low
Portland	97225	38	9.4	2.2	16	6	Moderate
Portland	97229	21	3.2	1.2	0	2	Low
Parkrose	97230	25	27.4	3.6	24	7	Moderate
Portland	97232	12	4.5	1.7	17	5	Moderate
E. Portland	97236	13	13.7	3.6	31	7	Moderate
Milwaukie	97267	15	3.0	1.4	0	2	Low

Other areas of high potential are in east Portland (zip codes 97206 and 97236), southern Hillsboro (97123), Tualatin (97062), and West Linn (97068).

The average indoor radon value map (Fig. 5) has fewer zip codes in the high potential class when compared to the maximum values map (Fig. 4). The high potential class has 18% of the zip codes, moderate has 40%, and low potential has 42%. The high potential areas are again Alameda Ridge in north Portland (zip codes 97211, 97212, 97213, 97217, 97218, and 97220), West Linn (zip code 97068), and Hillsboro to the west (zip code 97123).

The map of the percentage of homes with radon >4 pCi/l (Fig. 2) has fewer zip codes in the high potential class than either of the other two maps. This map is probably a more reliable indicator of radon potential than Figures 4 and 5. Seventeen percent of the zip codes are in the high potential class, 32% are in the moderate class, and 51% are in the low class. The high category

areas are mainly on Alameda Ridge in north Portland (zip codes 97211, 97212, 97213, 97217, 97218, and 97220).

The results of the overall radon potential based on the rank sums are mapped in Figure 3. The highest radon potential category has 17% of the zip codes (7 with a rank sum of 9 and 3 with a rank sum of 8). The moderate category has 39% of the zip codes (8 with a value of 7, 11 with 6, and 4 with a rank sum of 5). The low radon potential category has 46% of the zip codes (7 with a rank sum of 4, 3 with 3, and 17 with a rank sum of 2). The high values are located mainly on Alameda Ridge in north Portland (zip codes 97211, 97212, 97213, 97217, 97218, 97220), Hillsboro to the west (zip code 97123), and the West Linn area to the south (zip code 97068).

Presentation of data to public

As a result of our work we were covered in five newspapers, including the front page in our main newspaper, the Oregonian, in

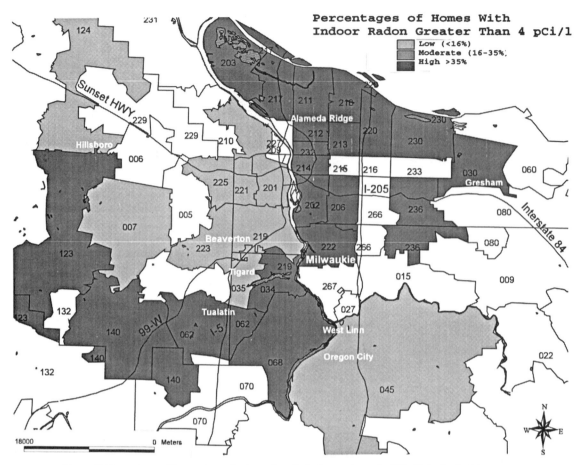

Figure 2. Percentage of homes in each zip code with indoor radon >4 pCi/l. Only the last three numbers of each zip code are given, and the first two zip code numbers are "97." Towns and geographic areas are written in white and highways in black. White mapping units lack enough data to summarize the zip code.

the evening edition. We had coverage on three television stations, including a half-hour program on one station the month following the initial press conferences. We also were covered on four radio stations that stress news.

DISCUSSION

Geological explanation for high values of indoor radon in Portland

It is difficult to determine unequivocally the reasons for the high values of radon in the Portland area and the reasons for the distribution of the high values because the data have been collected by zip codes that do not have natural geologic boundaries. Comparing the area of high soil permeability that is mapped as the Missoula flood gravels (Qfc of Beeson et al., 1991; Fig. 1) or the Multnomah soil series (Green, 1983) to the four radon potential maps, one sees that there is an overlap with the high potential zip codes on all maps.

The Alameda Ridge is a high radon potential area because the soils are highly permeable gravels with a sand matrix (Qfc)

deposited as a ribbon bar to the leeward side of Rocky Butte during the Missoula Floods 12,700 to 15,300 years ago (Waitt, 1985). The gravels contain abundant granitic gravel and sands that originated from the northwest part of Washington and Idaho and were brought to the Portland area during the catastrophic floods. Granite is usually a good source of radon. Homes with basements penetrate these gravels, and therefore there is a direct conduit for the gas to move into the basements. Also, there is little soil moisture in these well-drained soils that would reduce the flow of radon. Zip codes that contain some of the ridge are: 97203, 97211, 97212, 97213, 97217, 97218, and 97220. Homes built at the base of Alameda Ridge are of lower radon potential because they are built on thick deposits of silt that cover the gravels (Qff) and apparently protect the homes from radon.

The second area of highly permeable gravel soils that was deposited by the Missoula floods is in east Portland. Topographically, there are some high surfaces similar to the Alameda Ridge. These soils are found in zip codes 97030, 97232, 97233, and 97236. The soils are not quite as permeable as those of Alameda Ridge.

The third area with highly permeable gravel soils, also

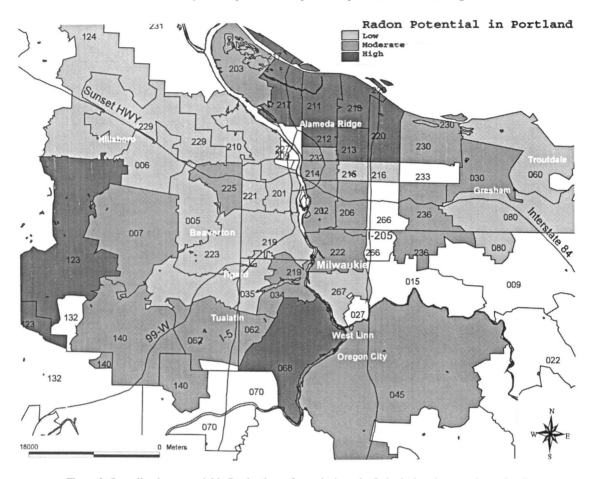

Figure 3. Overall radon potential in Portland area for each zip code. Only the last three numbers of each zip code are given, and the first two zip code numbers are "97." Towns and geographic areas are written in white and highways in black. White mapping units lack enough data to summarize the zip code.

deposited by the Missoula floods, is in southern Portland in the Eastmoreland and Milwaukie areas. Silts were deposited on top of the gravels by the floods, but water escaping from the Willamette Valley to the ocean after each of these floods carved out escape channels through this area exposing the gravels. The actual channels are narrow, and most of these zip code areas are blanketed with silt that protects the homes from radon. Zip codes of this area include 97202, 97206, 97214, and 97222.

The west Lake Oswego–Tualatin areas are other locations with highly permeable soils that are dry and contain granitic materials. Zip codes of these areas are 97034, 97035, and 97062. The Missoula floods carved out Lake Oswego and dumped the sediment onto a large fan at the west edge that extends into Durham and Tualatin. This alluvial fan of permeable soils occupies only a small percentage of these three zip code areas.

An enigma arose when we tried to explain the high radon values in the West Linn and Hillsboro areas. These places do not have highly permeable soils and are situated on basalt bedrock. We can only suggest that landslides and faults in those areas provide permeable ground for radon migration. We have attributed high indoor radon values in other studies in Salem, Clatskanie,

and Astoria, Oregon, to these geological conditions. Some of the rural areas to the west of Portland use ground water in the homes, which also could be the radon source. The zip codes associated with these regions are mainly 97068, 97140, 97123, 97007, 97006, and 97113.

At this point in the study of radon in Oregon, our hypothesis relating geology to indoor radon is based mainly on noticing similarities between areas of high indoor radon occurrence and areas of highly permeable soils containing granitic sediments. The correlation seems logical, but precise measurements need to be taken to prove our hypothesis. We have listed ways of achieving precise measurements in the recommendations section. To get people to participate in these types of studies is difficult, for many homeowners do not want to know their radon situation, or at least let others know it. They are more interested in the possibility of losing property value than learning about health hazards. The data used in this study were released to scientists only if the homeowners' addresses and names remained anonymous. Only their zip codes were used. Until we can get more cooperation from homeowners, radon potential maps must remain generalized.

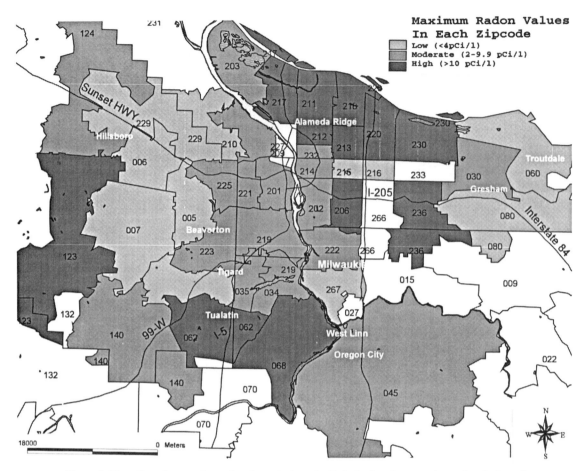

Figure 4. Map of maximum radon values in each zip code. Only the last three numbers of each zip code are given, and the first two zip code numbers are "97." Towns and geographic areas are written in white and highways in black. White mapping units lack enough data to summarize the zip code.

Evaluation of presentation of data to public

Overall, the response that we received from the media and the general public was positive. The Oregon Health Division received over 1,000 requests for further information on radon from telephone calls using the published number. We attributed our success to the fact that we were not alarming in our approach, although some members of the media did sensationalize the radon awareness. We did present data to the public, but we kept it simple (one radon map using zip codes and one simple table). We worked closely with professional public relations people on our staffs who opened many doors and gave good advice. We stressed that radon is a natural product that does create a health hazard in high concentrations and that it can be dealt with easily and cheaply.

RECOMMENDATIONS

Further sampling needed

It is recommended that another 200 indoor radon samples be taken to fill in holes in the data. Some of our classifications of

high and moderate potential categories we believe result from low numbers in the data set for the zip code. This is especially true for the suburbs of Portland. We recommend that the following zip codes have another 10 samples taken for each to give a minimal statistically significant rating: 97004, 97009, 97013, 97015, 97016, 97019, 97022, 97023, 97027, 97055, 97070, 97113, 97116, 97119, 97132, 97204, 97208, 97209, 97231, 97233, and 97266.

We also recommend that 10 or more samples be taken in zip code 97225 (West Slope) because we do not understand the geologic reasons for the high values in this area. More values for south Hillsboro (97123) would also confirm or disprove its high potential rating.

We also recommend that four areas be tested by comparing the permeable and nonpermeable soils. Twenty homes on one permeable soil surface (Qfc or Multnomah soil series) and 20 homes on a nonpermeable surface of silt-rich soils (Off) would be compared in each case (Beeson et al., 1991). The four test areas would be Alameda Ridge (Qfc) in north Portland compared to a lower terrace with Qff, east Portland high terrace gravels with Qfc compared to lower terraces covered with the silt-rich Qff, Eastmore-

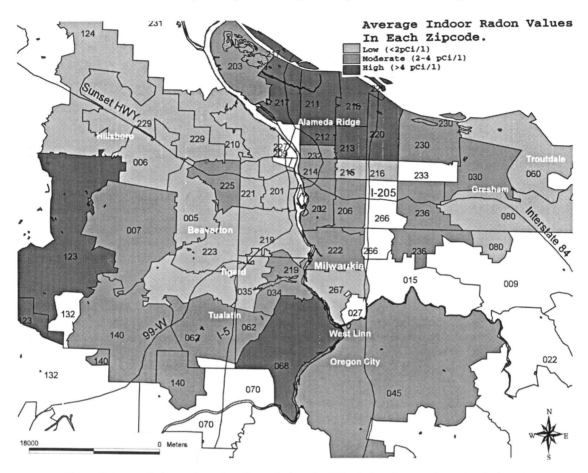

Figure 5. Average indoor radon values for each zip code. Only the last three numbers of each zip code are given, and the first two zip code numbers are "97." Towns and geographic areas are written in white and highways in black. White mapping units lack enough data to summarize the zip code.

land flood channel (Qfc) compared to nearby silt-covered uplands (Qff), and Tualatin and Durham gravel fans in southwest Portland compared to the surrounding silt soils (Qff). We would expect high indoor radon values on the highly permeable soils and low indoor radon values on the silt soils. This would be an excellent test for our hypothesis and would allow us to produce a very accurate radon potential map with natural boundaries based on the geological maps, not zip codes.

Homeowner recommendations

Homeowners are interested in what to do if a home has elevated levels of radon. Based on our experience in this area, we stress that radon detection can be accomplished easily and cheaply, and if mitigation is required, it can also be done inexpensively. Radon potential in most of Oregon is low, but a few zip codes in the Portland area show elevated levels. High soil permeability from Missoula flood gravels containing granitic sediments and landslides, plus homes located near faults or using well water in certain areas apparently can produce "hot spots" that can generate high radon values.

EPA and the Oregon Health Division both recommend that all homes should be tested for radon. The overall radon potential map for the Portland area (Fig. 3) provides guidance for evaluating radon potential in the Portland area. Homes in the high potential areas should be tested for radon. Zip codes included in the high potential category are 97211, 97212, 97213, 97217, 97218, 97220, 97068, and 97123. It is also recommended that people living in the moderate potential zones have their homes tested. Homes located in the low potential zones do have a chance for elevated indoor radon values, but the possibilities are much lower than the other two categories. The relatively low cost of testing with an alpha track detector (about $35, which includes the laboratory testing) makes feasible radon testing. The best time of the year to test for radon is in the winter when homes are closed, and maximum radon values can be measured. The alpha detector should be left in place for at least three months. If the house has a basement, the detector should be placed there; otherwise it should be placed in an area of poor air circulation on the first floor.

If the test results show more than 4 pCi/l, the action level for radon, mitigation generally can be easily and inexpensively accomplished by appropriate ventilation. Ventilation can be achieved by opening and closing windows often. Installation of a subslab depressurization system using electric fans is a bit more expensive, but it can be very efficient in removing the gases. High radon values might also necessitate sealing off the inside of the home from radon coming into the structure (EPA 1986a, 1988).

CONCLUSIONS

Even though Portland has been mapped on national radon potential maps as a low to moderate radon potential area, local geological conditions have created situations where one in every five houses has elevated radon values above the EPA action level of 4 pCi/l. This rate is more than twice the national average and over five times the rate for the rest of Oregon. The maximum indoor radon value recorded in the Portland area was 35.5 pCi/l. High soil permeability found on gravels deposited during the Missoula floods allows for radon to flow readily into basements. Homes built on faults or old landslides or rural homes using well water may also have increased indoor radon problems.

In this study 1,135 homes were tested for indoor concentrations of radon, and the values were recorded with zip codes. Using ranked sums of three characteristics of radon potential, eight zip codes have high indoor radon potential, 15 zip codes have moderate radon potential, 16 zip codes have low radon potential, and 21 zip codes need more data before trends can be established. Residents of Portland can consult the radon potential map of the region (Fig. 3) and the data (Table 1) to determine the radon potential for their zip code. Homes located in zip codes with moderate and high indoor radon potentials should have their homes tested.

This study led to our discovery that indoor radon was a problem in certain areas of Portland. We had to become the "voices of warning" to let the public know of the hazard. Awareness of a potential problem is an important key when one deals with a natural hazard that is invisible, odorless, and tasteless. By using reason and a noncatastrophic approach, we believe that we were successful in conveying our message and building public awareness of the problem without creating a panic. We stressed that there is a need to test for radon in some areas, that it is easy and cheap to do the test, that it is inexpensive to mitigate if one has a high indoor radon level, and that radon levels may vary from house to house in the same neighborhood. It is important for everyone to reduce the level of radiation exposure, and radon and its decay progeny are the largest sources of natural radiation in most of our lives (Nero et al., 1990).

ACKNOWLEDGMENTS

This project was supported by a grant from the Environmental Protection Agency through the Oregon Health Division to Portland State University. The geographical information system (GIS) maps were constructed by Mark Scott, a graduate student at Portland State University, through work at the Pacific Northwest Digital Data Clearinghouse of the Geology Department. The maps are available on the Internet at http://www.geol.edu/clearinghouse.

REFERENCES CITED

Ashbaugh, S. G., 1996, The distribution of naturally occurring soil radionuclides and radon potential of northwest Oregon [M.S. thesis]: Portland, Portland State University, 220 p.

Beeson, M. H., Tolan, T. L., and Madin, I. P., 1989, Geologic map of the Lake Oswego Quadrangle, Clackamas, Multnomah and Washington Counties, Oregon: Oregon Department of Geology and Mineral Industries, State of Oregon, Map GMS-59, scale 1:24,000, 1 sheet.

Beeson, M. H., Tolan, T. L., and Madin, I. P., 1991, Geologic map of the Portland Quadrangle, Multnomah and Washington Counties, Oregon and Clark County, Washington: Oregon Department of Geology and Mineral Industries, State of Oregon, Map GMS-75, scale 1:24,000, 1 sheet.

Bonneville Power Administration, 1993, Radon monitoring results from BPA's residential conservation programs: Portland, Oregon, Report No. 15, 17 p.

Duval, J. S., Riggle, F. B., Jones, W. J., and Pitkin, J. A., 1989, Equivalent uranium map of the conterminous United States: U.S. Geological Survey Open-File Report 89-478, scale 1:2,500,000.

Environmental Protection Agency, 1986a, Radon reduction techniques for detached houses: Washington, D.C., Environmental Protection Agency, EPA 625/5-86-019, 16 p.

Environmental Protection Agency, 1986b, A citizen's guide to radon: Washington, D.C., Environmental Protection Agency, EPA-86-004, 16 p.

Environmental Protection Agency, 1988, Radon-resistant residential new construction: Washington, D.C., Environmental Protection Agency, EPA 600/8-88-087, 24 p.

Environmental Protection Agency, 1993, Map of radon zone, United States: Washington, D.C., Environmental Protection Agency, EPA Map 402-R93-071.

Green, G. L., 1983, Soil survey of Multnomah County, Oregon: Washington, D.C., U.S.D.A. Soil Conservation Service, Government Printing Office, 225 p.

Henshaw, D. L., Eatough, J. P., and Richardson, R. B., 1990, Radon as a causative factor in induction of myeloid leukemia and other cancers: The Lancet, April 28, p. 1008–1012.

Hopke, P. K., 1987, Radon and its decay products: an overview, *in* Hopke, P. J., ed., Radon and its decay products: Occurrence, properties, and health effects: American Chemical Society, p. 1–8.

Keller, E. A., 1996, Environmental geology (seventh edition): New Jersey, Prentice Hall, 375 p.

Madin, I. P., 1990, Earthquake-hazard geology maps of the Portland metropolitan area, Oregon: text and explanation: State of Oregon, Department of Geology and Mineral Industries, Open-File Report 0-90-2, 27 p.

Miller, W. E., 1990, Radon hazard: a historical perspective, *in* Majumdar, S. K., Schmalz, R. F., and Miller, E. W., eds., Radon: Occurrence, control and health hazards: Easton, Pennsylvania, Pennsylvania Academy of Science, p. 1–12.

Nero, A. V., 1988, Radon and its decay products in indoor air, *in* Nazaroff, W. W., and Nero, A. V., eds., Radon and its decay products in indoor air: New York, John Wiley and Sons, p. 1–53.

Nero, A. V., Gadgil, A. J., Nazaroff, W. W., and Revzan, K. L., 1990, Indoor radon and decay products: concentrations, causes, and control strategies: Radon Technical Report Series, DOE/ER-0480P, 138 p.

Orr, E. L., Orr, W. N., and Baldwin, E. M., 1992, Geology of Oregon, (fourth edition): Dubuque, Iowa, Kendall/Hunt Publishing, 254 p.

Otton, J. K., 1992, The geology of radon: U.S. Geological Survey, 29 p.

Otton, J. K., Schumann, R. R., Owen, D. E., Thurman, N., and Duval, J. S., 1988, Map showing radon potential of rocks and soils in Fairfax County, Virginia: U.S. Geological Survey, Miscellaneous Field Studies Map, MF 2047, scale 1:62,500, 1 sheet.

Stone, R., 1993, Radon risk up in the air: Science, v. 261, p. 1515.

Waitt, R. B., Jr., 1985, Case for periodic, colossal jokulhlaups from Pleistocene Lake Missoula: Geological Society of America Bulletin, v. 96, no. 10, p. 1271–1286.

Manuscript Accepted by the Society June 5, 1997

Printed in U.S.A.

Geological Society of America
Reviews in Engineering Geology, Volume XII
1998

An outbreak of coccidioidomycosis (valley fever) caused by landslides triggered by the 1994 Northridge, California, earthquake

Randall W. Jibson and Edwin L. Harp
U.S. Geological Survey, Box 25046, MS 966, Denver Federal Center, Denver, Colorado 80225
Eileen Schneider, Rana A. Hajjeh, and Richard A. Spiegel
Centers for Disease Control and Prevention, 1600 Clifton Road, MS E-10 (E. S.) and MS C-23 (R. A. H. and R. A. S.), Atlanta, Georgia 30333

ABSTRACT

Following the January 17, 1994, Northridge, California, earthquake (M = 6.7), Ventura County, California, experienced a major outbreak of coccidioidomycosis (valley fever), a respiratory disease contracted by inhaling airborne fungal spores. In the eight weeks following the earthquake (January 24 through March 15), 203 outbreak-associated cases were reported, which is about an order of magnitude more than the expected number of cases, and 3 of these cases were fatal. Simi Valley, in easternmost Ventura County, had the highest attack rate in the county, and the attack rate decreased westward across the county. The temporal and spatial distribution of coccidioidomycosis cases indicates that the outbreak resulted from inhalation of spore-contaminated dust generated by earthquake-triggered landslides. Canyons northeast of Simi Valley produced many highly disrupted, dust-generating landslides during the earthquake and its aftershocks. Prevailing winds after the earthquake were from the northeast, which transported dust into Simi Valley and beyond to communities to the west. The 3 fatalities from the coccidioidomycosis epidemic accounted for 4% of the total earthquake-related fatalities.

INTRODUCTION

The M-6.7 Northridge, California, earthquake of January 17, 1994 caused widespread damage and at least 72 deaths. Strong shaking generated by the earthquake damaged or destroyed thousands of homes, buildings, and other structures and triggered tens of thousands of landslides over a broad area (Harp and Jibson, 1995, 1996). Following the earthquake, an outbreak of coccidioidomycosis (valley fever) occurred that caused three fatalities. Coccidioidomycosis is a systemic disease contracted by inhaling airborne dust containing fungal spores that trigger an infection. Schneider et al. (1997) detailed the epidemiology of the outbreak and the risk factors associated with it and noted the apparent relationship between the earthquake-triggered landslides and the outbreak. In this paper we summarize the findings of the epidemiologic investigation and present detailed evidence associating the outbreak with dust generated by earthquake-triggered landslides. This is the first documentation of an outbreak of coccidioidomycosis associated with an earthquake.

BACKGROUND ON THE EARTHQUAKE AND TRIGGERED LANDSLIDES

The Northridge earthquake (M-6.7) occurred at 4:31 a.m. local time on January 17, 1994. The hypocenter was 19 km beneath the Northridge area of the San Fernando Valley (Fig. 1) on a blind thrust fault striking N. 58° W. and dipping 42° south (Wald and Heaton, 1994). Free-field peak horizontal ground accelerations greater than 1 g were recorded at some sites, and high levels of ground shaking extended over a broad region. Thousands of structures were damaged or destroyed by the strong shaking, and total losses were estimated at more than $20 billion.

Jibson, R. W., Harp, E. L., Schneider, E., Hajjeh, R. A., and Spiegel, R. A., 1998, An outbreak of coccidioidomycosis (valley fever) caused by landslides triggered by the 1994 Northridge, California, earthquake, *in* Welby, C. W., and Gowan, M. E., eds., A Paradox of Power: Voices of Warning and Reason in the Geosciences: Boulder, Colorado, Geological Society of America Reviews in Engineering Geology, v. XII.

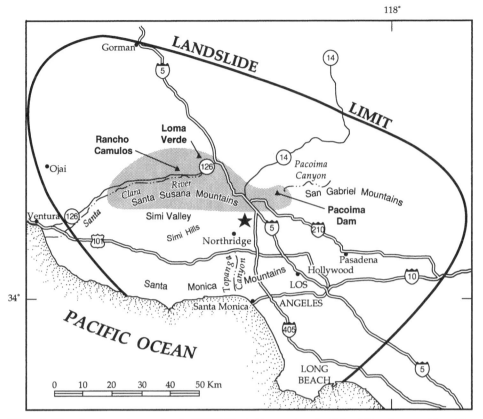

Figure 1. Map showing epicenter (star) of 1994 Northridge earthquake (**M** = 6.7) and areas affected by landslides. Heavy line shows maximum limit of triggered landslides; area of greatest landslide concentration is shaded.

The Northridge earthquake triggered more than 11,000 landslides over an area of about 10,000 km² (Harp and Jibson, 1995, 1996) that is roughly concentric about the epicenter (Fig. 1). Within this broad area of scattered landslide activity is a 1,000-km² area of much more concentrated landsliding that lies north and northwest of the epicenter, primarily in the Santa Susana Mountains and the mountains north of the Santa Clara River valley. Landslides were densest along the steep-walled canyons that are incised into the northern and southern flanks of the Santa Susana Mountains. In some of these areas more than 75% of the slope area was denuded by landslides triggered by strong shaking (Fig. 2). Characteristic landslides in such areas were several decimeters to a few meters deep and consisted of dry, highly disaggregated material that cascaded downslope to flatter areas at or near the base of the steep slopes (Fig. 3). These failures ranged in volume from a fraction of a cubic meter to a few hundred thousand cubic meters (Harp and Jibson, 1995, 1996).

The reason for this extraordinary concentration of landslides was twofold. First, the fault rupture extended directly beneath the mountains, which probably enhanced the strong ground motion there. Throughout the Santa Susana Mountains, pervasive shattered ridge tops and boulders thrown from their sockets attest to widespread high ground accelerations. Second, the Santa Susana Mountains consist primarily of late Miocene through Pleistocene clastic

sediment having little or no cementation; this sediment is being uplifted and folded by rapid tectonic deformation. The young, weak material lacks significant tensile strength and erodes readily to form steep-walled canyons that commonly head in nearly vertical slopes. The combination of young, weak sediment and steep relief reaching elevations of 1,000 m above sea level makes this area extremely susceptible to failure during seismic shaking.

BACKGROUND ON COCCIDIOIDOMYCOSIS

Coccidioidomycosis (locally known as valley fever, desert fever, or desert rheumatism) occurs only in the Western Hemisphere. It is endemic to parts of South and Central America as well as the semiarid southwest of North America, particularly parts of Arizona, California, Nevada, New Mexico, Texas, Utah, and northern Mexico (Drutz and Catanzaro, 1978; Pappagianis, 1988). Coccidioidomycosis is a reportable disease in California and several other states in which the disease is endemic. Within California it is highly endemic in the southern San Joaquin Valley and less endemic in the epicentral area of the Northridge earthquake (Edwards and Palmer, 1957; Fiese, 1958). Coccidioidomycosis is caused by infection with *Coccidioides immitis* spores, a dimorphic, saprophytic fungus that grows in the upper 10–20 cm of semiarid soils (Drutz and Catanzaro, 1978). Infec-

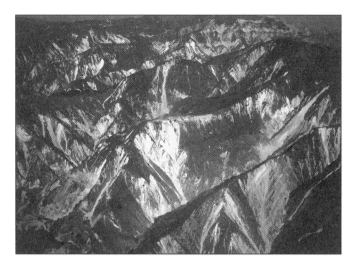

Figure 2. Slopes denuded by earthquake-triggered landslides in the Santa Susana Mountains. Virtually all the light-colored areas failed during the earthquake.

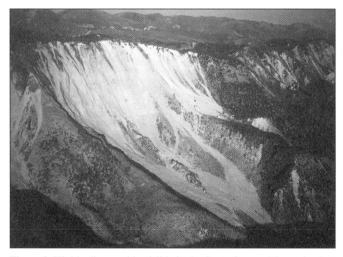

Figure 3. Highly disrupted landslide in the Santa Susana Mountains just north of Simi Valley. The weak sediment disaggregated into individual sediment grains and cascaded down the steep slopes.

tion results from inhaling airborne dust containing the spores, and coccidioidomycosis is not transmitted from person to person (Drutz and Catanzaro, 1978; Pappagianis, 1988). The incubation period for coccidioidomycosis ranges from 8–21 days; the average is 14 days (Smith et al., 1946; Stevens, 1995).

An estimated 100,000 coccidioidomycosis cases occur each year in the United States resulting in about $20 million in medical expenses and 50–70 fatalities (Stevens, 1995). About 60% of infected persons are asymptomatic, and the remaining 40% present with a flu-like respiratory illness. About 0.5% of infected persons develop disseminated coccidioidal disease, in which the infection spreads to different organs and body systems (Drutz and Catanzaro, 1978; Einstein and Johnson, 1993; Stevens, 1995).

Because coccidioidomycosis symptoms are similar to those of other common illnesses, definitive diagnosis requires isolation of the organism or serological testing. Therefore, the number of diagnosed cases probably underestimates of total actual cases because most infected persons are asymptomatic or have a mild, flu-like illness. For example, Einstein and Johnson (1993) estimated that the number of serologically confirmed cases represents only 8–10% of total infections. Almost all infected persons acquire lifetime immunity to the disease (Drutz and Catanzaro, 1978; Einstein and Johnson, 1993). Previous exposure to the infection can be determined by skin testing.

In endemic areas, people who are exposed to high levels of airborne dust in their work environments are at higher risk for infection with *C. immitis*. People working in agriculture, construction (particularly excavation), archaeology, and field geology are particularly at high risk for contracting coccidioidomycosis (Pappagianis, 1988).

Even within highly endemic areas, *C. immitis* distribution in soils is spotty. The fungal spores thrive in sandy, alkaline soils rich in carbonized organic material and salts (Elconin et al., 1967; Swatek et al., 1967; Drutz and Catanzaro, 1978; Einstein and Johnson, 1993). Pappagianis (1988) noted a particular affinity of *C. immitis* to soils developed on marine sediment. Endemic areas are characterized by a semiarid climate that facilitates the airborne distribution of *C. immitis* spores: rainy winters having few freezes enhance germination and fungal growth, and hot, dry summers cause the fungal growths to become brittle and easily detached by surface winds (Smith et al., 1946; Drutz and Catanzaro, 1978; Pappagianis, 1988). Previously reported epidemics of coccidioidomycosis in the San Joaquin Valley of California have been linked to periods of drought and periods of increased dust from disturbance of the ground surface (Smith et al., 1946; Centers for Disease Control and Prevention, 1994). Arroyos and dry washes are especially conducive to *C. immitis* concentration because they have prolonged periods of moist soil conditions during the rainy season (Pappagianis, 1988); furthermore, *C. immitis* is hydrophobic and thus floats, which enhances transport and deposition along arroyo walls during seasonal runoff periods (Swatek et al., 1967).

EPIDEMIOLOGY OF THE COCCIDIOIDOMYCOSIS OUTBREAK

During the first five weeks following the earthquake, Ventura County public health officials noted a large increase in reporting of coccidioidomycosis cases as compared to previous years. Between January 24 and March 15, 1994, 203 outbreak-associated cases of coccidioidomycosis were identified (Schneider et al., 1997). By contrast, fewer than 60 coccidioidomycosis cases were reported annually in both 1992 and 1993 in Ventura County. Fifty-five (27%) of the diagnosed patients required hospitalization, the median duration of which was 7.5 days. Six patients (3%) developed disseminated coccidioidal disease, and three persons (1.5%) died (Schneider et al., 1997).

TEMPORAL CORRELATION OF EPIDEMIC WITH THE EARTHQUAKE

The temporal correlation between the abrupt increase in coccidioidomycosis cases and the occurrence of the earthquake is striking. Figure 4 shows the temporal distribution of the onset of coccidioidomycosis symptoms for 213 cases in Ventura County diagnosed from January 1 through March 15, 1994; 203 of these cases meet the case definition for being outbreak associated. From January 1, through January 17 (the day of the earthquake), one case was reported, which is consistent with similar time periods in 1991 and 1992. Immediately after the earthquake, an increase in reporting of coccidioidomycosis cases occurred. A sharp peak in the temporal distribution occurred two weeks after the earthquake; this time interval corresponded exactly to the median incubation period of coccidioidomycosis (Smith et al., 1946; Stevens, 1995). Following this peak, cases tailed off through March 15.

Figure 4 shows a clear temporal relationship between the onset of the epidemic and the time of the earthquake. The question that remains to be answered, however, is what the earthquake did that triggered the epidemic. We address this question by analyzing the spatial distribution of the reported coccidioidomycosis cases.

SPATIAL DISTRIBUTION OF COCCIDIOIDOMYCOSIS CASES

Although the temporal association of the earthquake and the onset of the coccidioidomycosis epidemic is evident, the spatial distribution of the cases is more complex. The earthquake was cen-tered in the San Fernando Valley of Los Angeles County (Fig. 1), and strong ground shaking and damage were greatest there. The coccidioidomycosis outbreak, however, occurred in Ventura County and was concentrated primarily in Simi Valley, which lies at the eastern edge of the county and tens of kilometers west of the epicenter. Figure 5 shows the distribution of postearthquake coc-cidioidomycosis cases, and the distribution is clearly nonrandom.

Simi Valley, located near the base of the Santa Susana Moun-tains, had 56% of the reported outbreak-associated (January 24–March 15) coccidioidomycosis cases despite having less than 15% of the county's population. The attack rate (number of per-sons who had coccidioidomycosis divided by the number of per-sons at risk for infection) in Simi Valley was 114 cases per 100,000 people as compared to 30 cases per 100,000 in Ventura County as a whole. Figure 6 shows the attack rate for several communities; Simi Valley had by far the highest attack rate, and rates decreased in communities to the west and south. In westernmost Ventura County, the attack rate was only 3 per 100,000 population. Analy-sis of the attack rate by census tract showed large variability even within Simi Valley, where the attack rate ranged from 27 to 473 cases per 100,000 population (median: 97 per 100,000). The high-est attack rate was in the census tract located closest to the moun-tain front (Schneider et al., 1997) and the triggered landslides.

The distribution of cases is elongated in a northeast-south-west direction (Fig. 5). The overall pattern forms a cone having its apex at the northern edge of the Simi Valley at the foot of the Santa Susana Mountains, and the density of cases decreases out-ward from the apex. As noted previously, coccidioidomycosis is contracted almost exclusively through inhaling airborne fungal spores; therefore, this highly nonrandom distribution of coccid-

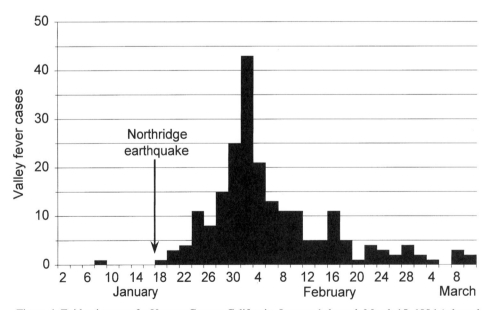

Figure 4. Epidemic curve for Ventura County, California, January 1 through March 15, 1994 (adapted from Schneider et al., 1997). The epidemic curve is a histogram showing the temporal distribution of diagnosed coccidioidomycosis cases; the peak of the histogram is two weeks following the earthquake, which is the median incubation period for coccidioidomycosis.

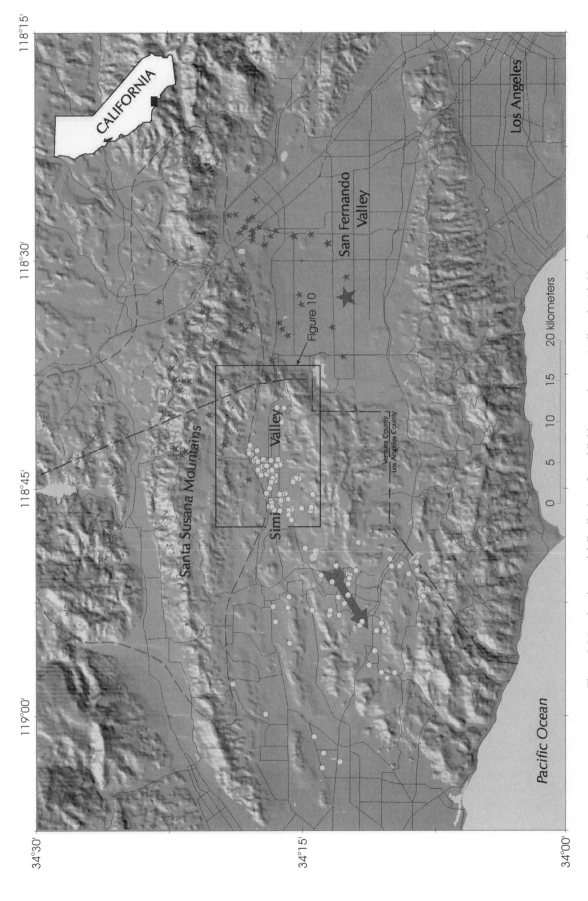

Figure 5. Map showing spatial distribution of coccidioidomycosis cases (yellow dots) in Ventura County following the Northridge earthquake. Triggered landslides are in red, and the area of greatest landslide concentration is outlined (dashed red line). Green arrow shows the prevailing wind direction during the three days following the earthquake as measured by a National Weather Service anemometer in Thousand Oaks. Large blue star is mainshock epicenter; small blue stars are prominent aftershocks (adapted from Schneider et al., 1997). Area shown in Figure 10 is outlined.

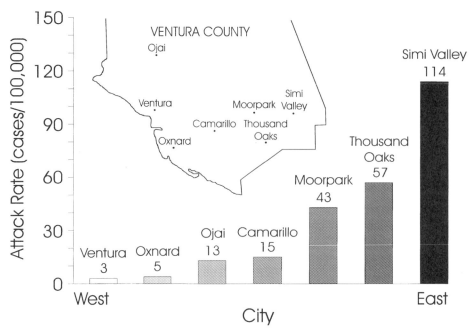

Figure 6. Coccidioidomycosis attack rate (infections per 100,000 people) by city in Ventura County (data from Schneider et al., 1997). Attack rate decreased markedly from east to west.

ioidomycosis cases likely resulted from a dust-generating source near the densest part of the distribution. The likely source for that dust is a dense concentration of earthquake-triggered landslides northeast of the apex of the conical distribution (Fig. 5).

Results of the case-control study conducted by the Centers for Disease Control and Prevention (Schneider et al., 1997) showed that persons who reported being physically in a dust cloud generated by an earthquake-triggered landslide were three times more likely to be diagnosed with acute coccidioidomycosis as those who were not in dust clouds. Among persons physically in a dust cloud, risk increased with duration of exposure. These landslides are thus the most likely source of the dust causing the densely concentrated epidemic. Validating this hypothesis requires showing that the earthquake-triggered landslides generated large amounts of airborne dust and that the predominant wind direction after the earthquake would have transported the dust southwestward from the landslide area into the outbreak area.

TRIGGERED LANDSLIDES AS A DUST SOURCE

As noted previously, the Santa Susana Mountains consist of young, weak, uncemented or very weakly cemented granular sediment. In the steeply incised canyons on the flanks of the mountains, the strong shaking from the Northridge earthquake triggered abundant landslides. The landslides involved fairly shallow masses (generally 1–2 m thick) of weathered material that failed by disaggregating into individual sediment grains and cascading down the steep slopes. As documented by numerous photographs taken soon after the earthquake (Fig. 7), these failures generated very dense dust clouds.

The U.S. Air Force flew high-altitude (nominal scale 1:60,000) reconnaissance photos of the region about 6 hours after the earthquake, and dust plumes are clearly visible in landslide areas on many of these photos (Fig. 8). Likewise, sequential National Weather Service satellite photos of Southern California documented earthquake-generated dust. Figure 9A is a satellite image taken a few minutes before the 3:33 p.m. aftershock on January 17. Cloud banks offshore are visible, but no clouds are present over land areas. Figure 9B shows the same area 30 minutes later (following the aftershock); the offshore cloud banks have not moved, but in the area of the Santa Susana Mountains

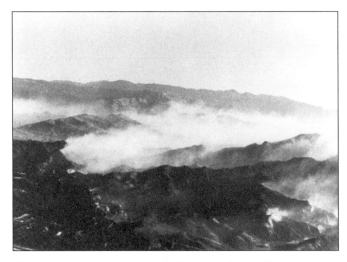

Figure 7. Oblique airphoto taken within a few hours of the earthquake showing dust from earthquake-triggered landslides.

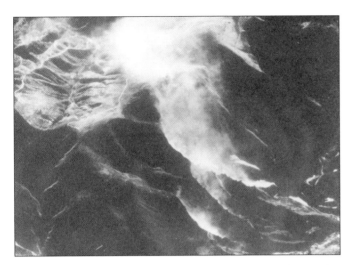

Figure 8. High-altitude U.S. Air Force airphoto taken about 6 hours after the earthquake showing dust plumes from triggered landslides.

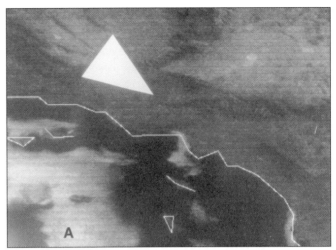

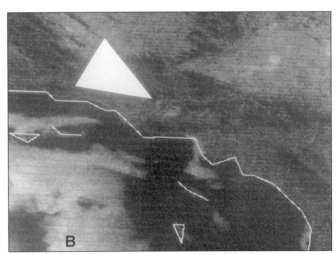

Figure 9. National Weather Service satellite photos taken (A) just before and (B) just after the 3:33 p.m. aftershock of January 17. Jagged line denotes approximate location of shoreline. Arrow in photo B shows cloud mass not visible in photo A, which presumably is dust from triggered landslides. Note that offshore cloud masses visible in photo A have not moved in photo B.

and Simi Valley, clouds are clearly visible. These clouds were probably dust clouds because they appeared in the areas of intense landslide activity, and no nearby cloud masses are visible in the previous photo that could have moved to that location during the 30-minute interval between photos.

Even moderate-sized landslides in the weak material of the Santa Susana Mountains generated extraordinarily dense dust plumes. People in Simi Valley at the time of the earthquake reported that automobile drivers were using headlights while driving because of the thick dust in the air. Even days after the earthquake, individual landslides continued to ravel or were reactivated by aftershocks and sent thick dust plumes into the air.

WEATHER CONDITIONS DURING AND AFTER THE EARTHQUAKE

Weather conditions at the time of the earthquake were particularly favorable for dust transport from the Santa Susana Mountains into Simi Valley and beyond to communities to the west and southwest. Little seasonal rainfall had accumulated in the region before the earthquake, and the coarse-granular surficial materials that failed were very dry. No rain fell after the earthquake for several days; thus, the dust remained dry and was easily suspended in the air.

A mild Santa Ana wind condition prevailed at the time of the earthquake and for the next few days. This weather pattern was characterized by moderate surface winds of 15–40 km/hr blowing from the east and northeast to the west and southwest. Such a wind condition favored suspended-dust transport from the Santa Susana Mountains into Simi Valley. At the same time, clearing of the dust clouds from the valleys was inhibited by a mild westerly sea breeze along the coast, which caused stagnation of air in the affected valleys (Schneider et al., 1997). This weather pattern persisted through January 20.

The arrow in Figure 5 shows the predominant wind direction at the time of the earthquake at the National Weather Service Thousand Oaks anemometer, the closest operating instrument to the densest concentration of coccidioidomycosis cases. The wind direction aligned exactly with the elongation direction of the coccidioidomycosis cases, and directly upwind from this cluster of outbreaks is the densest concentration of landslides on the south side of the mountain crest.

DISCUSSION

The postearthquake investigation by the Centers for Disease Control and Prevention (Schneider et al., 1997) indicated that the Ventura County coccidioidomycosis outbreak was associated with the earthquake. This conclusion was based on (1) the epidemic curve (Fig. 4); (2) distribution of outbreak-associated cases in

Simi Valley; (3) the occurrence of seismically triggered, dust-generating landslides; and (4) weather conditions at the time of the earthquake. More detailed examination of some specific geologic conditions provides insight into how they may have affected the outbreak.

The sharply conical distribution of coccidioidomycosis cases in Simi Valley that decreased in density away from the apex indicates a point source for the dust containing the spores. Close examination of the map of triggered landslides (Fig. 10) upwind from the coccidioidomycosis outbreaks shows that most of the dust probably originated in Chivo and Las Llajas Canyons, which extend parallel to the prevailing wind direction and the alignment of outbreaks. These canyons produced very high concentrations of disrupted landslides, and the orientation of these canyons parallel to the northeasterly winds probably enhanced airborne particulate transport into Simi Valley. The other canyons along the south flank of the Santa Susana Mountains are oriented in a more north-south direction, at an angle of about 50–60° to the

wind direction. Chivo and Las Llajas Canyons are arroyos incised in sandy, silty, salt-rich marine sediment, conditions that, as noted above, have been associated with enhanced *C. immitis* growth (Elconin et al., 1967; Swatek et al., 1967; Drutz and Catanzaro, 1978; Pappagianis, 1988; Einstein and Johnson, 1993).

Los Angeles County, where the earthquake was centered and where most of the damage occurred, did not experience a similar increase in coccidioidomycosis cases following the earthquake. So why did an outbreak not occur in the more densely populated, strongly shaken San Fernando Valley? Several factors are most likely responsible. Two geologic factors include the highly variable spore concentration in surficial soils (Elconin et al., 1967; Drutz and Catanzaro, 1978; Pappagianis, 1988) and the geographic distribution of triggered landslides (Fig. 5). The San Gabriel Mountains, which lie northeast—upwind—of the San Fernando Valley, produced only very sparse, scattered landslides, with the exception of Pacoima Canyon. Also, the San Gabriel Mountains consist of much older and somewhat stronger rock

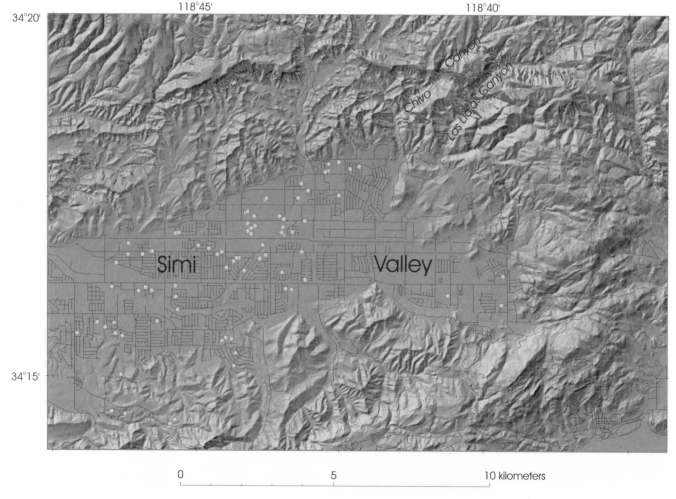

Figure 10. Map showing triggered landslides (red areas) in canyons immediately upwind of the apex of the coccidioidomycosis concentration in Simi Valley. Chivo and Las Llajas Canyons are aligned parallel with the wind direction and the elongation direction of the coccidioidomycosis distribution (yellow dots). Location shown in Figure 5.

than the Santa Susana Mountains. These rocks are primarily granitic and metamorphic, and they weather to produce thinner, coarser grained soils that are likely to produce less dust than the deep, silty soils in the Santa Susana Mountains. More importantly, soils developed on granitic rocks are highly acidic and thus far less compatible with *C. immitis* growth (Pappagianis, 1988) than the alkaline soils of the Santa Susanas. Both the much sparser landslide concentration and the radically different lithology and soil chemistry of the San Gabriel Mountains might account for the absence of a similar outbreak in the San Fernando Valley.

Some measures can be taken to reduce the likelihood of contracting coccidioidomycosis. Dust-control measures, including planting vegetation, wetting soil, paving dirt roads, and using face masks, have, in some instances, reduced infection rates, but the benefits of such preventive measures are temporary and incomplete (Smith et al., 1946). After a single dust-generating event such as an earthquake, instructing the public to avoid dust clouds may be beneficial in reducing exposure. Perhaps most important is educating both the general public and health-care providers regarding the risks posed by coccidioidomycosis, ways to minimize exposure to infection, and how to recognize possible symptoms so that the disease can be rapidly diagnosed and treated. Such increased awareness of coccidioidomycosis is particularly important for earth scientists, who are at increased risk for infection because of occupational exposure. Earth scientists should be aware that conducting field activities in endemic areas places them at risk for contracting coccidioidomycosis, and activities that disturb surficial materials and generate dust (such as trenching and collecting rock, soil, and fossil samples) increase risk in particular. Because initial infection confers lifelong immunity, people engaging in such work can undergo skin testing to determine if they have been infected previously or if they are at risk for initial infection.

SUMMARY AND CONCLUSIONS

Strong shaking from the Northridge earthquake triggered abundant landslides in the very weak slopes of the Santa Susana Mountains. These landslides generated dense dust clouds that were transported by prevailing northeasterly winds into the Simi Valley and beyond to Thousand Oaks and other communities to the west and south. Analysis of the epidemiological data indicated a strong relationship between the earthquake, the triggered landslides, and the coccidioidomycosis outbreak (Schneider et al., 1997). The earthquake-triggered outbreak led to three coccidioidomycosis fatalities, which accounted for 4% of the total earthquake fatalities.

The results of this investigation are significant for earthquake hazard assessment and emergency preparedness in areas where coccidioidomycosis is endemic and where landslide-generated dust clouds could occur. Public-health officials and health-care providers must be aware of the risk factors for coccidioidomycosis, and they should be better integrated into earthquake-preparedness planning. If such epidemics are anticipated, closer and more rapid screening of patients with coccidioidomycosis symptoms can take place, and more rapid medical treatment may reduce the number of serious or fatal cases.

ACKNOWLEDGMENTS

The findings of this study are the result of collaboration of several organizations: Public health officials from the Ventura County Health Department and the California Department of Health Services provided epidemiological data, the University of California provided background information concerning the occurrence of coccidioidomycosis, airphotos were taken by the U.S. Air Force, satellite photos were provided by the National Aeronautics and Space Administration, and weather data were provided by the National Weather Service. Grant Marshall, Ross Stein, and John Michael of the U.S. Geological Survey compiled the map of coccidioidomycosis outbreaks. Jim Dewey, Lynn Highland, Neil Gilbert, David Garrett, and Charles Welby reviewed the manuscript.

REFERENCES CITED

Centers for Disease Control and Prevention, 1994, Update: Coccidioidomycosis—California, 1991–1993: Morbidity and Mortality Weekly Report, v. 43, no. 23, p. 421–423.

Drutz, D. J., and Catanzaro, A., 1978, Coccidioidomycosis [Parts I and II]: American Review of Respiratory Disease, v. 117, p. 559–585, 727–771.

Edwards, P. Q., and Palmer, C. E., 1957, Prevalence of sensitivity to coccidioidin, with special reference to specific and nonspecific reactions to coccidioidin and to histoplasmin: Diseases of the Chest, v. 31, p. 35–60.

Einstein, H. E., and Johnson, R. H., 1993, Coccidioidomycosis: New aspects of epidemiology and therapy: Clinical Infectious Diseases, v. 16, p. 349–356.

Elconin, A. F., Egeberg, M. C., Bald, J. G., Matkin, A. O., and Egeberg, R. O., 1967, A fungicide effective against *Coccidioides immitis* in the soil, *in* Ajello, L., ed., Coccidioidomycosis: Tucson, Arizona, University of Arizona Press, p. 319–321.

Fiese, M. J., 1958, Geographic distribution of *Coccidioides immitis*, *in* Coccidioidomycosis: Springfield, Illinois, Charles C. Thomas, p. 53–76.

Harp, E. L., and Jibson, R. W., 1995, Inventory of landslides triggered by the 1994 Northridge, California, earthquake: U.S. Geological Survey Open-File Report 95-213, 17 p., 2 pl.

Harp, E. L., and Jibson, R. W., 1996, Landslides triggered by the 1994 Northridge, California, earthquake: Seismological Society of America Bulletin, v. 86, no. 1B, p. S319–S332.

Pappagianis, D., 1988, Epidemiology of coccidioidomycosis: Current Topics in Medical Mycology, v. 2, p. 199–238.

Schneider, E., Hajjeh, R. A., Spiegel, R. A., Jibson, R. W., Harp, E. L., Marshall, G. A., Gunn, R. A., McNeil, M. M., Pinner, R. W., Baron, R. C., Burger, R. C., Hutwanger, L. C., Crump, C., Kaufman, L., Reef, S. E., Feldman, G. M., Pappagianis, D., and Werner, S. B., 1997, A coccidioidomycosis outbreak following the Northridge earthquake, Ventura County, California, January–March 1994: Journal of the American Medical Association, v. 277, no. 11, p. 904–908.

Smith, C. E., Beard, R. R., Rosenberger, H. G., and Whiting, E. G., 1946, Effect of season and dust control on coccidioidomycosis: Journal of the American Medical Association, v. 132, p. 833–838.

Stevens, D. A., 1995, Coccidioidomycosis: New England Journal of Medicine, v. 332, p. 1077–1082.

Swatek, F. E., Omieczynski, D. T., and Plunkett, O. A., 1967, *Coccidioides immitis* in California, *in* Ajello, L., ed., Coccidioidomycosis: Tucson, Arizona, University of Arizona Press, p. 255–264.

Wald, D. J., and Heaton, T. H., 1994, A dislocation model of the 1994 Northridge, California, earthquake determined from strong ground motions: U.S. Geological Survey Open-File Report 94-278, 53 p.

Manuscript Accepted by the Society June 5, 1997

Geological Society of America
Reviews in Engineering Geology, Volume XII
1998

Sewage sludge (biosolids) land disposal in a southeastern U.S. Piedmont setting: Ground-water pollution potential

Charles W. Welby
Department of Marine, Earth, and Atmospheric Sciences, North Carolina State University, Raleigh, North Carolina 27695-8208

ABSTRACT

A multiyear study of the effect on ground water of land disposal of sewage sludge (biosolids) provides insight into the risk of nitrate pollution of ground water in a southeastern U.S. Piedmont Province setting. Two fields used for biosolid disposal and growth of row crops provided information about potential rates of nitrate movement to shallow ground water and possibly to ground water in the crystalline rocks underlying the saprolite. Initial studies based on semiannual sampling of a limited number of monitoring wells suggested that nitrate from a given biosolids application might take 200 to 300 days to reach the water table once a minimum cumulative nitrate loading had been reached after several years of biosolids application. In the longer used of two fields studied nitrate-nitrogen (NO3-N) concentrations of greater than 50 mg/l extended downward from the water table 6.1 m (20 ft) or more nearly to the crystalline bedrock surface.

Ground-water monitoring at a field to which biosolids were first applied during the study suggests that in some cases only 90 to 100 days may elapse before biosolids-derived nitrate reaches the water table. Water-table depths ranged from less than 3.05 m (10 ft) near a stream to over 9.2 m (30 ft) in the higher portions of the field.

Stable nitrogen isotopes were used to identify the appearance of nitrate in the ground water. These were also used to determine that nitrate from biosolids was entering a stream through baseflow and thereby contributing to nitrate buildup in surface waters.

The study also demonstrates that during biosolid application to fields nitrate accumulates to form a nitrate reservoir in the soil and saprolite. Nitrate in this reservoir can be moved to the saturated zone during periods of precipitation when precipitation exceeds evapotranspiration and use of the nitrate by crops. The ground water is especially vulnerable to nitrate buildup when a field lies fallow during the ground-water recharge period during winter and spring months. Evidence from this study as well as others suggests that nitrate concentrations in ground water will decline once biosolids application ceases.

In considering use of land disposal and cropping for handling municipal sewage sludge, decision-makers need to contemplate future possible uses of the land and whether or not nitrate-enriched ground water may be a limiting factor in future uses. Trade offs must be made between the risk of significant ground-water pollution and additional costs for nitrate removal.

Welby, C. W., 1998, Sewage sludge (biosolids) land disposal in a southeastern U.S. Piedmont setting: Ground-water pollution potential, *in* Welby, C. W., and Gowan, M. E., eds., A Paradox of Power: Voices of Warning and Reason in the Geosciences: Boulder, Colorado, Geological Society of America Reviews in Engineering Geology, v. XII.

PURPOSE

The investigation's purpose has been to develop an improved understanding of how effective the cropping practices have been in the removal of nitrate from the biosolids and to learn about the risk of shallow ground-water contamination from leaching of nitrate from the applied biosolids. Included in the second part of the purpose is the development of an understanding of the maximum volume of biosolids that should be applied and the application pattern that best limits the amount of nitrate-nitrogen (NO3-N) that can reach the shallow ground water.

The objective of this report is to summarize what has been learned about land application of municipal biosolids and the potential for ground-water pollution in a southeastern U.S. Piedmont Province setting.

BACKGROUND

Introduction

Approximately 20 years ago the City of Raleigh, North Carolina, began construction of a new sewage treatment plant. The facility was based upon land disposal of the sewage sludge (biosolids) left after treatment of the sewage, the effluent being discharged to the Neuse River. Historically, studies of possible ground-water contamination from agricultural land uses have been concentrated in areas dominated by sediments and sedimentary rocks (Gerhart, 1986; Higgins, 1984; Powlson et al., 1989; Spalding et al., 1993; Walther, 1989; Weil et al., 1990). The current study area is situated in the North Carolina Piedmont Province and is underlain by granitic bedrock covered by varying thicknesses of saprolite derived from it.

Three studies of fields on which the sludge was to be applied or has been applied have been conducted at the site. The original study in 1974–1975 examined the recharge potential and groundwater quality in selected fields prior to the application of any sewage sludge (Anderson, 1975). Incorporated in this study was acreage that had been farmed using artificial fertilizers and acreage covered by second-growth forest.

The second study, completed in 1989, concentrated on analysis of ground-water chemical data collected from various fields during semiannual, state-mandated monitoring from 1981 through 1987. In addition, selected wells were sampled more frequently during the 1987–1989 interval. A third study began in 1990 as an outgrowth of the second study. Attention in this study was concentrated on two fields, one to which biosolids had been applied since the beginning of the facility's operation and a second field to which biosolids were first applied in the fall of 1990.

The Neuse River Waste Water Treatment Plant (NRWWTP) lies about 32 km (20 mi) southeast of Raleigh, North Carolina (Fig. 1), and is located in rolling terrane underlain by the Rolesville Granite (Parker, 1979). Saprolite varies in thickness from zero to over 15.3 m (50 ft) in the area. Soils tend to be sandy and silty loams, and beneath a clay-rich subsoil the saprolite is gener-

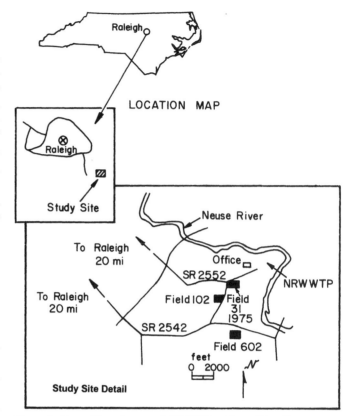

Figure 1. General location map. NRWWTP = Neuse River Waste Water Treatment Plant.

ally in the fine clayey and silty sand class. Weathered feldspar bands as well as quartz cobbles and pebbles are common. The locations of Field 102 and Field 602 are shown in Figure 1.

Rainfall measured at the NRWWTP site has averaged 1,067 mm (42 in) per year since the study started in the fall of 1990. The highest monthly rainfall of 287 mm (11.3 in) occurred in June 1995; during dry periods monthly rainfall may be less than 2.5 cm (1 in). The winter and spring monthly precipitation generally falls between 10.2 to 20.4 mm (4 to 8 in). As a general rule, precipitation is evenly distributed through the year, but evapotranspiration exceeds precipitation beginning in late spring and continuing through late fall. The climate is humid subtropical (Koppen Class Cfa; Muller and Oberlander, 1984, Table 8.1, p. 195).

1974–1975 study

The 1974–1975 study (Anderson, 1975) conducted as the NRWWTP facilities were being constructed provides limited background water quality data. Wells were constructed in fields that had been cropped for a number of years as well as in a wooded area. The position of one of the fields used in this study (Field 31) is indicated on Figure 1.

Modified Stiff diagrams of water-quality data from the cropped fields suggest that shallow ground water underlying the upland areas where row crops had been grown with artificial fertilizers had been impacted by downward leaching of nitrate from the artificial fertilizers used. Figure 2 compares the ground-water quality of one of the fields with a nearby forested area. The upper two diagrams are from wells in the forested area, and the lower two are from wells located in the field. Most notable is the higher nitrate concentrations exhibited by the ground water beneath Field 31 when compared with ground water from the forested area. The higher concentrations of sodium and calcium and magnesium are also suggestive of an impact from the artificial fertilizer. Based upon the 1974–1975 work, it was anticipated that application of biosolids from the treatment plant would result in a buildup of NO3-N, as well as possibly other highly soluble chemicals, in the shallow ground water.

1987–1989 study of monitoring data

The ground-water monitoring data collected from 1981 through 1988 were evaluated in relation to the biosolids loading history (King et al., 1989; Welby, 1989). For the two fields in which crops had been grown prior to the beginning of the 1974–1975 study, it was found that the nitrate-nitrogen (NO3-N) and chloride (Cl) concentrations in the ground water had increased cumulatively. Figure 3 records this buildup at the field described by the lower two Stiff diagrams of Figure 2.

Among the observations resulting from this study is that the elapsed time between the last application of biosolids for a given loading event and the beginning of a rise in NO3-N and Cl concentrations in the ground water was on the order of 200 to 300 days. The increases in NO3-N occurred once a minimum mass of NO3-N had been applied over a period of several years. A given loading of biosolids prior to the planting of a crop consists of two or more applications over a period of several weeks. Biosolids loadings in Field 31 averaged 287 kg/acre (631 lbs/acre) of Plant Available Nitrogen (PAN). Figure 4 summarizes 1983–1988 data from Field 102, showing the cumulative application of NO3-N as well as the increase of Cl and NO3-N. A minimum cumulative NO3-N loading over a period of several years seemed required before NO3-N began to increase in the ground water. This minimum mass appears to vary from field to field.

At this point it should be noted that the application rates are based upon the assumption that the biosolids contain 20% PAN. This nitrogen is available to plants and for transport into the subsurface. The assumption made is that the other 80% of the nitrogen is organically bound and unavailable for transport. However, Walther (1989) suggests that as much as 50% of the nitrogen in sewage sludge may leach to ground water.

Because of the infrequency of sampling (semiannual) it was not possible to relate downward migration of NO3-N to the saturated zone to the precipitation pattern at the NRWWTP. However, in a semiquantitative way it was observed that the crops were not absorbing all of the applied NO3-N and that some was escaping to the ground water. The 1974–1975 study (Anderson, 1975) had anticipated this fact; also information from the literature indicates that ground-water contamination by NO3-N could

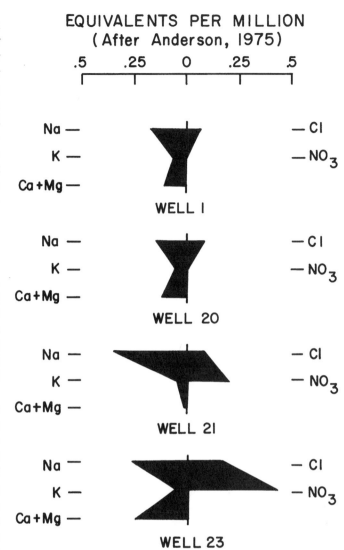

Figure 2. Modified Stiff diagrams after Anderson (1975). Well 1 and Well 20 were located in a forested area; Well 21 and Well 23 were located in a field used for corn and other row crops.

be anticipated with the application of the biosolids (Hall, 1992; Milburn et al., 1990).

The system of monitoring wells that existed at the NRWWTP facility during the 1980s did not allow for construction of water-table maps for estimation of ground-water flow directions. Some of the monitoring wells did not show any NO3-N buildup, and evaluation of their placement suggested that the water-table configuration in the adjacent fields was such that ground-water flow directions were away from the wells. Some of the monitoring wells showing the effects of NO3-N application were at the toe of slopes, and others were in the theoretical recharge areas of their respective fields.

CURRENT (1990–1995) STUDY

The most recent study at the NRWWTP was designed to compare the ground-water quality beneath a field that had been

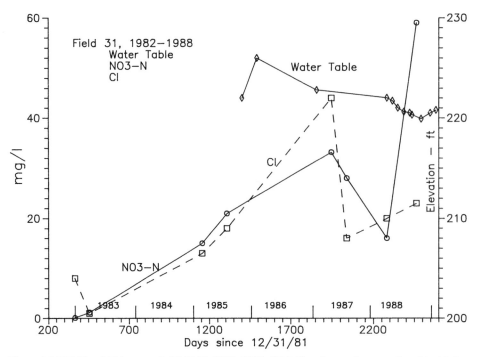

Figure 3. NO3-N and Cl increase in Field 31, 1982–1988. NO3-N = nitrate-nitrogen; Cl = chloride ion.

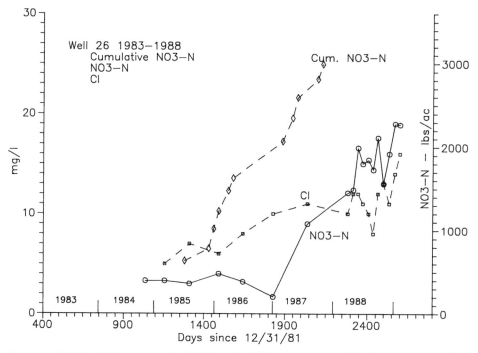

Figure 4. NO3-N and Cl increase in Field 102, 1983–1988 and cumulative NO3-N application. NO3-N = nitrate-nitrogen; Cl = Chloride ion.

used for biosolids disposal since 1981 (Field 102) and one that was to come on line in the fall of 1990 (Field 602). Each field slopes toward a stream along its lower edge, and Field 102 has an irrigation/fishing pond adjacent to its western edge (Fig. 5).

Monitoring wells were installed within the fields and along their downslope edges. In Field 102 a monitoring well installed

shortly after the field was first used was incorporated into the monitoring scheme for the latest study (Well 26).

Monitoring well locations

Figure 6 illustrates the location of the monitoring wells and typical water table configurations for the two fields. Monitoring well stations constructed in 1990 consisted of one well with a 1.53 m (5 ft) screen set a foot or so below the ambient water table and a second well with a 0.6 m (2 ft) screen placed approximately 3.05 m (10 ft) below the base of the first well. Two state-mandated wells at Field 602 that were constructed prior to commencement of the study have 3.05-m (10-ft) screens, and one well within Field 602 was constructed with a 3.05-m (10-ft) screen.

A series of shallow monitoring wells with 0.31 m (1 ft) screens were installed at Field 602 adjacent to the small stream at its lower edge. Some were installed along the upper edge of the flood plain, and others were installed above the flood plain (Fig. 6B, P Wells). These wells have proved useful in supplying information about baseflow to the stream and insight into probable baseflow transport of biosolids-derived NO3-N to the stream. A series of shallow piezometers were also installed in the stream bed (W wells; Fig. 6B) to assess baseflow and possible head differences beneath the stream bed and within the flood plain of the stream.

Sampling procedures

The monitoring wells were sampled by bailing. Preparation for sampling consisted of bailing a well dry, or in those cases where a well could not be bailed dry, a volume of water equivalent to two volumes of the water column was removed. The wells were then allowed to recover for approximately 24 hours prior to sampling. Field measurements consisting of water level, specific conductivity, temperature, and pH were made at the time of sampling. Samples were returned to the Water Quality Laboratory at the NRWWTP for analysis.

Background water quality

Background water quality data collected in the fall of 1990 at Field 602 show that the ground water had average NO3-N concentrations of 4.1 mg/l and Cl concentrations of 3.3 mg/l, respectively. By way of contrast, the state-mandated well with a 3.05 m (10 ft) screen upgradient from Field 602 (Well 31) had NO3-N and Cl concentrations of 2.91 and 6.3 mg/l, respectively. The background well from the 1987–1989 study, located near the NRWWTP office complex exhibited an average of 5.7 mg/l NO3-N and 11.9 mg/l Cl from 17 analyses made between October 1987 and February 1988.

The background NO3-N and Cl concentrations for the deeper portions of the saturated zone were less than for the portions nearer the water table. With the application of the biosolids and the passage of time the NO3-N and Cl concentrations in Field 602 began to increase in the wells located near the center of the field (Well 32; Fig. 6B). The nonparametric Cox-Stuart test (Conover, 1970) was used to test for trends of increasing NO3-N and Cl concentrations. This test demonstrated presence of an increase in both chemical parameters within about two years time following initial biosolids application. Wells located at the lower edge of the field and along the side of the field did not show the

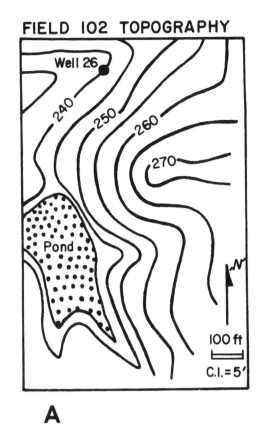

FIELD 102 TOPOGRAPHY

A

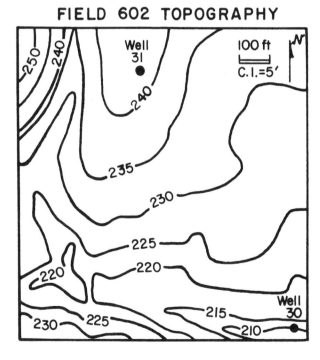

FIELD 602 TOPOGRAPHY

B

Figure 5. Topography of, A, Field 102; and B, Field 602.

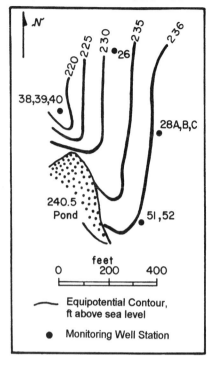

NRWWTP FIELD 102
NOV. 15, 1993
EQUIPOTENTIAL SURFACE

A

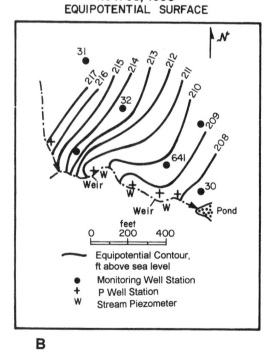

NRWWTP FIELD 602
NOV. 08, 1993
EQUIPOTENTIAL SURFACE

B

Figure 6. Water-table configuration and monitoring well locations: A, Field 102; and B, Field 602. NRWWTP = Neuse River Waste Water Treatment plant.

same systematic buildup of NO3-N that was exhibited by the wells near the center of the field until late 1994 when the wells located at the southwest corner of the field began to exhibit a slight upward trend in the NO3-N concentrations. However, the NO3-N concentrations still remained below the drinking water standard of 10 mg/l NO3-N.

Field 102

Water-quality data from Field 102 record what are considered to be elevated concentrations of NO3-N in the wells located at the top of the hill (Figs. 5A, 6A). Wells constructed later and located midway down the slope also show elevated NO3-N concentrations (e.g., Well 51). On the other hand, wells located at what was thought to be in a down-gradient position exhibit comparatively low concentrations of NO3-N (Table 1). Well 26, used in the 1987–1989 study as well as the current study (Fig. 6A), provides evidence for NO3-N pollution of the shallow ground water. Nitrate-nitrogen concentrations in 1984 were less than 5 mg/l, and by 1994 they had reached over 20 mg/l in Well 26 (Table 1; Fig. 4).

The data from Field 102 also record the fact that the NO3-N, and to a lesser extent the Cl, has migrated downward toward the underlying bedrock. Wells 28B and 52 are completed in the weathered zone immediately above the granitic bedrock (Table 1; Fig. 6A).

Time-series study

Time-series plots of NO3-N and Cl provide insight into the behavior of these two chemicals with respect to potential ground-water contamination. For Field 602 the shallower wells exhibit increases in NO3-N during the study period. Timing of precipitation also plays a role in the NO3-N movement. Figure 7 shows the approximate parallelism of a well hydrograph and the increasing and decreasing values of NO3-N in the shallow ground water. Curve-fitting, both linear and polynomial, as well as the Cox-Stuart test (Conover, 1970) indicate an overall increase of NO3-N with time. Comparison of the biosolids application cumulative curve with the NO3-N and Cl plots suggests that the NO3-N begins to appear in the ground water four to five months after biosolids application. Precise timing is probably controlled by cropping practices and the relation between the

TABLE 1. FIELD 102 NITRATE-NITROGEN

	26	28B	28C	38	39	40	51	52
				Well				
1980 Average of Four Analyses = Background								
NO3-N (mg/l)	20.2	18.1	31.2	0.34	0.063	0.36	....	....
Cl (mg/l)	14	8.8	10.9	2.1	4.3	3.8	....	....
Fall 1993								
NO3-N (mg/l)	19.5	36.0	38.4	0.29	....	0.66	45.4	30.8
Cl (mg/l)	15	64.0	18.5	4.8	....	5.0	11.3	9.5

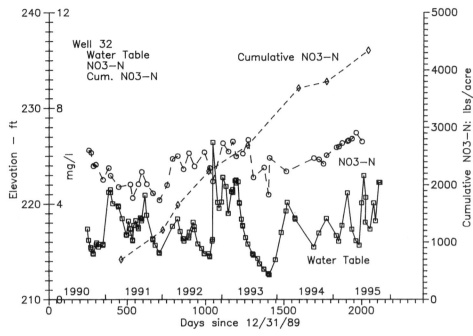

Figure 7. Pattern of NO3-N increase in Well 32, Field 602. NO3-N = nitrate-nitrogen.

time of biosolids application, occurrence of precipitation, and the ground-water recharge pattern (Otomo and Kuboi, 1988).

Stable isotope studies

The stable isotopes of nitrogen, N^{14} and N^{15}, provide a means of identifying sources of NO3-N. *Del* N^{15} values exceeding +10‰ point to sewage-derived biosolids as a source of the NO3-N (Kreitler, 1975, 1979; Gormly and Spalding, 1979). Samples from Field 102 show clearly that the ground water has been impacted by the biosolids application with *del* N^{15} values exceeding +10‰ (Table 2).

In the case of Field 602 the picture is not so clear. The *del* N^{15} values for the wells within the field are less than +10‰ (Wells 32, 33, 641). However, in the case of Well 642 with its 0.61-m (2-ft) screen placed at the water table the *del* N^{15} value is +9.5‰. The position of the screen taken together with the *del* N^{15} value probably indicates that biosolids-derived NO3-N has reached the uppermost part of the saturated zone at this location. Its companion well (Well 641) with a 6.1-m (10-ft) screen placed 1.53 to 4.58 m (5 to 15 ft) below the water table, has a *del* N^{15} value of +3‰ in a 1993 analysis. Only in late 1994 did the NO3-N concentrations in this well begin to increase. The deeper wells in Field 602 provide *del* N^{15} values consistent with natural or artificial fertilizer sources of NO3-N. For comparison, *del* N^{15} values for two fields to which only artificial fertilizer has been applied in recent years are also given in Table 2.

The several shallow monitoring wells along the creek at the base of the slope in Field 602 (Fig. 6B) include one pair of wells in which the *del* N^{15} values indicate a biosolids impact on the ground water. These wells were constructed to monitor baseflow

to the stream. The water table configuration in Field 602 is illustrated in Figure 8 along with the probable direction of ground-water flow to the stream. Comparison of this figure with Figure 6B brings out the nature of the water table configuration variability and possible time-related variations in flow directions beneath Field 602.

The elevated *del* N^{15} values found in wells P1 and P2 (Table 2; Fig. 6B) together with the *del* N^{15} values found in Well 642 suggest that the NO3-N contamination in the case of this field is moving through the uppermost part of the saturated zone. The screen of P1 is set 0.46 m (1.5 ft) below that of P2, which samples the uppermost 0.31-m (1-ft) interval of the water table. These data indicate that the biosolids-derived NO3-N apparently has not yet moved extensively downward toward the underlying bedrock in Field 602. Yet at the toe of the slope in Field 602 the contamination has reached at least 1.22 m (4 ft) below the water table (Table 2). This relationship is in contrast to the situation in Field 102 where relatively high concentrations of NO3-N extend downward more than 6.1 m (20 ft).

Three water samples collected from within the stream and the stream bed for stable isotope analyses provided evidence that biosolids-derived NO3-N is reaching the stream. The actual NO3-N concentration of stream water derived from baseflow in the summer of 1995 ranged from 4.2 to 6.5 mg/l. These concentrations are lower than those found in samples from wells P1 and P2, which are located approximately 6.1 m (20 ft) laterally from the stream (Fig. 8). Yet the *del* N^{15} values of two samples from the stream water were +11.2 and +11.4‰, respectively. Whether the total NO3-N value was affected by dilution from upstream water with lower NO3-N or whether the NO3-N value is affected by denitrification cannot be determined with the evidence at hand.

TABLE 2. ISOTOPE RESULTS

Well	Screen Midpoint- ft below surface	NO3-N (mg/l)	Del-N15 (‰)
Field 102			
28B	52.6	45	+11.2
28C	39.8	56	+10.8
51	26.5	54	+12.3
52	33.0	36	+11.0
Field 602			
32	24.5	5.0	+ 3.2
33	34.0	5.6	+ 3.2
36	21.0	3.4	+ 3.3
641	25.0	4.2	+ 3.0
		4.2	+ 2.5
642	13.0	3.4	+ 9.5
P-1	5.7	8.1	+10.8
P-2	7.0		+15.6
Other Fields (No biosolids applied)			
64A	33.0	3.8	+ 3.3
R2	27.0	13	+ 4.5
29	32.0	6.4	+ 6.7

Biosolids loading

Theoretically, for ground-water protection at least, some optimal pattern of biosolids loading of the fields should exist. This pattern should include the total mass of the NO3-N that is available for plant uptake and the frequency of biosolids application. The frequency is controlled in large measure by the nature of the crops grown on the land and the demand for biosolids disposal arising from the treatment of Raleigh's sewage. Thus it is necessary to look to the mass of biosolids applied to a field between crops to understand the potential for downward migration of NO3-N.

Since the fall of 1990 biosolids have been applied to Field 602 in five application and cropping cycles. The average of these loadings has been 245 kg (538 lbs) of plant available nitrogen (PAN)/acre, or an average of 3,056 kg (6,724 lbs) PAN on the 12.5-acre field. As noted earlier, these values assume that the biosolids contain 20% PAN and that the rest of the nitrogen is bound organically and is thus unavailable to the plants or for conversion to NO3-N. A similar relationship exists for Field 102 where seven cycles of crops and biosolids have occurred during the current study. The average loading has been 233 kg (512 lbs) PAN/acre or a total of 2,792 kg (6,144 lbs) PAN for the field per application. It appears from the increase in NO3-N in the ground water that this loading is in excess of what the plants use. It is also possible that the PAN exceeds 20% or that the organically bound nitrogen is freed by soil processes, becoming available for conversion to nitrate. The approximate parallelism of the well hydrographs and the pattern of increase and decrease of NO3-N concentrations in the ground water (Fig. 7) suggests that the timing of the biosolids applications may be critical.

Estimates made from the data used in the 1989 study indicate

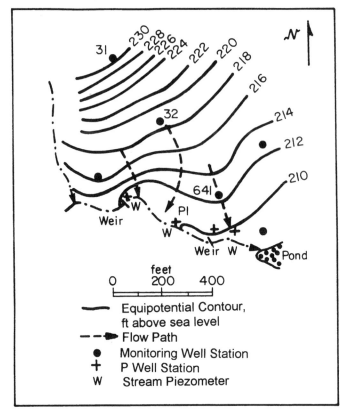

NRWWTP FIELD 602
NOV. 08, 1994
EQUIPOTENTIAL SURFACE

Figure 8. Field 602, November 8, 1994, equipotential surface and flow lines. NRWWTP = Neuse River Waste Water Treatment Plant.

that it may take from 200 to 300 days for the effects of the biosolids application to be recognized in the ground-water quality data. The post-1990 data suggest a lag of from 3 to 4 months between the peak of the well hydrographs and the appearance of an upward trend in the NO3-N content of the ground water (Fig. 7).

If application occurs late in the fall and early winter at the beginning or during the period of ground-water recharge, the NO3-N can be mobilized and move downward. As a case in point, Herbel and Spalding (1993) concluded that nitrate in fertility plots moved downward in response to percolation caused by irregularly spaced heavy spring rains on fallow fields. If nitrate is applied closer to the time that the crops are utilizing the nitrogen and when evapotranspiration limits downward flux of infiltrating precipitation, then less of the PAN has the opportunity to move downward. On the other hand, PAN not used as well as nitrogen freed from the organic matter has the opportunity to become nitrate and to migrate downward during times of ground-water recharge (Walther, 1989).

Resting of fields

Within the literature discussing the impact of biosolids application and cropping on ground-water quality there is evidence that the resting of a field may permit denitrification within the saturated zone (Higgins, 1984). In both Field 102 and Field 602 the dissolved oxygen content of the ground water drops below 10 mg/l, and conditions are apparently conducive to denitrification. However, the buildup of NO3-N in the shallow ground water beneath Field 102 to depths of 6.1 m (20 ft) or more indicate that denitrification processes present are inadequate to eliminate totally the nitrate available for transport to the saturated zone. A study in New Jersey (Higgins, 1984) noted that 15 to 18 months elapsed before NO3-N concentration began dropping toward background values.

From detailed evaluation of the NO3-N time-series curves for Field 102 and Field 602 it appears that the NO3-N concentrations in the ground water decrease after reaching a peak following a biosolids application event. The concentrations then rise again after a new application of biosolids. The drop of the NO3-N concentrations appears to take place during times less favorable for ground-water recharge (Fig. 7). The total amount of NO3-N that has accumulated in the vadose zone over a period of years may be the ultimate control on when ground-water concentrations of NO3-N may start to decrease following cessation of biosolids application. In essence, a reservoir of NO3-N accumulates while a field is being cropped and biosolids applied. With cessation of biosolids application it takes time for the reservoir to be depleted, and downward movement of NO3-N can be expected to continue until the NO3-N reservoir is depleted by migration and denitrification.

Comparison of water quality

Table 3 lists the NO3-N background data for the shallow ground water beneath Field 102, Field 602, and Field 61A. The latter field has been used to study the migration of NO3-N from artificial fertilizers to the shallow ground water. For comparison purposes, the NO3-N concentrations found in the drinking water of the City of Raleigh, the effluent discharged to the Neuse River, and selected water wells in Wake County (May and Thomas, 1968) are listed in Table 4.

The background water quality in Field 602 and Field 61A probably reflects their long use for row crops and use of artificial fertilizer; the elevated NO3-N content of the ground water beneath Field 102 appears to reflect approximately eight years of biosolids application. The nitrate content of the finished Raleigh drinking water is very low. The median value of ground-water NO3-N from the Raleigh area reflects the high nitrate content of ground water derived from some wells in the Triassic sedimentary rocks where the ground water may be highly mineralized. In general, however, the NO3-N levels of water from the crystalline rocks is low.

Baseflow contributions of NO3-N

Two V-notch weirs installed at opposite ends of a 122-m (400-ft) stretch of the stream at Field 602 provided data on baseflow contributions to the stream. Ground-water seepage into the

TABLE 3. BACKGROUND CONCENTRATIONS NO3-N, 1990

Well		NO3-N (mg/l)
Average of First Four Analyses		
Field 102		
28C		31.2
28B		18.1
38		0.34
51		45.4
52		11.3
Field 602		
31	Background Well	2.9
32		5.9
33		5.3
34		8.9
36		3.2
37		1.9
Field 61A		
62		4.0
64		3.3

TABLE 4. COMPARISON OF WATER QUALITY

	NO3-N (mg/l)
Raleigh Raw Water (Falls Lake/Neuse River)	0.3
Raleigh Finished Water	<0.1–0.48
Raleigh Waste Water Treatment Plant Effluent	±13
Water Wells (after May and Thomas, 1968)	
Median value	0.81
Hornblende Gneiss	0.02
Mica Gneiss	3.8

stream was observed along the 122-m (400-ft) stretch early in the investigation. Flow measurements during low-flow stages of the stream indicated an average baseflow of 8.21 E-4 cu m/sec (0.029 cfs) from measurements made during a 2-yr period. If the average NO3-N concentration in the baseflow falls between the average values of 2.9 and 5.9 mg/l found in wells P1 and P2, then the NO3-N contributions from baseflow along the 122-m (400-ft) stream reach is between 1,640 and 3,440 mg/l/d/m of stream (500 and 1,050 mg/l/d/ft).

CONCLUSIONS AND COMMENTS

It is apparent that at the loading rates used on the NRWWTP facility acreage there has been NO3-N pollution of the shallow ground water. In the field used since 1980 nitrate has migrated down to the vicinity of the bedrock at depths of 9.2 to 15.3 m (30 to 50 ft). In Field 602 the downward migration of the NO3-N is apparent in the time-series plots of NO3-N for some of the wells and is clearly documented in at least one well (Well 642) in addition to wells placed along the lower edge of the field. It can be anticipated that if biosolids loading of Field 602 continues as in the past that a pattern of increased NO3-N pollution will appear beneath the field. Some of the nitrate moves in shallow ground-water flow toward streams adjacent to the fields.

Baseflow measurements in the stream at Field 602 combined with knowledge of the NO3-N concentrations in the shallow ground water adjacent to the stream provide a basis for estimating NO3-N contributions to surface water. It appears that at those times when the stream is being fed by baseflow along the 122 m (400 ft) between weirs that between 1 to 3 kg of NO3-N per day per meter of stream length may be provided to the surface waters.

It is also evident that past, and probably current, NO3-N application rates are higher than the plants can absorb or remove from the soil. In addition, application of the biosolids immediately before or during the recharge season permits NO3-N to move downward to the water table. Whether the excess of the NO3-N can be attributed to an underestimation of the amount of plant available nitrogen (PAN) or simply to an overloading of the biosolids onto the fields has not been determined at this time. In any event, the present study of the NRWWTP biosolids application and cropping program points to the necessity of examining the loading rates and assumed plant availability of the nitrogen along with the cropping pattern and the local water budget. Consideration should be given to the best way of meshing these four factors so that migration of the NO3-N to the shallow ground water is minimized.

Factors that also need to be considered in evaluating the necessity of a land application system for disposing of the biosolids include the question of surface water quality and cost of disposal. The number of acres available for application are a factor in determining the loading rate. The City of Raleigh has about 1,600 acres available through ownership or lease. One must also consider whether or not the ground water is apt to be used as a drinking water source of any importance at some time in the future. Thus we have the question of cost for additional acreage over and above that required by normal urban growth versus the risk to public health from nitrate contamination of the ground water versus the cost of additional treatment to remove the NO3-N from the biosolids.

The work done so far at the NRWWTP indicates that in the southeastern Piedmont Province the nitrate from biosolids cannot be completely removed by cropping or by denitrification in the vadose zone. Some NO3-N pollution of the ground water must be anticipated if land disposal of biosolids by municipalities is to be used. The extent to which the NO3-N may reach into the fractures of the underlying crystalline rocks is an as yet unanswered question. However, given the hydrology of the piedmont in general and the fact that the saprolite serves as a reservoir for the ground water in the bedrock, water withdrawal from the fractured bedrock can be anticipated to cause nitrate-rich water to move downward into the fractures and eventually to water supply wells. The hazards and risks are site specific.

Those concerned with ground-water quality must also recognize that there is some indication that given enough time ground water polluted with significant levels of NO3-N will eventually recover through denitrification once the source of NO3-N is no longer available. A reasonable way of handling the situation would seem to be to zone an area where biosolids are to be applied so that ground water will not be a factor in utilization of the land. The most obvious way to handle the problem is to zone the land to an agricultural use alone and to allow sufficient time for denitrification and dilution to occur before uses dependent upon ground water with less than 10 mg/l nitrogen are placed on the land at some future time. Other approaches to the water supply are also possible if a decision should be made to utilize another method of sewage treatment that does not require land disposal of the biosolids, thus freeing the land for uses other than agricultural.

ACKNOWLEDGMENTS

Financial support of this study came from the City of Raleigh, North Carolina, through grants made to the University of North Carolina Water Resources Institute. Chemical analyses were carried out in the Water Quality Laboratory at the City of Raleigh's Neuse River Waste Water Treatment Plant (NRWWTP) under the direction of Thomas Smith. City of Raleigh personnel who contributed to the study in one way or another include Carl Simmons and Dale Crisp, director and assistant director of public utilities, respectively; Billy Ray Creech and John Kivineimi, superintendents at the NRWWTP during the period of the study; and Ahktar Paktiwal, soil scientist at the NRWWTP. Numerous students from the Department of Marine, Earth, and Atmospheric Sciences, North Carolina State University, helped at one time or another with well installation, data collection, and data analysis. Robert Holman, associate director of the University of North Carolina Water Resources Research Institute, served as a sounding board for ideas. The author gratefully acknowledges the contributions others have made.

REFERENCES CITED

Anderson, M. B., 1975, The hydrogeology of the Neuse Wastewater Treatment site [M.S. thesis]: Raleigh, North Carolina State University, 83 p., plus maps.

Conover, W. J., 1970, Practical nonparametric statistics: New York, John Wiley and Sons Inc., 462 p.

Gerhart, J. A., 1986, Ground-water recharge and its effects on nitrate concentration beneath a manured field site in Pennsylvania: Ground Water, v. 24, p. 483–489.

Gormly, J. R., and Spalding, R. F., 1979, Sources and concentrations of nitrate-nitrogen in ground water of the Central Platte region, Nebraska: Ground Water, v. 17, p. 291–301.

Hall, D., 1992, Effects of nutrient management on nitrate levels in ground water near Ephrata, Pennsylvania: Ground Water, v. 30, p. 720–730.

Herbal, M. G., and Spalding, R. F., 1993, Vadose zone fertilizer-derived nitrate and $\delta^{15}N$ extracts: Ground Water, v. 31, p. 376–382.

Higgins, A. J., 1984, Impacts on ground water due to land application of sewage sludge: Water Resources Bulletin, v. 20, p. 425–434.

King, L. D., Welby, C. W., Safley, L. M., Hoover, M., Heath, R., and Borden, R., 1989, Evaluation of land application of sewage sludge at the Neuse River Wastewater Treatment Plant, Raleigh, North Carolina, Vol. 1: North Carolina State University, Raleigh, University of North Carolina Water Resources Institute, unpaged.

Kreitler, C. W., 1975, Determining the source of nitrate in ground water by nitrogen isotope studies: University of Texas Austin, Texas Bureau of Economic Geology Report of Investigations 83, 57 p.

Kreitler, C. W., 1979, Nitrogen-isotope ratio studies of soils and ground water nitrate from alluvial fan aquifers in Texas: Journal of Hydrology, v. 42, p. 147–170.

May, V. J., and Thomas, J. D., 1968, Geology and ground-water resources in the Raleigh area, North Carolina: North Carolina Department of Water Resources Ground Water Bulletin 15, 135 p.

Milburn, P., Richards, J. E., Gartley, C., Pollock, T., O'Neil, H., and Bailey, H., 1990, Nitrate leaching from systematically tiled potato fields in New Brunswick, Canada: Journal of Environmental Quality, v. 19, p. 448–454.

Muller, R. A., and Oberlander, T. M., 1984, Physical geography today: New York, Random House, 591 p.

Otomo, S., and Kuboi, T., 1988, Prediction of time variation in water and chloride profiles in soil subject to cropping and annual application of sewage sludge: Journal of Hydrology, v. 99, p. 1–17.

Parker, J. M., III, 1979, Geology and mineral resources of Wake County: North Carolina Department Natural Resources and Community Development, Geological Survey Division, Bulletin 86, 122 p., plus maps.

Powlson, D. S., Poulton, P., Addiscott, T. M., and McCann, D. S., 1989, Leaching of nitrate from soils receiving organic and inorganic fertilizers continuously for 135 years, *in* Hansen, J. A. A., and Henriksen, K., eds., Nitrogen in organic wastes applied to soils: San Diego, Academic Press, 375 p.

Spalding, R. F., Erner, M. E., Martin, G. E., and Snow, D. D., 1993, Effects of sludge disposal on ground water nitrate concentrations: Journal of Hydrology, v. 142, p. 213–218.

Walther, W., 1989, Nitrate leaching out of soils and their significance for ground water, results of long-term tests, *in* Hansen, J. A. A., and Henriksen, K., eds., Nitrogen in organic wastes applied to soils: San Diego, Academic Press, p. 346–356.

Weil, R. R., Weismiller, R. A., and Turner, R. S., 1990, Nitrate contamination of ground water under irrigated coastal plain soils: Journal of Environmental Quality, v. 19, p. 441–448.

Welby, C. W., 1989, Agriculture to agriculture—History of nitrate in ground water at a sewage sludge site: Association of Engineering Geologists, Abstracts with Program, 32nd Annual Meeting, Vail, Colorado, Oct 1–6, p. 118–119.

MANUSCRIPT ACCEPTED BY THE SOCIETY JUNE 5, 1997

Geological Society of America
Reviews in Engineering Geology, Volume XII
1998

Seismic microzonation in the Pacific Northwest, with an example of earthquake hazard mapping in southwest British Columbia

Victor M. Levson, Patrick A. Monahan, and Daniel G. Meldrum
British Columbia Geological Survey, 1810 Blanshard Street, Victoria, British Columbia V8V 1X4, Canada
Bryan D. Watts, Alex Sy, and Li Yan
Klohn-Crippen Consultants Limited, 10200 Shellbridge Way, Richmond, British Columbia V6X 2W7, Canada

ABSTRACT

Due to a general lack of exposed faults it is difficult to predict the location and timing of future earthquakes in the Pacific Northwest region. Other geologic and geotechnical site conditions that control soil behavior and consequent surface damage can, however, be readily identified. Earthquake-hazard maps that reflect these conditions thus can be used as a predictive tool for seismic policy development and emergency planning. Many seismically prone jurisdictions have not yet implemented earthquake hazard mapping programs, largely reflecting a lack of awareness of the utility of these maps. Demonstrated applications of the maps include identification of geologically vulnerable areas with critical facilities and selection of suitable areas for new facilities, prioritization of seismic upgrading programs, recognition of high hazard areas requiring special study or restricted development, assessment of property insurance, estimation of risk, and establishment of more stringent regulatory requirements where needed.

A pilot program in southwest British Columbia illustrates the methodology used to develop an earthquake-hazard map. Existing and new geotechnical data are integrated with surficial geology mapping in a geographic information system (GIS) format. Liquefaction and ground motion amplification hazards within each geological map unit are assessed both qualitatively and quantitatively.

Probabilistic assessments of liquefaction potential, using ground acceleration data from the National Building Code of Canada, include a measure of the severity of potential surface disruption that in turn is a function of the geotechnical characteristics, thickness, and depth of each liquefiable unit. Potential for ground-motion amplification was estimated by comparison of geological map units with soil classes adopted by the U.S. National Earthquake Hazards Reduction Program. The hazard for each map unit was expressed as a range that reflects observed geological variation. The final hazard map, designed for land use and emergency planning purposes, shows a conservative default to the highest rating of either the liquefaction or amplification hazard.

Levson, V. M., Monahan, P. A., Meldrum, D. G., Watts, B. D., Sy, A., and Yan, L., 1998, Seismic microzonation in the Pacific Northwest, with an example of earthquake hazard mapping in southwest British Columbia, *in* Welby, C. W., and Gowan, M. E., eds., A Paradox of Power: Voices of Warning and Reason in the Geosciences: Boulder, Colorado, Geological Society of America Reviews in Engineering Geology, v. XII.

INTRODUCTION

Earthquake-hazard maps, also referred to as seismic microzonation maps, are detailed (generally 1:20,000 to 1:50,000 scale) maps that identify the relative potential for ground disturbance during an earthquake. In this paper we describe the major types and elements of earthquake hazard maps and discuss their applications. Emphasis is placed on work being conducted in the Pacific Northwest region, extending from northern California to Alaska, and an example of a recent mapping program from southwest British Columbia is used to illustrate the procedures involved.

Earthquake-hazard maps are compiled from geologic and geotechnical data to reflect local site conditions, which, in addition to earthquake source and magnitude, exert a major control on potential ground disruption. Records of historical earthquakes show that damage is largely controlled by mappable site characteristics. Earthquake hazard maps based on site geology, therefore, can be used for mitigative planning in seismically active regions. They are intended for regional purposes such as land use and emergency planning. They do not replace the need for site-specific geotechnical evaluations.

Earthquake-hazard maps can depict any of several hazards including liquefaction, amplification, landslides, tsunamis/seiches, subsidence, and ground rupture. Liquefaction, resulting from loss of strength in loose, saturated, cohesionless soils during an earthquake, is emphasized in this paper because it is one of the most commonly mapped earthquake hazards. It is particularly important in southwest British Columbia where extensive urban development has occurred on soils highly susceptible to liquefaction (Watts, et al. 1992).

Terminology

Earthquake *hazards* refer to the menace or threat imposed by potential earthquakes and associated phenomena (such as ground shaking, liquefaction, and landslides) but they are not related to the amount of adverse consequences. The latter are defined by the earthquake *risk*, which refers to the chance or probability that damage, economic loss, injury, or death will occur as a result of the hazard (Sauter, 1996). Earthquake-hazard maps may show, for example, areas where liquefiable soils are present and result in a greater hazard, compared to areas with nonliquefiable soils. Seismic microzonation is defined as "the process of determining absolute or relative seismic hazard at many sites accounting for the effects of geologic and topographic amplification of motion and of soil stability and liquefaction, for the purpose of delineating seismic microzones" (Earthquake Engineering Research Institute, Committee on Seismic Risk, 1984, p. 39).

Liquefaction-induced ground movement can vary from minor ground settling to large lateral displacements due to flow slides or spreads. Liquefaction *susceptibility* as used here refers to a soil's resistance to liquefaction when subjected to seismic loading. It depends on soil gradation, density, age, and depth to water table but not on regional seismicity. Liquefaction *potential*

is a measure of a soil's propensity to liquefy, and thus it is a function of not only liquefaction susceptibility but also of the seismic activity in the region (Klohn-Crippen Consultants Ltd., 1994). A discussion of liquefaction terminology for engineering applications has been provided by Robertson (1994).

EARTHQUAKE-HAZARD MAPS

Description

Earthquake-hazard maps are based on the local geology and geotechnical characteristics of the ground. They depict the severity of earthquake hazard that is expected in a map unit relative to other units. Although the size and location of future earthquakes are difficult to predict, the behavior of the soil at any one location relative to another can be estimated by evaluating local geologic and geotechnical site conditions. For example, certain types of soils may be susceptible to liquefaction during an earthquake or prone to landsliding whereas others may be relatively stable. Thus, many areas that are susceptible to ground disruption can be identified and quantitatively assessed, even in the absence of data regarding when and where the next earthquake will occur.

Earthquake-hazard maps may include one or more of the earthquake hazards mentioned above, but the most common hazards evaluated are liquefaction, amplification of ground motion, and landslides. Although most earthquake-hazard maps focus only on one hazard type, some mapping programs have integrated several hazards into one map (e.g., Mabey and Madin, 1993; Mabey et al., 1994, 1995; Levson et al., 1996c). Maps of this type are developed to show the relative earthquake hazard in different areas due to variations in local geologic conditions at a city block or neighborhood scale. These maps are often produced for the purposes of providing information that can be used more effectively by land use and emergency planners and the general public.

Methods

Excellent reviews of earthquake hazard mapping methods have been provided by Aki and Irikura (1991), Finn (1991, 1994), Hansen and Franks (1991), the International Society for Soil Mechanics and Foundation Engineering (1993), and Youd (1991). Earthquake hazards can be mapped using a number of different methods, usually reflecting different levels of certainty or degrees of quantification of the data. The amount, quality, and cost of information required for mapping generally increases with increasing levels of certainty (Klohn-Crippen Consultants, Ltd. 1994). For example, liquefaction hazard maps can be grouped into liquefaction susceptibility, liquefaction potential, and liquefaction-induced ground displacement maps (Youd and Perkins, 1978; Youd, 1991; Finn, 1994). Liquefaction susceptibility maps (level 1) are based on surficial geology data such as sediment type, geomorphologic characteristics, relative density, deposit age, water-table depth, and geologic or historical evidence of liquefaction. Deposits most susceptible to liquefaction generally are young, loose, saturated, coarse silt- to sand-sized sediments that occur in areas where the water table is shallow. Gravels may also liquefy under some conditions such as the presence of capping silts or clays of low permeability. Since liquefaction susceptibility is dependent on the physical characteristics of the soil, it does not account for variations in regional seismicity. Liquefaction potential (level 2) maps, however, indicate the probability of liquefaction actually occurring by accounting for the expected intensity of seismic shaking (based, for example, on past records of earthquakes) as well as soil conditions. Liquefaction-induced ground displacement or lateral displacement maps (level 3) can be produced by accounting for ground movement (lateral spreading) on slopes and towards free faces such as a river banks (e.g., Youd and Perkins, 1987; Mabey and Youd, 1991; Bartlett and Youd, 1992; Youd and Jones, 1993). The example mapping project, described below, combined levels 1 and 2 liquefaction assessments.

Applications and limitations

General applications of earthquake-hazard maps to planning include: (1) identification of vulnerable lifeline systems (e.g., water, gas, and power lines); (2) planning transportation and utility corridors; (3) setting priorities for seismic upgrading or remedial work on schools, hospitals, fire halls, and other structures; (4) identifying good sites for new essential facilities (e.g., schools, hospitals, bridges, and toxic waste containment facilities); (5) identifying areas requiring special study or high hazard areas in which development restrictions may be required; (6) evaluating property insurance; (7) assessment of risk for financing new projects; (8) providing information on site effects for design of new structures; and (9) establishing more stringent design requirements where needed. Excellent examples of how earthquake hazard maps can be used for land-use planning and other applications have been presented by the Earthquake Engineering Research Institute (1991; see, for example, Mader, 1991; Power et al., 1991; Kuroiwa and Alva, 1991), the Portland Metro Advisory Committee for Mitigating Earthquake Damage (Metro, 1996), and Geohazards International (Escuela Politécnica Nacional et al., 1994).

Due to the site-specific and facility-specific nature of seismic evaluations and upgrading programs in many jurisdictions, there is potential for duplication, poor regional coverage, and inadequate prioritization of mitigation activities. Large amounts of effort and funds are currently being spent by numerous public agencies in seismic retrofitting and site-specific engineering evaluations, but prioritization of these activities often is not based on geological criteria. The result is that large areas are erroneously considered to have equal susceptibility to disturbance during an earthquake. A better regional understanding of geologic and geotechnical conditions through the production of earthquake hazard maps would alleviate this problem, particularly for land-use and emergency planning purposes. A regional

approach is also more cost effective (Klohn-Crippen Consultants Ltd., 1994).

The evaluation and compilation procedures used to develop earthquake-hazard maps impose several limitations on their applicability. The maps are regional in scope and indicate general areas where earthquake hazards are greatest. The earthquake hazard at any one site, however, may be higher or lower than predicted due to geological variations within map units, gradational map unit boundaries, and the regional scale of these maps. In addition, map-unit boundaries are based on geological criteria and on limited borehole information and, as such, they are approximate and may change with additional data. For these reasons a low hazard rating cannot be interpreted as freedom from the earthquake hazards mapped at any specific locality. Site-specific geotechnical investigations, therefore, should be performed to evaluate the hazard rating for individual sites, particularly near zone boundaries. Furthermore, a low hazard rating does not mean that ground shaking will not occur, but rather that the hazard due to ground shaking is expected to be less than in areas with a higher hazard rating.

Earthquake-hazard maps can be used to estimate the relative hazard due to geological controls, but they can not be used solely to predict the amount of damage that will occur because many other factors such as building design, for example, must be considered. Likewise, earthquake-hazard maps can not be used to estimate risk, as this is dependent on many other factors such as the number of people present in the area at any one time and the types of facilities that are there. For example, although the earthquake hazard may be high in a farmer's field, the risk of damage is obviously low, compared to the same level of hazard in a developed area of a city.

Examples

Earthquake-hazard mapping has been completed and successfully applied in numerous parts of the United States including California (Youd et al., 1975, 1978; Nilson and Brabb, 1979; Dupré and Tinsley, 1980; Power et al., 1982, 1986; Kavazanjian et al., 1985; Wieczorek et al., 1985; Tinsley et al., 1985; Youd and Perkins, 1987; Dupré, 1990; Leighton and Associates; 1990; Sanchez et al., 1991), Utah (Mabey and Youd, 1989; Anderson et al., 1994a, b, c, d, e), central Mississippi valley (Obermeier, 1984, 1988), Missouri (Higgins and Rockaway, 1986), Tennessee (Sharma and Kovacs, 1980), South Carolina (Elton and Hadj-Hamou, 1990), New York (Budhu et al., 1987), and Alaska (Combellick, 1984). More generalized earthquake-hazard maps, showing areas of higher and lower potential for liquefaction or enhanced ground shaking, are currently being produced for California and for states that fall within the New Madrid seismic zone (DuMontelle, 1995).

Of particular relevance to the Pacific Northwest is recent mapping in the Seattle–Tacoma region in Washington State (Grant et al., 1991; Grant and Perkins, 1993; Palmer et al., 1994, 1995; Dragovich and Pringle, 1995), in the Portland, Oregon–Vancouver,

Washington, region (Madin, 1990; Mabey and Madin, 1993; Youd and Jones, 1993; Mabey et al., 1994, 1995), in Salem, Oregon (Wang and Leonard, 1996), and in Greater Vancouver (Watts et al., 1992; British Columbia Hydro and Power Authority, 1992) and Chilliwack (Levson et al., 1995, 1996a, 1996c, 1997), British Columbia. Also of relevance in British Columbia are paleoseismic and geological studies by Clague et al. (1992), Hunter et al. (1992), and Luternauer et al. (1993, 1994). Earthquake-hazard maps have also been produced in many other countries throughout the world including Japan (Ishihara and Ogawa, 1978; Kotoda et al., 1988; Kusano et al., 1989; Ishihara and Yasuda, 1991; Wakamatsu, 1992), Indonesia (Thenhaus et al., 1993), Greece (Pitilakis et al., 1982; Pitilakis, 1995), Italy (Marcellini et al., 1991), Puerto Rico (Soto, 1987), Yugoslavia (Talaganov and Aleksovski, 1984), Algeria (Power et al., 1991), China (Fang et al., 1980), Peru (Kuroiwa and Alva, 1991), and Argentina (INPRES, 1982, 1987). Numerous other case study examples of earthquake-hazard mapping have been provided by the Earthquake Engineering Research Institute (1991) and by the International Society for Soil Mechanics and Foundation Engineering (1993).

EARTHQUAKES AND EARTHQUAKE-HAZARD MAPPING IN THE PACIFIC NORTHWEST

The Pacific Northwest region of North America is a seismically active area subject to crustal, subcrustal, and great subduction earthquakes (Shedlock and Weaver, 1991; Rogers, 1992, 1994; Atwater et al., 1995). One of the world's largest earthquakes was a subduction zone event that occurred along the Aleutian subduction zone in southern Alaska in 1964. The largest historic earthquake in Canada (M 8.1) occurred in 1949 near the Queen Charlotte Islands. The most destructive in western Canada occurred in 1946 near Courtenay, on Vancouver Island (M 7.3). The largest earthquake in the Puget Sound region was the 1949 Olympia earthquake (M 7.1). Although these and other large damaging earthquakes in the region occurred in historic times, most were prior to extensive urban development. One of the most recent earthquakes in the area occurred more than 30 years ago in the Seattle–Tacoma area in 1965, and caused $12 to $50 million in damage. The recently estimated potential economic impact of a similar (M 6.5) earthquake on the Lower Mainland in British Columbia was $14.3 to $32.1 billion (Munich Reinsurance Company of Canada, 1992).

Earthquakes in the Pacific Northwest region are controlled largely by tectonic processes along offshore subduction zones. Unlike southern California, these processes are seldom reflected in surface faults on land, making it especially difficult to predict the location and timing of future earthquakes. However, since variations in soil behavior and consequent surface damage are largely controlled by other mappable geologic and geotechnical site conditions, earthquake-hazard maps can be effectively used as a predictive tool for emergency and land-use planning in this region. As a result, earthquake hazard mapping programs are currently being conducted by government geological surveys in

Washington, Oregon, and British Columbia (Madin, 1990; Mabey and Madin, 1993; Youd and Jones, 1993; Palmer et al., 1994, 1995; Mabey et al., 1994, 1995; Dragovich and Pringle, 1995; Levson et al., 1995, 1996a, c; Wang and Leonard, 1996). In general, planning departments in large cities are well advanced in their use of this earthquake hazard mapping information for land use and emergency planning (e.g. City of Seattle, 1992; Metro, 1993, 1996).

A CASE-STUDY EXAMPLE OF EARTHQUAKE-HAZARD MAPPING IN SOUTHWESTERN BRITISH COLUMBIA

A pilot earthquake hazard mapping program was conducted by the British Columbia Geological Survey in 1995 in the Chilliwack region (Levson et al., 1995, 1996a). The project area included the entire Chilliwack District and parts of the Fraser Valley Regional District (contained within National Topographic System map sheets 92 G/1E and H/4W, south of the Fraser River and north of 49° 3′ N lat.). The area mapped covers nearly 30,000 ha and is located approximately 100 km east of Vancouver.

Methodology

The methodology used included the following: (1) collection of existing data from more than 1,700 geotechnical test holes from 390 locations (Fig. 1), including approximately 250 standard penetration tests, 50 cone penetration tests, 200 dynamic cone penetration tests, and 60 Becker penetration tests, as well as 700 water wells; shear-wave data were available for only a few sites (for a description of the sources and types of data collected see Levson et al., 1996a); (2) surficial geology mapping at a scale of 1:20,000 focusing on the Fraser River valley lowland and Ryder Lake upland area (Fig. 2; Levson et al., 1996b; data collected for each map unit included: type of sediment, age, genesis, grain-size characteristics, thickness, subsurface stratigraphy, and hydrogeologic and geotechnical properties); (3) collection of new, high-quality, geotechnical data at sites selected to fill gaps in the existing database, including seismic cone penetration tests (SCPT) at eight sites (Fig. 3) and spectral analysis of surface waves (SASW) and Becker penetration tests at gravel-rich sites; (4) input of surficial geology and geotechnical data, representing a wide geographic distribution and reflecting the geological and geotechnical variations of the area, into a geographic information system (GIS; Fig. 4; Meldrum et al., 1997); (5) development of a three-dimensional geologic model for the area; (6) integration of surficial geology, geotechnical borehole data, and geophysical information, to compile a Quaternary geology map that reflects sedimentary facies in the upper 20 m of the section (Monahan and Levson, 1997); (7) qualitative evaluation of liquefaction susceptibility within each map unit; (8) quantitative evaluation of liquefaction potential at specific sites within the map area with good quality geotechnical data; (9) integration of liquefaction susceptibility and liquefaction potential assessments to produce the final

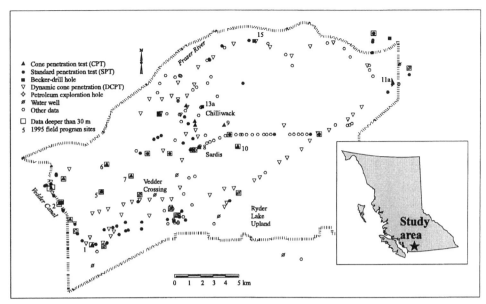

Figure 1. Distribution and type of geotechnical borehole data collected for the study area.

liquefaction hazard map (Fig. 5; Levson et al., 1997); (10) an assessment of ground motion amplification hazards (Monahan et al., 1997); and (11) development of a combined liquefaction and amplification hazard map (Levson et al., 1996c). The methods used generally follow those recommended by the Seismic Microzonation Task Group (Klohn-Crippen Consultants Ltd., 1994).

Liquefaction susceptibility

Since the susceptibility of a soil to liquefaction is dependent on geologic parameters such as grain-size distribution, density, deposit age, and water-table depth, a first approximation of the liquefaction hazard for this area was made by an analysis of the surficial geology. The first step in the production of a liquefaction susceptibility map was the integration of surficial geology data with geotechnical borehole data and other subsurface data such as water-well logs. Three-dimensional geologic models of the area and a Quaternary geology map representing the upper 20 m of the surficial geology (Monahan and Levson, 1997) were constructed from this information. Liquefaction susceptibility of each unit on the Quaternary geology map was then estimated based on correlations between surficial geology and liquefaction (Youd and Perkins, 1978), with local modifications introduced for the Lower Mainland (Watts et al., 1992) and Chilliwack (Levson et al., 1995, 1996a) areas. Table 1 is a summary of the estimated liquefaction susceptibility of the main types of surficial geologic deposits in the area.

Probabilistic assessment of liquefaction potential and severity

Liquefaction potential was estimated for different map units using a modified version of PROLIQ2 (Atkinson et al., 1986), originally developed by Klohn-Crippen Consultants Ltd. and the University of British Columbia. The program combines a SPT-based method of liquefaction assessment (Seed, 1979; Seed and Idriss, 1982), with a probabilistic method of evaluating the seismic hazard (Cornell, 1968). The probability of liquefaction occurring in a 50-year period at specified depths at a given site was calculated for 69 test holes at 27 different sites. Of these test holes, 58 were standard penetration tests at mud rotary drill-hole sites, and 11 were cone-penetration tests. The assessment was based on the National Building Code of Canada (NBCC) seismic model with the mean attenuation curve of Hasegawa et al. (1981) and the ground amplification chart of Idriss (1991).

The PROLIQ2 computer model generates the probability of liquefaction occurring at specific depths at a given site, but it does not provide a measure of liquefaction-induced damage potential, which is a more useful parameter for regional hazard mapping and land-use planning purposes. A measure of damage potential should include not only the probability of liquefaction occurring but also the thickness and depth of the liquefiable zones. In a liquefaction event the severity of surface disruption is a function of the depth and thickness of each liquefiable unit, with shallow liquefaction causing more ground disruption and potential structural damage than liquefaction at greater depths. To account for this, the concept of Probability of Liquefaction Severity (PLS) was introduced by Klohn-Crippen Consultants Ltd. PLS (formerly referred to as LHI, Levson et al., 1996c) is a weighted average of probabilities determined for each layer of sediment to a depth of 20 m. PLS is determined by the following equation:

$$PLS = \frac{\sum(W_iH_iPl_i)}{\sum(W_iH_i)}$$

where Pl_i is the probability of liquefaction at depth i (expressed as a percentage), H_i is the layer thickness, and W_i is the value of a

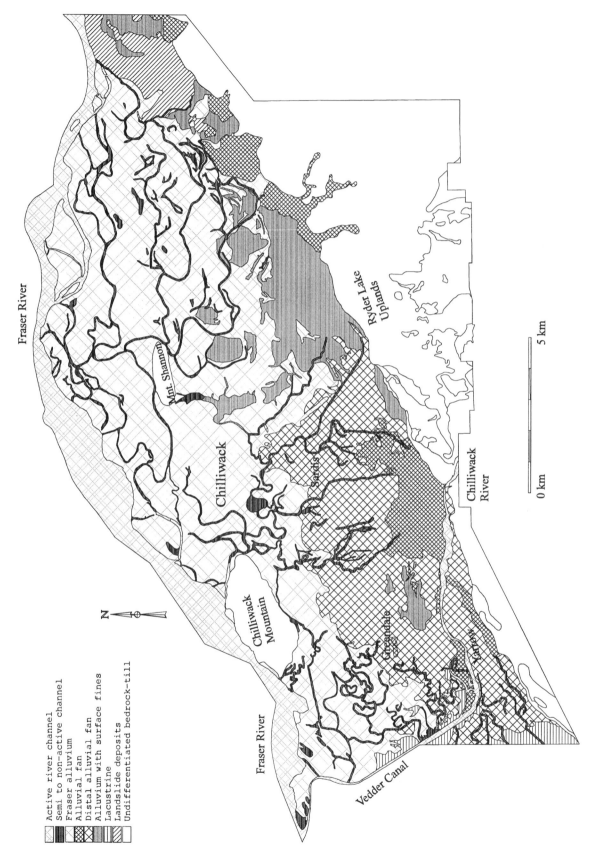

Figure 2. Generalized surficial geology of the study area.

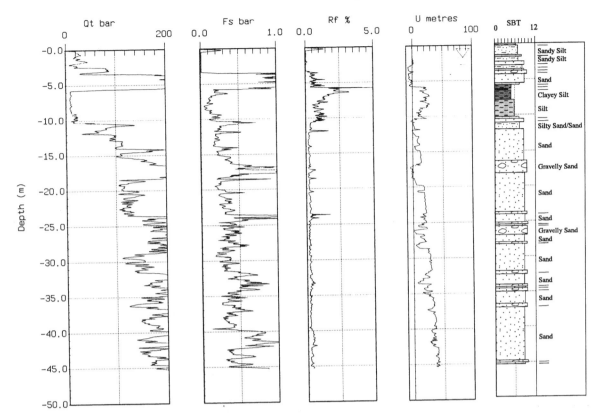

Figure 3. Cone penetration test results: example from location 7 (Fig. 1) showing cone-bearing (Qt), sleeve friction (Fs), friction ratio (Rf), and pore pressure (U) data (interpretive geologic profile on right using soil behavior type, SBT, of Robertson and Campanella, 1988). Alluvial fan sediments in the upper 5 m of the profile overlie flood-plain silts and clayey silts (at 5–10 m depth) and older Fraser River alluvium (below 10 m depth).

weighting function. The weighting function has a value of 0.1 at the ground surface and zero at 20 m depth, similar to the deterministic calculation introduced by Iwasaki et al. (1981). Sites where PLS determinations were made are shown on Figure 5.

The relationship of Quaternary geology map units to liquefaction potential as expressed by PLS values, is shown in Figure 6. Sediments within active and semiactive channels on the Fraser River flood plain have the highest PLS. Other sandy deposits of lacustrine, alluvial fan, and fluvial origin exhibit moderate to high PLS values. Gravelly Fraser River alluvium, large paleochannel deposits, and lacustrine sediments overlain by thin fan alluvium show low to moderate PLS values. Coarse alluvial fan deposits and Fraser River alluvium overlain by thick sequences of fine sediments and organics have the lowest PLS in the map area. Liquefaction hazard ratings for each geological map unit (Fig. 5) were based on the corresponding range in PLS values. For map units with no available PLS determinations, the liquefaction hazard was estimated on the basis of available geological and geotechnical data, particularly water-table depth, sediment type, and density (Table 1). Map units lacking PLS data are mainly those with low or very low liquefaction susceptibilities, such as colluvial fan deposits, till, and other Pleistocene sediments.

The PLS, as used here, does not quantify the effects or con-

sequences of liquefaction such as lateral ground displacement on slopes and toward free faces. However, lateral movements are qualitatively considered in this evaluation since areas along free faces, including the margins of active and semiactive channels, are given a relatively high hazard rating.

Ground motion amplification hazard mapping

Potential ground motion amplification was estimated by comparison of the characteristics of each Quaternary geology map unit with soil classes adopted by the U.S. National Earthquake Hazards Reduction Program (Finn, 1996). The categories for susceptibility to amplification were defined on the basis of shear wave velocity data (derived from SCPTs and SASWs) and of the physical properties of the soils (moisture content, plasticity index, and undrained shear strength). The amplification hazard map was compiled using soils data from the upper 30 m. The effects of deeper soils and bedrock topography on amplification are important but these factors are poorly understood in the map area and therefore could not be included in the assessment. As with the liquefaction map, the hazard for each map unit was expressed as a range that reflects observed geological variation (Monahan et al., 1997).

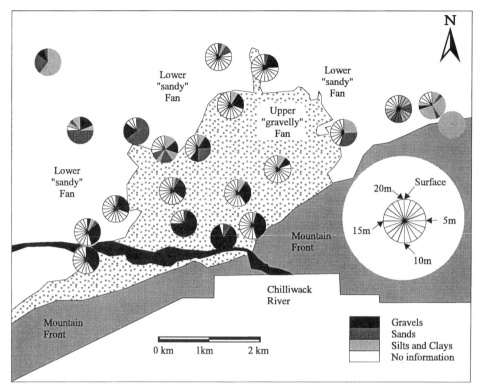

Figure 4. Simplified pie plots, generated from a geographic information system (GIS), used for rapid visualization of three-dimensional geotechnical and water well borehole data, in the southwest part of the study area. The pie plots represent the dominant sediment type in each meter of the bore holes down to a depth of 20 m. Map unit boundaries were constructed using both surficial geology and borehole data. Note, for example, the greater thickness and coarser texture of sediments in the proximal versus distal parts of the Chilliwack River alluvial fan, with gravels occurring mainly in the upper fan and thick silt and clay beds restricted to the lower fan.

Combining liquefaction and ground motion amplification hazards

A simple, objective approach was used to combine earthquake-induced liquefaction and ground-motion amplification hazards into one map for land use and emergency planning purposes (Fig. 7). The approach is conservative in that it reflects the highest rating from either of the two types of hazards. For map units with liquefaction and amplification hazard ratings that span different ranges, the higher ends of the ranges were selected. For example, a map unit with a low to high liquefaction hazard rating and a moderate amplification rating is presented as a moderate to high hazard (i.e., the composite rating reflects the highest bounding values, in this case the moderate amplification hazard at the bottom end and the high liquefaction hazard at the top end).

No attempt is made to add or average the two hazards to develop a combined relative hazard rating because the two types of hazards are distinct and are not simply additive. In the approach used here, a high rating in either type of hazard will result in an overall high earthquake hazard even though the rating

in the other type of hazard may be lower. Therefore, if significant damage may result from one type of hazard, such as high amplification of ground motion, this will not be minimized by the possibility that minor liquefaction will occur in the area. Although ground motion amplification may increase the liquefaction hazard, this possibility has been considered in the assessment of liquefaction potential. Furthermore, an increased liquefaction hazard generally does not increase the amplification hazard. The approach used here has the advantage that other distinct types of earthquake hazards, such as seismically induced landslides, can readily be incorporated in a composite map.

CONCLUSIONS

Earthquake hazard maps are essential tools for effective emergency and land-use planning. These maps can be used to aid in setting priorities for seismic upgrading or remedial work on existing facilities. For emergency planners they are useful for identifying critical facilities (e.g., lifeline systems, transportation corridors, and emergency centers such as fire halls or medical

TABLE 1. LIQUEFACTION SUSCEPTIBILITY OF CHILLIWACK REGION SOILS

Surficial Geology	Age	Distribution	Sediment Type	Water Table	Liquefaction Susceptibility
River channel	Very recent	Along rivers and streams	Sand and gravel	At surface	High to very high
Fraser alluvium	Holocene	Widespread on flood plain	Sand, silt, and gravel	Near surface	Moderate to high
Sandy alluvial fan	Holocene	Lower Vedder River fan	Sand, silty-sand, and gravelly silty-sand	Variable	Moderate to high
Gravelly alluvial fan	Holocene	At mouth of mountain streams	Gravel, sand, and silty-sand	Variable	Low to moderate
Alluvium with near surface fines	Holocene	Abandoned channels and other lows on flood plain	Silt, clay, and organics over sand and gravel	At surface	Low to moderate
Bog	Holocene	Widespread	Peat and organic silts	At surface	Nil at surface
Lacustrine deposits	Holocene/Late Pleistocene	Sumas valley, Vedder Canal area	Sand, silt, and/or clay	Near surface	Low to high
Eolian	Holocene	Small areas, Ryder Upland	Silt and sand	Variable	Low to high
Till	Pleistocene	Ryder Upland	Diamicton	Variable	Very low
Glaciofluvial	Pleistocene	Ryder Upland	Gravel and sand	Variable	Very low
Bedrock	Pre-Pleistocene	Mountainous areas	Rock	Variable	None

facilities) that are geologically the most likely to be affected adversely during an earthquake. Relative earthquake hazard maps can be produced from surficial geology data and from the large geotechnical database that exists for most urban areas. Earthquake hazard maps may reflect one or more hazards, most commonly liquefaction and amplification hazards.

A pilot earthquake mapping program in the Chilliwack area in British Columbia included compilation of existing data from more than 2,400 subsurface test holes, 1:20,000-scale surficial geology mapping, a field program of seismic cone and Becker penetration tests, and integration of geologic and geotechnical data to produce a liquefaction susceptibility (level 1) map. Probabilistic assessments of liquefaction that reflect the relative severity of ground disruption at a number of sites in the region demonstrate the relationship between geology and the liquefaction hazard and provide a more quantitative determination of the liquefaction hazard in each map unit (level 2 map). Liquefaction potential and ground motion amplification hazards are combined onto one map using a conservative, nonaveraging, default approach that reflects the highest rating of the two hazards investigated.

Although standards and methods for earthquake hazard mapping exist, many seismically active jurisdictions in the Pacific Northwest, as well as in other regions, have not implemented mapping programs. Earthquake hazard mapping programs should initially emphasize liquefaction, amplification, and landslide hazards, although other hazard types will also be important in some regions. Comprehensive earthquake hazard mapping programs provide the information necessary for effective land-use and emergency planning, allow for better allocation of funds for seismic upgrading programs, and, through policy development and mitigative measures, may help prevent loss of life, injury, and property damage due to earthquakes.

ACKNOWLEDGMENTS

Support for this project was provided by the British Columbia Resource Inventory Committee, the Ministry of Transportation and Highways, Fraser Valley Regional District, Chilliwack District, Thurber Engineering Ltd., Klohn-Crippen Consultants Ltd., and the Joint Emergency Preparedness Program. The manuscript was improved by the comments of Drs. M. A. Mabey and P. E. Malin.

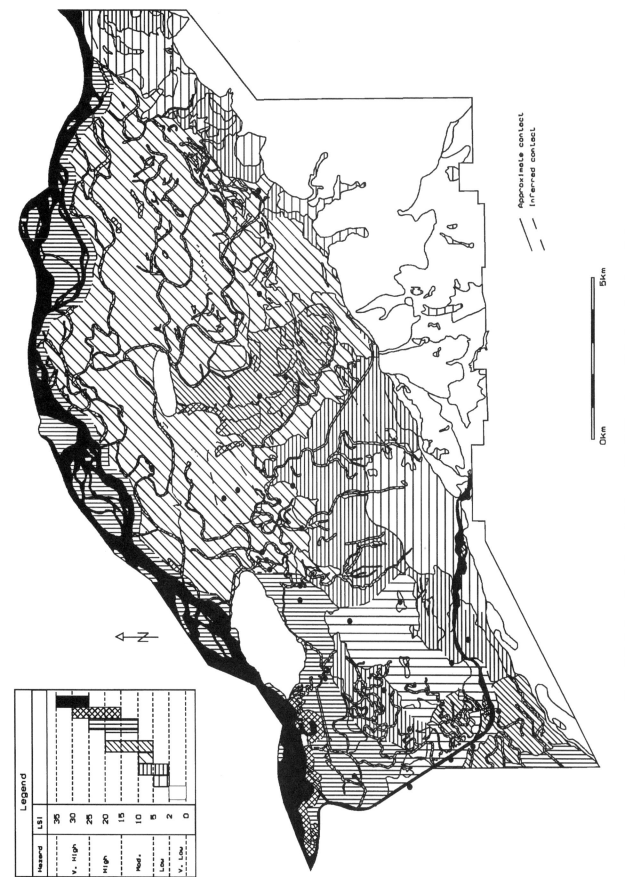

Figure 5. Preliminary liquefaction potential map of the Chilliwack area. Dots show sites where a Probability of Liquefaction Severity (PLS) value was determined (see text for explanation).

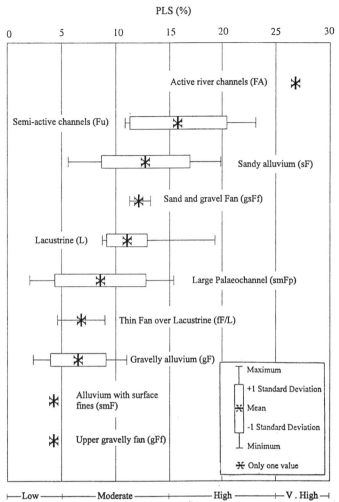

Figure 6. Relationship of liquefaction potential and Quaternary geology. Abbreviations in brackets refer to the genesis of the sediments (F = fluvial, L = lacustrine) preceded by grain-size information (g = gravelly, s = sandy, m = muddy) and followed by landform information (p = floodplain, f = alluvial fan). (E.g., smFp is a sandy to muddy fluvial floodplain.)

REFERENCES CITED

Aki, K., and Irikura, K., 1991, Characterization and mapping of earthquake shaking for seismic zonation, *in* Proceedings, Fourth International Conference on Seismic Zonation, Stanford, California, Volume 1: Oakland, California, Earthquake Engineering Research Institute, p. 61–110.

Anderson, L. R., Keaton, J. R., and Bay, J. A., 1994a, Liquefaction potential map for the northern Wasatch Front, Utah: Utah Geological Survey Contract Report 94-6, scale 1:48,000, 150 p. text.

Anderson, L. R., Keaton, J. R., and Bischoff, J. E., 1994b, Liquefaction potential map for Utah County, Utah: Utah Geological Survey Contract Report 94-8, scale 1:48,000, 1 sheet, 46 p. text.

Anderson, L. R., Keaton, J. R., Ellis, S. J., and Aubry, K., 1994c, Liquefaction potential map for Davis County, Utah: Utah Geological Survey Contract Report 94-7, scale 1:48,000, 6 sheets, 50 p. text.

Anderson, L. R., Keaton, J. R., and Rice, J. D., 1994d, Liquefaction potential map for central Utah: Utah Geological Survey Contract Report 94-10, scale 1:48,000, 1 sheet, 134 p. text.

Anderson, L. R., Keaton, J. R., Spitzley, J. E., and Allen, A. C., 1994e, Liquefaction potential map for Salt Lake County, Utah: Utah Geological Survey Contract Report 94-9, scale 1:48,000, 1 sheet, 48 p. text.

Atkinson, G. M., Finn, W. D. L., and Charlwood, R. G., 1986, PROLIQ2—A computer program for estimating the probability of seismic liquefaction including both aerial and fault sources: Vancouver, British Columbia, Department of Civil Engineering, University of British Columbia, 78 p.

Atwater, B. F., and 15 others, 1995, Summary of coastal geologic evidence for past great earthquakes at the Cascadia subduction zone: Earthquake Spectra, v. 11, p. 1–18.

Bartlett, S. F., and Youd, T. L., 1992, Empirical analysis of horizontal ground displacement generated by liquefaction-induced lateral spreads: National Center for Earthquake Engineering Research, Technical Report NCEER-92-0021, 63 p.

British Columbia Hydro and Power Authority, 1992, Liquefaction hazard assessment for the Lower Mainland region: Report No. H24747, includes 1:75,000-scale liquefaction hazard map, 1 sheet.

Budhu, M., Jihayakumar, V., Giese, F. F., and Baumgras, L., 1987, Liquefaction potential for New York State—a preliminary report on sites in Manhattan and Buffalo: National Center for Earthquake Engineering Research, Technical Report, NCEER-87-0009, 38 p.

City of Seattle, 1992, Seismic hazards in Seattle: City of Seattle, Planning Department, 53 p.

Clague, J. J., Naesgaard, E., and Sy, A., 1992, Liquefaction features on the Fraser River delta: evidence for prehistoric earthquakes?: Canadian Journal of Earth Sciences, v. 29, p. 1734–1745.

Combellick, R. A., 1984, Potential for earthquake-induced liquefaction in the Fairbanks–Ninana area, Alaska: Alaska Division of Geology and Geophysical Surveys, Report of Investigations 84-5, 10 p., plus maps and figs.

Cornell, C. A., 1968, Engineering seismic risk analysis: Seismological Society of America, Bulletin, v. 58, p. 1583–1606.

Dragovich, J. D., and Pringle, P. T., 1995, Liquefaction susceptibility for the Sumner 7.5-minute Quadrangle, Washington, with a section on liquefaction susceptibility by S. P. Palmer: Washington Division of Geology and Earth Resources, Geologic Map GM44, scale 1:24,000, 1 sheet, 26 p. text.

DuMontelle, P. B., 1995, Earthquake hazards map showing areas of relative potential for shaking and/or liquefaction: Central United States Earthquake Consortium, compiled by Illinois State Geological Survey, scale 1:2,000,000, 1 sheet.

Dupré, W. R., 1990, Map showing geologic and liquefaction susceptibility of Quaternary deposits in the Monterey, Seaside, Spreckles, and Carmel Valley Quadrangles, Monterey County, California: U.S. Geological Survey, Miscellaneous Field Studies Map MF-2096, scale 1:24,000.

Dupré, W. R., and Tinsley, J. C., 1980, Maps showing geology and liquefaction potential of northern Monterey and southern Santa Cruz counties, California: U.S. Geological Survey, Miscellaneous Field Studies, Map MF-1199, scale 1:62,500.

Earthquake Engineering Research Institute, Committee on Seismic Risk, 1984, Glossary of terms for probabilistic seismic risk and hazard analysis: Earthquake Spectra, v. 1, Number 1, p. 33–40.

Earthquake Engineering Research Institute, 1991, Fourth International Conference on Seismic Zonation: Oakland, California, Earthquake Engineering Research Institute, v. 1, 876 p.

Elton, D. J., and Hadj-Hamou, T., 1990, Liquefaction potential map for Charleston, South Carolina: Journal of Geotechnical Engineering ASCE 116, no. 2, p. 244–265.

Escuela Politécnica Nacional, Geohazards International, Illustre Municipio de Quito, ORSTOM, OYO Corporation, 1994, The Quito, Ecuador, Earthquake Risk Management Project: Stanford, Geohazards International, 34 p.

Fang, H. Q., Wang Z. Y., Zhao, S. D., Huang, Z. L., and Miao, X. K., 1980, Approach to Tangshan earthquake engineering geological problems: Beijing, China, Geotechnical Investigation Institute, Chinese Academy of Building Research, 353 p.

Finn, L. W. D., 1991, Geotechnical engineering aspects of microzonation, *in* Proceedings, Fourth International Conference on Seismic Zonation, Stanford, California, Volume 1: Oakland, California, Earthquake Engineering Research Institute, p. 199–259.

Finn, L. W. D., 1994, Geotechnical aspects of the estimation and mitigation of

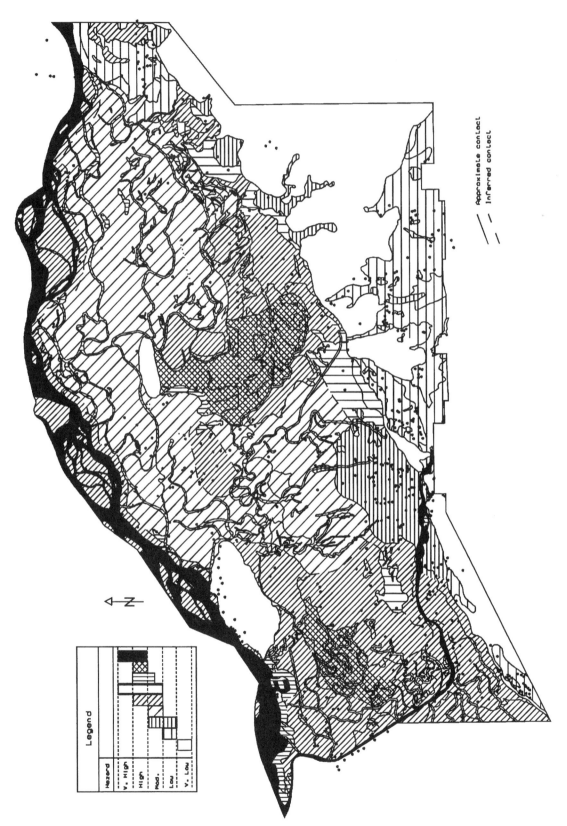

Figure 7. Preliminary relative earthquake hazard map of the Chilliwack area showing areas of relative potential for liquefaction or amplification of ground motion. Dots show locations of subsurface data.

earthquake risk, *in* Tucker, B. E., Erdik, M., and Hwang, C. N., eds., Issues in earthquake risk: Dordrecht, The Netherlands; Kluwer Academic Publishers, p. 35–77.

Finn, L. W. D., 1996, Ground motion amplification factors for use in building codes, *in* Proceedings, International Workshop on Site Response, Japan: Port and Harbour Research Institute, v. 2, p. 105–117.

Grant, W. P., and Perkins, W. J., 1993, Evaluation of liquefaction potential, Tacoma, Washington: Shannon and Wilson, Inc. (under contract to U.S. Geological Survey), Final Technical Report, v. 1, 3 maps, scale 1:48,000.

Grant, W. P., Perkins, W. J., and Youd, T. L., 1991, Evaluation of liquefaction potential, Seattle, Washington: U.S. Geological Survey Open-File Report 91-441-T, 44 p.

Hansen, A., and Franks, C. A. M., 1991, Characterization and mapping of earthquake-triggered landslides for seismic zonation, *in* Proceedings, Fourth International Conference on Seismic Zonation, Stanford, California, Volume 1: Oakland, California, Earthquake Engineering Research Institute, p. 149–195.

Hasegawa, H. S., Basham, P. W., and Berry, M. J., 1981, Attenuation relations for strong seismic ground motions in Canada: Seismological Society of America Bulletin, v. 71, p. 1943–1962.

Higgins, J. D., and Rockaway, J. D., 1986, Graphics system for seismic response mapping: Association of Engineering Geologists Bulletin, v. 23, p. 77–91.

Hunter, J. A., Luternauer, J. L., Neave, K. G., Pullan, S. E., Good, R. L., Burns, R. A., and Douma, M., 1992, Shallow shear-wave velocity-depth data in the Fraser River delta from surface refraction methods, 1989, 1990, 1991: Geological Survey of Canada-Open File 2504, 271 p.

Idriss, I. M., 1991, Earthquake ground motions at soft soil sites, *in* Proceedings, Second International Conference on Recent Advances in Geotechnical Earthquake Engineering and Soil Dynamics, Rolla, Missouri, University of Missouri-Rolla: v. 3, p. 2265–2272.

INPRES, 1982, Seismic microzonation of the Tulum Valley, San Juan Province, Argentina: San Juan, Argentina, Instituto Nacional de Prevencion Sismica, 3 volumes.

INPRES, 1987, Microzonificacion sismica Del Gran Mendoza: San Juan, Argentina Instituto Nacional de Prevencion Sismica (in Spanish).

International Society for Soil Mechanics and Foundation Engineering, 1993, Manual for zonation on seismic geotechnical hazards, report of the Technical Committee for Earthquake Geotechnical Engineering, TC4: Tokyo, Japan, Japanese Society of Soil Mechanics and Foundation Engineering, 149 p.

Ishihara, K., and Ogawa, K., 1978, Liquefaction susceptibility map of downtown Tokyo, *in* Proceedings, Second International Conference on Microzonation for Safer Construction, San Francisco, California: National Science Foundation, v. 2, p. 897–910.

Ishihara, K., and Yasuda, S., 1991, Microzonation for liquefaction potential during earthquakes in Japan, *in* Proceedings, Fourth International Conference on Seismic Zonation, Stanford, California, Volume 1: Oakland, California, Earthquake Engineering Research Institute, p. 703–724.

Iwasaki, T., Tokida, K., and Taksuoka, F., 1981, Soil liquefaction potential evaluation with use of the simplified procedure, *in* Proceedings, First International Conference on Recent Advances in Geotechnical Earthquake Engineering and Soil Dynamics: Rolla, Missouri, University of Missouri-Rolla, v. 1, p 209–214.

Kavazanjian, E., Roth, R. A., and Heriberto, E., 1985, Liquefaction potential mapping for San Francisco: Journal of Geotechnical Engineering, v. 111, p. 54–76.

Klohn-Crippen Consultants Ltd., 1994, Preliminary seismic microzonation assessment for British Columbia: B.C. Resource Inventory Committee Report 17, 108 p.

Kotoda, K., Wakamatsu, W., and Midorikawa, S., 1988, Seismic microzoning on soil liquefaction potential based on geomorphological land classification: Soils and Foundations, v. 28, p. 127–143.

Kuroiwa, J., and Alva, J., 1991, Microzonation and its application to urban and regional planning for disaster mitigation in Peru, *in* Proceedings, Fourth International Conference on Seismic Zonation, Stanford, California, Volume 1: Oakland, California, Earthquake Engineering Research Institute, p. 771–794.

Kusano, K., Abe, H., Odawa, Y., and Nakayama, T., 1989, Liquefaction potential map in Tokyo lowland, *in* Proceedings, Ninth World Conference on Earthquake Engineering, Tokyo: Japan Association For Earthquake Disaster Prevention, v. 2, Paper 2-2-6, p. 157–162.

Leighton and Associates, 1990, Liquefaction susceptibility: Los Angeles County Department of Regional Planning, Unpublished Map, Project 287 1855-16, scale 1:125,000.

Levson, V. M., Monahan, P. A., Meldrum, D. G., Matysek, P. F., Watts, B. D., Yan, L., and Sy, A., 1995, Seismic microzonation mapping in southwestern British Columbia: a pilot project, *in* Proceedings, 48th Canadian Geotechnical Conference, Trends in Geotechnique, September, 1995, Vancouver: Canadian Geotechnical Society, v. 2, p. 927–936.

Levson, V. M., Monahan, P. A., Meldrum, D. G., Matysek, P. F., Gerath, R. F., Watts, B. D., Sy, A., and Yan, L., 1996a, Surficial geology and earthquake hazard mapping, Chilliwack, British Columbia (92G/1 and H/4), *in* Grant, B. M., and Newell, J. M., eds., Geological fieldwork 1995: British Columbia Geological Survey Paper 1996-1, p. 191–203.

Levson, V. M., Gerath, R. F., Meldrum, D. G., and Monahan, P. A., 1996b, Surficial geology of the Chilliwack area, NTS 92G/1E and H/4W: British Columbia Geological Survey Open-File 1996-12, scale 1:50,000, 1 sheet.

Levson, V. M., Monahan, P. A., Meldrum, D. G., Matysek, P. F., Sy, A., Watts, B. D., Yan, L., and Gerath, R. F., 1996c, Preliminary relative earthquake hazard map of the Chilliwack area showing areas of relative potential for liquefaction and/or amplification of ground motion: British Columbia Geological Survey Open-File 1996-25, scale 1:50,000, 1 sheet.

Levson, V. M., Monahan, P. A., Meldrum, D. G., Sy, A., Yan, L., Watts, B. D., and Gerath, R. F., 1997, Relative liquefaction susceptibility and liquefaction potential of the Chilliwack area, preliminary map: British Columbia Geological Survey Open-File Map, scale 1:40,000, 1 sheet, text (in press).

Luternauer, J. L., and nine others, 1993, The Fraser River delta architecture, geological dynamics and human impact, *in* Proceedings, Eighth Symposium on Coastal and Ocean Management, Deltas of the World: New Orleans, American Society of Civil Engineers, p. 99–113.

Luternauer, J. L., and 19 others, 1994, Fraser River delta: geology, geohazards and human impact, *in* Monger, J. W. H., ed., Geology and geological hazards of the Vancouver region, southwestern British Columbia: Geological Survey of Canada Bulletin 481, p. 197–220.

Mabey, M. A., and Madin, I. P., 1993, Relative earthquake hazard map of the Portland, Oregon 7-1/2 Minute Quadrangle: Oregon Department of Geology and Mineral Industries and Metro, scale 1:24,000, 1 sheet, 10 p. text.

Mabey, M. A., and Youd, T. L., 1989, Liquefaction severity index maps of the state of Utah, *in* Watters, R. J., ed., Proceedings, 25th Symposium on Engineering Geology and Geotechnical Engineering, Reno, Nevada: Rotterdam, The Netherlands, A. A. Balkema Company, p. 305–312.

Mabey, M. A., and Youd, T. L., 1991, Liquefaction hazard mapping for the Seattle, Washington, urban region using LSI (liquefaction severity index): Brigham Young University Technical Report CEG-91-01, under contract to U.S. Geological Survey, 64 p.

Mabey, M. A., Madin, I. P., and Palmer, S. P., 1994, Relative earthquake hazard map for the Vancouver, Washington, urban region: Washington Division of Geology and Earth Resources Geologic Map GM-42, scale 1:24,000, 2 sheets, 5 p. text.

Mabey, M. A., Meier, D. B., and Palmer, S. P., 1995, Relative earthquake hazard map of the Mount Tabor Quadrangle, Multnomah County, Oregon, and Clark County, Washington: Oregon Department of Geology and Mineral Industries Geological Map Series, GMS-89, scale 1:24,000, 1 sheet, 5 p. text.

Mader, G. G., 1991, The use of seismic zonation in land use planning, zoning and code implementation, *in* Proceedings, Fourth International Conference on Seismic Zonation, Stanford, California, Volume 1: Oakland, California, Earthquake Engineering Research Institute, p. 357–384.

Madin, I. P., 1990, Earthquake-hazard geology maps of the Portland metropolitan area, Oregon—text and map explanation: Oregon Department of Geology and Mineral Industries Open-File Report 90-2, scale 1:24,000, 21 p. text.

Marcellini, A., and 21 others, 1991, Benevento seismic risk project: progress report, *in* Proceedings, Fourth International Conference on Seismic Zonation, Stanford, California, Volume 1: Oakland, California, Earthquake Engineering Research Institute, p. 605–669.

Meldrum, D. G., Monahan, P. A., and Levson, V. M., 1997, Lithological data from geotechnical test holes and water wells in the Chilliwack area, British Columbia (92G/1 and H/4): British Columbia Geological Survey Open-File (in press).

Metro, 1993, Earthquake scenario pilot project: assessment of damage and losses: Metro and the Oregon Department of Geology and Mineral Industries, 19 p.

Metro, 1996, Using earthquake hazard maps for land use planning and building permit administration, Portland metropolitan area: Report of the Metro Advisory Committee for Mitigating Earthquake Damage, 38 p.

Monahan, P. A., and Levson, V. M., 1997, Quaternary geology map (upper 20 meters), Chilliwack, British Columbia (92G/1 and H/4): British Columbia Geological Survey Open File (in press).

Monahan, P. A., Levson, V. M., Meldrum, D. G., Watts, B. D., Sy, A., and Yan, L., 1997, Ground motion amplification hazard map, Chilliwack, British Columbia (92G/1 and H/4): British Columbia Geological Survey Open-File (in press).

Munich Reinsurance Company of Canada, 1992, A study of the economic impact of a severe earthquake in the lower mainland of British Columbia: 99 p.

Nilson, T. H., and Brabb, E. E., 1979, Landslides: U.S. Geological Survey Professional Paper 941-A, p. A75–A87.

Obermeier, S. F., 1984, Liquefaction potential for the central Mississippi valley, *in* Proceedings, Symposium on the New Madrid Seismic Zone: U.S. Geological Survey, Open-File Report 84-770, p. 391–446.

Obermeier, S. F., 1988, Liquefaction potential in the Central Mississippi Valley: U.S. Geological Survey, Bulletin 1832, 21 p.

Palmer, S. P., Schasse, H. W., and Norman, D. K., 1994, Liquefaction susceptibility for the Des Moines and Renton 7.5-minute Quadrangles, Washington: Washington Division of Geology and Earth Resources, Geologic Map GM-41, scale 1:24,000, 2 sheets, 15 p. text.

Palmer, S. P., Walsh, T. J., Logan, R. L., and Gerstel, W. J., 1995, Liquefaction susceptibility for the Auborn and Poverty Bay 7.5-minute Quadrangles, Washington: Washington Division of Geology and Earth Resources Geologic Map GM43, scale 1:24,000, 2 sheets, 15 p. text.

Pitilakis, K. D., 1995, Seismic microzonation practice in Greece: a critical review of some important factors, *in* Proceedings, European Conference on Earthquake Engineering, 10th: A. A. Balkema, Rotterdam, v. 4, p. 2537–2545.

Pitilakis, K., Tsotsos, S., and Hatzigogos, T., 1982, Study of liquefaction potential in the area of Thessaloniki, *in* Proceedings, Symposium on Earthquake Engineering, 7th, Roorkee, India: University of Roorkee and Indian Society of Earthquake Technology, v. 1, p. 375–380.

Power, M. S., Dawson, A. W., Streiff, D. W., Perman, R. C., and Berger, V., 1982, Evaluation of liquefaction susceptibility in the San Diego, California, urban area: Woodward-Clyde Consultants, San Diego, California, Unpublished Final Technical Report, U.S. Geological Survey Contract No. 14-08-0001-19110, 33 p., plus figures and tables.

Power, M. S., Berger, V., Youngs, R. R., Coppersmith, K. J., and Streiff, D. W., 1986, Evaluation of liquefaction opportunity and liquefaction potential in the San Diego, California, urban area: Woodward-Clyde Consultants, San Diego, California, Unpublished Final Technical Report, U.S. Geological Survey Contract No. 14-08-0001-20407, 89 p., plus figures and tables.

Power, M. S., and eight others, 1991, Seismic microzonation of the Ech Cheliff region, Algeria, *in* Proceedings, Fourth International Conference on Seismic Zonation, Stanford, California, Volume 1: Oakland, California, Earthquake Engineering Research Institute, p. 771–794.

Robertson, P. K., 1994, Suggested terminology for liquefaction, *in* Proceedings, 47th Canadian Geotechnical Conference, Halifax, Nova Scotia: Canadian Geotechnical Society, p. 277–286.

Robertson, P. K., and Campanella, R. G., 1988, Guidelines for geotechnical design using CPT and CPTU: University of British Columbia, Department of Civil Engineering, Soil Mechanics Series Number 120, 192 p.

Rogers, G. C., 1992, The earthquake threat in southwest British Columbia, *in* Proceedings, Vancouver Geotechnical Society and Canadian Geotechnical Society, 1992 Symposium, Geotechnique and Natural Hazards: Vancouver, Canada, BiTech Publishers Ltd., p. 63–69.

Rogers, G. C., 1994, Earthquakes in the Vancouver area, *in* Monger, J. W. H., ed., Geology and geological hazards of the Vancouver region, southwestern

British Columbia: Geological Survey of Canada Bulletin 481, p. 221-229.

Sanchez, P. E., Ziony, J. I., McKnight, J. S., Clark, B. R., and Gath, E. M., 1991, Seismic zonation of the Los Angeles region, *in* Proceedings, Fourth International Conference on Seismic Zonation, Stanford, California, Volume 1: Oakland, California, Earthquake Engineering Research Institute, p. 797–844.

Sauter, F. F., 1996, Redefining terms in the field of seismic safety and risk mitigation: Earthquake Spectra, v. 12, p. 315–326.

Seed, H. B., 1979, Soil liquefaction and cyclic mobility evaluation for level ground during earthquakes: Journal of Geotechnical Engineering, v. 105, p. 201–255.

Seed, H. B., and Idriss, I. M., 1982, Ground motions and soil liquefaction during earthquakes: Earthquake Engineering Research Institute Monograph 5, 134 p.

Sharma, S., and Kovacs, W. D., 1980, Microzonation of the Memphis, Tennessee, area: School of Civil Engineering, Purdue University, Unpublished Research Report, U.S. Geological Survey Contract Number 14-08-0002-17752, 129 p.

Shedlock, K. M. and Weaver, C. S., 1991, Program for earthquake hazard assessment in the Pacific Northwest: U.S. Geological Survey Circular 1067, 29 p.

Soto, A. E., 1987, San Juan [Puerto Rico] metropolitan area liquefaction potential map: U.S. Geological Survey Open-File Report 87-0008, p. 162–164.

Talaganov, K., and Aleksovski, D., 1984, Soil stability and urban design case study, *in* Proceedings, 8th World Conference on Earthquake Engineering: Englewood Cliffs, New Jersey, Prentice-Hall, Inc., v. 3, p. 453–460.

Thenhaus, P. C., Hanson, S. L., Effendi, I., Kertapati, E. K., and Algermissen, S. T., 1993, Pilot studies of seismic hazard and risk in north Sulawesi Province, Indonesia: Earthquake Spectra, v. 9, p. 97–120.

Tinsley, J. C., Youd, T. L., Perkins, D. M., and Chen, A. T. F., 1985, Evaluating liquefaction potential, *in* Ziony, J. I., ed., Evaluating earthquake hazards in the Los Angeles region: U.S. Geological Survey Professional Paper 1360, p. 263–316.

Wakamatsu, K., 1992, Evaluation of liquefaction susceptibility based on detailed geomorphological classification, *in* Proceedings, Architectural Institute of Japan Annual Meeting: Architectural Institute of Japan, v. B, p. 1443–1444.

Wang, Y., and Leonard, W. J., 1996, Relative earthquake hazard maps of the Salem East and Salem West Quadrangles, Marion and Polk Counties, Oregon: Oregon Department of Geology and Mineral Industries Geological Map Series, GMS-105, scale 1:24,000, 4 sheets, 10 p. text.

Watts, B. D., Seyers, W. D., and Stewart, R. A., 1992, Liquefaction susceptibility of greater Vancouver area soils, *in* Proceedings, Vancouver Geotechnical Society and Canadian Geotechnical Society, 1992 Symposium, Geotechnique and Natural Hazards: Vancouver, Canada, BiTech Publishers Ltd., p. 145–157.

Wieczorek, G. F., Wilson, R. C., and Harp, E. L., 1985, Map showing slope stability during earthquakes in San Mateo County, California: U.S. Geological Survey Map I-1257-E, scale 1:62,500.

Youd, T. L., 1991, Mapping of earthquake-induced liquefaction for seismic zonation, *in* Proceedings, Fourth International Conference on Seismic Zonation, Stanford, California, Volume 1: Oakland, California, Earthquake Engineering Research Institute, p. 111–147.

Youd, T. L., and Jones, C. F., 1993, Liquefaction hazard maps for the Portland Quadrangle, Oregon: Oregon Department of Geology and Mineral Industries, Geological Map Series Map GMS-79, scale 1:24,000, 17 p. text.

Youd, T. L., and Perkins, J. B., 1978, Mapping of liquefaction-induced ground failure potential: Journal of the Geotechnical Engineering, ASCE 104 (GT4), p. 433–446.

Youd, T. L., and Perkins, J. B., 1987, Map showing liquefaction susceptibility of San Mateo County, California: U.S. Geological Survey, Miscellaneous Investigations Map I-1257-G, scale 1:62,500.

Youd, T. L., Nichols D. R., Halley, E. J., and Lajoie, K. R., 1975, Liquefaction potential, *in* Studies for seismic zonation of the San Francisco Bay region: U.S. Geological Survey Professional Paper 941-A, p. A68–A74.

Youd, T. L., Tinsley, J. C., Perkins D. M., King, E. J., and Preston, R. F., 1978, Liquefaction potential map of San Fernando Valley, California, *in* Proceedings, International Conference on Microzonation for Safer Construction, San Francisco: National Science Foundation, v. 1, p. 267–278.

Manuscript Accepted by the Society June 5, 1997

Printed in U.S.A.

Geological Society of America
Reviews in Engineering Geology, Volume XII
1998

Asbestos monitoring and regulation in public drinking-water supplies: A case history from North Carolina

Jeffrey C. Reid and Robert H. Carpenter
North Carolina Geological Survey, 512 N. Salisbury Street, Raleigh, North Carolina 27611

ABSTRACT

Vulnerability assessments of the potential for asbestos contamination in public water supplies provide a basis for states to grant waivers from compliance monitoring requirements of public water supply systems if they can demonstrate they are not vulnerable under final U.S. Environmental Protection Agency (EPA) rulings published in the Federal Register.

Land area of geologic units of North Carolina as represented on the 1:500,000-scale state geologic map in digital format and published geologic maps provide the technical basis for waivers for compliance monitoring and associated expensive analytical laboratory testing. These data show that only 3.68% of North Carolina's land area of 18,790 square km (48,666 square mi) is underlain by rocks that are potentially hosts for asbestiform minerals. We assumed the EPA would follow the initiative of the Occupational Safety and Health Administration (OSHA) and remove nonasbestiform anthophyllite, tremolite, and actinolite from inclusion in the definition of asbestos. We concluded that the portion of North Carolina likely to contain any chrysotile asbestos would be reduced to 0.77% of land area. Ultramafic rocks that have a higher probability of chrysotile occurrences comprise only 0.07%, or 33.8 square mi of land surface in North Carolina.

With additional investigation to delineate watersheds in which chrysotile susceptible rocks occur, the regulatory agency exempted 73 of North Carolina's 100 counties from asbestos testing of surface water supply intakes. Sixty-eight percent (3,493) of the state's surface water supply intakes were exempted from unnecessary testing, saving taxpayers at least $368,000; this is about one-third of the North Carolina Geological Survey's annual appropriated budget. Author staff time to perform the work leading to the conclusion was about two person-weeks at a taxpayer cost of about $2,000.

INTRODUCTION

This investigation resulted from a service request in July 1992 to the North Carolina Geological Survey from the Department of Environment, Health, and Natural Resources' Public Water Supply Section for technical advice on how to deal with U.S. Environmental Protection Agency (EPA) regulations (Carpenter and Reid, 1994). It demonstrates how application of basic geologic relationships such as mineral and rock associations can preclude expensive and unnecessary environmental and public health assessments.

Definition of asbestos

Prior to June 8, 1992, the following fibrous minerals were defined as asbestos by the Occupational Safety and Health Administration (OSHA) (29 CFR 1910.1001 and 29 CFR 1928.56): chrysotile, crocidolite, amosite (grunerite), cum-

Reid, J. C., and Carpenter, R. H., 1998, Asbestos monitoring and regulation in public drinking-water supplies: A case history from North Carolina, *in* Welby, C. W., and Gowan, M. E., eds., A Paradox of Power: Voices of Warning and Reason in the Geosciences: Boulder, Colorado, Geological Society of America Reviews in Engineering Geology, v. XII.

mingtonite, tremolite, anthophyllite, and actinolite. On June 8, 1992, OSHA revised the asbestos standards and removed nonasbestiform tremolite, anthophyllite, and actinolite from this list (Federal Register, 1992, p. 24310). The EPA's drinking water standards do not define asbestos, but the report, "Drinking Water Criteria Document for Asbestos" (U.S. Environmental Protection Agency, 1988), includes a list of minerals similar to that in OSHA's pre-1992 list. The regulatory status of other acicular minerals such as kyanite, sillimanite, and andalusite is uncertain and has not been addressed by the EPA. Drinking water standards were published in the Federal Register on January 30, 1991. Several studies have addressed issues related to asbestos in drinking water including Toft et al. (1984), Levy et al. (1976), and Van Baalen (1995). Lamarche (1981) reviewed the geology of asbestos deposits.

OCCURRENCES OF ASBESTOS IN NORTH CAROLINA

Figure 1 shows North Carolina counties containing ultramafic and mafic rocks (with amphibole). The areal extent of various rock units that probably contain asbestiform minerals is summarized in Table 1 (North Carolina Geological Survey, 1988). Amosite and crocidolite are rare asbestiform minerals that are not reported to occur in North Carolina. Resolution of

regulatory treatment of asbestiform varieties of the amphiboles, tremolite, actinolite, and anthophyllite is beyond the scope of this paper.

Based on worldwide lithologic associations, chrysotile is essentially confined to altered or metamorphosed peridotites (Virta and Mann, 1994). Ultramafic rocks in North Carolina are designated as PzZu on the Geologic Map of North Carolina (North Carolina Geological Survey, 1985). All are magnesium-rich and consist of dunite, serpentinite, soapstone, and pyroxenite. Specimens of chrysotile have been ". . . found at the Baker mine, and near Patterson in Caldwell County; at the Buck Creek mine, Clay County; also at Webster, Jackson County; and Corundum Hill mine, Macon County" (Pratt and Lewis, 1905); other chrysotile occurrences cannot be precluded. There has been no commercial production of chysotile in the state. Anthophyllite is locally abundant in ultramafic rocks and has been mined at a number of sites in western North Carolina (Conrad et al., 1963). The aggregate surface area of these rocks in North Carolina is 33.8 square mi, or 0.07% of the total surface area of the state (Table 1).

Metamorphic rocks (map symbol PzZm) in the central portion of North Carolina include metagabbro and metadiorite (Fig. 1). These types of rocks commonly contain tremolite or actinolite, and rarely, anthophyllite. Compared to ultramafic rocks, the probability of chrysotile occurrence is much lower in

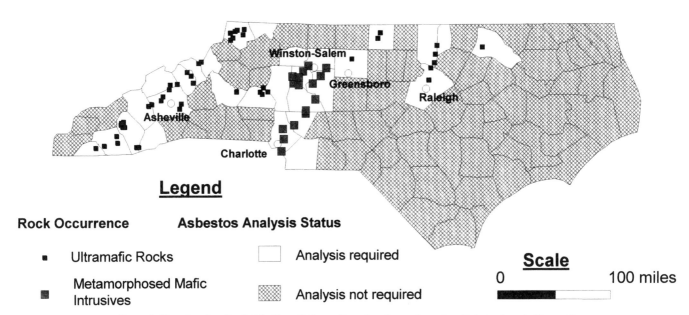

Status of Requirements for Analysis of Asbestos in North Carolina Public Water Supply Systems

Figure 1. Map showing the distribution of ultramafic and metamorphosed mafic intrusives (with amphibole) in North Carolina and the status of requirements for analysis of asbestos in North Carolina public water supply systems.

metamafic rocks. These rocks underlie an area of 130 square km (338 square mi), or 0.69% of the state's surface area.

Other metamorphosed magnesium-rich rocks may contain tremolite, actinolite, or anthophyllite but are not likely to contain chrysotile, include amphibolites, mafic metavolcanic rocks, greenstone, and dolomitic marble. The aggregate surface area of these units is 505 square km (1,310 square mi), or 3.5% of the total surface area of the state (Table 1).

RESULTS

Vulnerability assessments of the potential for asbestos contamination provide a basis for states to grant waivers from compliance monitoring requirements (Federal Register, January 30, 1991, p. 3565, Item #3, and Section 141.23 (5)(b)(2); See Appendix A) to those water-supply systems that can demonstrate they are not vulnerable. From a geological standpoint, waivers from monitoring requirements are justified for most of the state since only 3.68% of the surface of North Carolina is underlain by rocks that are possible hosts of asbestiform minerals. Assuming that EPA follows the initiative of OSHA and removes anthophyllite, tremolite, and actinolite from inclusion in the definition of asbestos, that portion of the state in which some occurrences of chrysotile are possible is reduced to 0.77%. Ultramafic rocks having the highest probability of chrysotile occurrence comprise only 0.07%, or 13 square km (33.8 square mi), of the surface of North Carolina. On the basis of this information, 50 of North Carolina's 100 counties were exempted from asbestos-testing of surface water supply intakes (Fig. 1).

After additional investigation in which watersheds with chrysotile-susceptible rocks were delineated, 68% (3,493) of the state's surface water supply intakes were exempted from testing. The resulting savings in analytical costs were at least $368,000; this is about one-third of the North Carolina Geological Survey's annual appropriated budget. Staff time to perform the work leading to this conclusion was about two person-weeks at a taxpayer cost of about $2,000. Ultimately the state regulatory agency decided to exempt 73 counties.

SUMMARY

This study exempted 73 of North Carolina's 100 counties from unnecessary expensive testing of surface water supply intakes for asbestos. Sixty-eight percent (3,493) of the state's surface water supply intakes were exempted saving taxpayers at least $368,000 compared with the study cost of about $2,000 over two weeks. This study had a high benefit to cost ratio of 184:1.

ACKNOWLEDGMENTS

Charles Welby encouraged this article. Kelly Eguakun helped in manuscript preparation. This article benefited from reviews from Edward F. Stoddard, Malcom Ross, and Charles Welby.

APPENDIX A. INTRODUCTION AND REGULATORY BACKGROUND

On January 30, 1991, the U.S. Environmental Protection Agency (EPA) published in the Federal Register 40 CFR Parts 141, 142, and 143 otherwise known as "Part II" on National Primary Drinking Water Regulations; Final Rule (Federal Register, 1991, p. 3525–3597). In this document the EPA promulgated Maximum Contaminant Level Goals (MCLGs) and National Primary Drinking Water Regulations (NPDWRs) for 26 synthetic organic chemicals (SOCs) and 7 inorganic chemicals (IOCs) including asbestos.

The NPDWRs also include monitoring, reporting, and public notification for these compounds. The EPA document includes the Best Available Technology (BAT) upon which the MCLGs are based and the BAT for the purpose of issuing a variance (Federal Register, 1991, p. 3526).

The EPA report lists MCLG for asbestos of "7 million fibers/liter (longer than 10μm)" and a "MCL of 7 million fibers/liter longer than 10μm" (Federal Register, 1991, Table 1, p. 3528). The EPA report lists the BAT to remove asbestos as "Coagulation/filtration (Not 1415 BAT for small systems for variances unless treatment is currently in place), corrosion control, direct filtration, or diatomite filtration" (Federal Register, 1991, Table 2, p. 3528.)

Basis for exclusion

Table 8 (Federal Register, 1991, p. 3529) provides compliance monitoring requirements. For asbestos the base requirement is "1 sample every 9 years." The trigger that would increase monitoring is >MCL. However, this table *introduces waivers for sampling based on vulnerability assessments* (Federal Register, 1991, Table 8, p. 3529). Table 9 (Federal Register, 1991, p. 3529) indicates transmission electron microscopy (TEM) for the required analytical method.

The Final Rules discusses in more detail "initial and repeat base requirements." EPA (Federal Register, 1991, p. 3565) also proposed an alternative approach. This approach required all water supply systems to monitor for asbestos unless the system conducted a vulnerability assessment.

The Final Rules state "The base repeat frequency is once in the first three-year monitoring period of each nine-year cycle, which means that after the initial base monitoring requirement is completed, systems would not be required to monitor again until the 2002 to 2005 compliance period. EPA has not eliminated the repeat base requirement because of the concern that there may be occurrence in a limited number of systems. Systems that are not vulnerable would continue to be eligible to receive waivers. EPA is requiring infrequent base monitoring requirements because of the low probability of occurrence, the limited analytic capabilities to measure asbestos, and the high analytical costs. Also, the EPA believes that regulatory activities such as the corrosion control activities and asbestos/cement pipe ban will reduce the future occurrence of this contaminant" (Federal Register, 1991).

Item (3) (Federal Register, 1991, p. 3565) "allows States to grant waivers based on a vulnerability assessment by systems that considers contamination in the raw water supply and/or from the corrosion of asbestos/cement pipe . . . in the distribution system. Systems not receiving a *waiver must monitor at* the base frequency. Because monitoring is not required for the second and third three-year periods, no waiver is needed in those monitoring periods" (emphasis added).

Specific language for a waiver is found in Section §141.23(5) (Federal Register, 1991, p. 3579) concerning the frequency of monitoring asbestos which states the frequency of asbestos monitoring §141.23(5)(b) (Federal Register, 1991, p. 3580). Explicit provision is provided in paragraph §141.23 (5)(b)(2) for a waiver. It states "(2) *If the system believes it is not vulnerable to either asbestos contamination in*

J. C. Reid and R. H. Carpenter

TABLE 1. LIST BY COUNTY, ACRES, SQUARE MILES, AND PERCENT OF STATE UNDERLAIN BY ULTRAMAFIC AND MAFIC ROCK UNITS SHOWN ON THE 1985 GEOLOGIC MAP OF NORTH CAROLINA

Geologic Location	Rock Type	Symbol	Alamance	Alexander	Alleghany	Ashe	Avery	Buncombe	Burke	Cabarrus	Caldwell
Inner Piedmont, etc.	Amphibolite, etc.	CZab		12259.4					5465.8		
Murphy belt	Amphibolite	CZam									
Inner Piedmont, etc.	Amphibolite	CZma1									
Charlotte/Milton belts	Mafic metavolcanic	CZmv	21987.1								
Charlotte/Milton belts	Meta-gabbro and diorite	PzZg	47726.4								
Carolina State Belt	Meta-mafic rock	PzZm								18746.7	
Blue Ridge Belt	Meta-ultramafic	PzZu			395.0	4240.3	42.6	719.5	308.8		250.2
Blue Ridge Belt	Amphibolite	Ybam									
Blue Ridge Belt	Amphibolite	Yman									
Blue Ridge Belt	Amphibolite	Zaba					44.9				
Blue Ridge Belt	Amphibolite	Zata			8066.1	58429.0	13904.5				
Blue Ridge Belt	Greenstone	Zgmg					4886.3		247.3		688.3
Blue Ridge Belt	Amphibolite	ZYba									
Totals	**Acres**		69713.5	12259.4	8461.1	62669.3	19278.3	719.5	6021.9	18746.7	938.5
	Square miles		108.9	19.2	13.2	97.9	30.1	1.1	9.4	29.3	1.5
	Percent of state		0.2	0.04	0.03	0.20	0.06	0.00	0.02	0.06	0.00

Geologic Location	Rock Type	Symbol	Caswell	Catawaba	Chatham	Cherokee	Clay	Davidson	Davie	Durham	Forsyth
Inner Piedmont, etc.	Amphibolite, etc.	CZab		88489.5							
Murphy belt	Amphibolite	CZam									
Inner Piedmont, etc.	Amphibolite	CZma1				151.8					
Charlotte/Milton belts	Mafic metavolcanic	CZmv	8456.2		29233.0			3428.9			
Charlotte/Milton belts	Meta-gabbro and diorite	PzZg	35033.7		477.6			7500.6			
Carolina State Belt	Meta-mafic rock	PzZm	987.6					35577.5		1847.3	
Blue Ridge Belt	Meta-ultramafic	PzZu		1843.8			804.9		60892.9		16626.9
Blue Ridge Belt	Amphibolite	Ybam									
Blue Ridge Belt	Amphibolite	Yman				10219.0	434.5				
Blue Ridge Belt	Amphibolite	Zaba									
Blue Ridge Belt	Amphibolite	Zata									
Blue Ridge Belt	Greenstone	Zgmg									
Blue Ridge Belt	Amphibolite	ZYba					5493.5				
Totals	**Acres**		44477.5	90333.3	29710.6	10370.8	6732.9	46507.0	60892.9	1847.3	16626.9
	Square miles		69.5	141.1	46.4	16.2	10.5	72.7	95.1	2.9	26.0
	Percent of state		0.14	0.29	0.10	0.03	0.02	0.15	0.20	0.01	0.05

TABLE 1. LIST BY COUNTY, ACRES, SQUARE MILES, AND PERCENT OF STATE UNDERLAIN BY ULTRAMAFIC AND MAFIC ROCK UNITS SHOWN ON THE 1985 GEOLOGIC MAP OF NORTH CAROLINA (continued - page 2)

Geologic Location	Rock Type	Symbol	County								
			Franklin	Gaston	Granville	Guilford	Halifax	Haywood	Henderson	Iredell	Jackson
Inner Piedmont, etc.	Amphibolite, etc.	CZab		2848.4					2131.5	91238.6	
Murphy belt	Amphibolite	CZam	2497.3		79.3					611.2	
Inner Piedmont, etc.	Amphibolite	CZma1									
Charlotte/Milton belts	Mafic metavolcanic	CZmv				15012.9	6833.7			7438.5	
Charlotte/Milton belts	Meta-gabbro and diorite	PzZg			27592.9	53414.6					
Carolina State Belt	Meta-mafic rock	PzZm								5166.1	
Blue Ridge Belt	Meta-ultramafic	PzZu			876.6	233.4	215.6	151.7		4469.8	2620.7
Blue Ridge Belt	Amphibolite	Ybam									
Blue Ridge Belt	Amphibolite	Yman									
Blue Ridge Belt	Amphibolite	Zaba									
Blue Ridge Belt	Amphibolite	Zata									4870.0
Blue Ridge Belt	Greenstone	Zgmg									
Blue Ridge Belt	Amphibolite	ZYba									
Totals		**Acres**	2497.3	2848.4	28548.8	68660.9	7049.3	151.7	2131.5	108924.2	7490.7
		Square miles	3.9	4.5	44.6	107.3	11.0	0.2	3.3	170.2	11.7
		Percent of state	0.01	0.01	0.09	0.22	0.02	0.00	0.01	0.35	0.02

Geologic Location	Rock Type	Symbol	County								
			Johnston	Lincoln	Macon	Madison	McDowell	Mecklenburg	Mitchell	Montgomery	Moore
Inner Piedmont, etc.	Amphibolite, etc.	CZab		34397.4			14505.9				
Murphy belt	Amphibolite	CZam	144.7								
Inner Piedmont, etc.	Amphibolite	CZma1									
Charlotte/Milton belts	Mafic metavolcanic	CZmv								1308.1	562.9
Charlotte/Milton belts	Meta-gabbro and diorite	PzZg									
Carolina State Belt	Meta-mafic rock	PzZm						28663.4			
Blue Ridge Belt	Meta-ultramafic	PzZu			523.8	243.7	78.2				
Blue Ridge Belt	Amphibolite	Ybam				1441.6			155.9		
Blue Ridge Belt	Amphibolite	Yman			349.6						
Blue Ridge Belt	Amphibolite	Zaba									
Blue Ridge Belt	Amphibolite	Zata			1751.5		1138.7		10022.9		
Blue Ridge Belt	Greenstone	Zgmg							16188.5		
Blue Ridge Belt	Amphibolite	ZYba									
Totals		**Acres**	144.7	34397.4	2624.9	1685.3	15722.8	28663.4	26367.3	1308.1	562.9
		Square miles	0.2	53.7	4.1	2.6	24.6	44.8	41.2	2.0	0.9
		Percent of state	0.00	0.11	0.01	0.01	0.05	0.09	0.08	0.00	0.00

TABLE 1. LIST BY COUNTY, ACRES, SQUARE MILES, AND PERCENT OF STATE UNDERLAIN BY ULTRAMAFIC AND MAFIC ROCK UNITS SHOWN ON THE 1985 GEOLOGIC MAP OF NORTH CAROLINA (continued - page 3)

Geologic Location	Rock Type	Symbol	Nash	Orange	Person	Polk	County Randolph	Rockingham	Rowan	Rutherford	Stanley
Inner Piedmont, etc.	Amphibolite, etc.	CZab								43106.3	
Murphy belt	Amphibolite	CZam				0.6		729.0			
Inner Piedmont, etc.	Amphibolite	CZma1									
Charlotte/Milton belts	Mafic metavolcanic	CZmv	6584.9	3329.2				5702.5			5934.4
Charlotte/Milton belts	Meta-gabbro and diorite	PzZg		44768.2	23084.5		25204.1		1135.1		
Carolina State Belt	Meta-mafic rock	PzZm					9942.8		36483.8		
Blue Ridge Belt	Meta-ultramafic	PzZu							148.0		
Blue Ridge Belt	Amphibolite	Ybam									
Blue Ridge Belt	Amphibolite	Yman									
Blue Ridge Belt	Amphibolite	Zaba									
Blue Ridge Belt	Amphibolite	Zata									
Blue Ridge Belt	Greenstone	Zgmg									
Blue Ridge Belt	Amphibolite	ZYba									
Totals	**Acres**		6584.9	48097.4	23084.5	0.6	35146.9	6431.5	37766.9	43106.3	5934.4
	Square miles		10.3	75.2	36.1	0.0	54.9	10.0	59.0	67.4	9.3
	Percent of state		0.02	0.15	0.07	0.00	0.11	0.02	0.12	0.14	0.02

Geologic Location	Rock Type	Symbol	Stokes	Surry	Swain	Transylvania	County Union	Wake	Warren	Watuga	Wilkes
Inner Piedmont, etc.	Amphibolite, etc.	CZab									
Murphy belt	Amphibolite	CZam	4799.5	3365.5	379.7			8487.8	2669.4		
Inner Piedmont, etc.	Amphibolite	CZma1									
Charlotte/Milton belts	Mafic metavolcanic	CZmv						5821.3			
Charlotte/Milton belts	Meta-gabbro and diorite	PzZg									
Carolina State Belt	Meta-mafic rock	PzZm					5908.3				
Blue Ridge Belt	Meta-ultramafic	PzZu						1755.6			119.7
Blue Ridge Belt	Amphibolite	Ybam									
Blue Ridge Belt	Amphibolite	Yman				170.5					
Blue Ridge Belt	Amphibolite	Zaba		128.8	633.9						
Blue Ridge Belt	Amphibolite	Zata				6325.4				535.3	
Blue Ridge Belt	Greenstone	Zgmg								28154.7	3420.1
Blue Ridge Belt	Amphibolite	ZYba								4252.2	
Totals	**Acres**		4799.5	3494.3	1013.6	6495.9	5908.3	16064.7	2669.4	32942.2	3539.8
	Square miles		7.5	5.5	1.6	10.1	9.2	25.1	4.2	51.5	5.5
	Percent of state		0.02	0.01	0.00	0.02	0.02	0.05	0.01	0.11	0.01

TABLE 1. LIST BY COUNTY, ACRES, SQUARE MILES, AND PERCENT OF STATE UNDERLAIN BY ULTRAMAFIC AND MAFIC ROCK UNITS SHOWN ON THE 1985 GEOLOGIC MAP OF NORTH CAROLINA (continued - page 4)

Geologic Location	Rock Type	Symbol	County Yadkin	County Yancey	Statewide Totals Acres	Statewide Totals Square Miles	Statewide Totals Percent of State
Inner Piedmont, etc.	Amphibolite, etc.	CZab			294443.4	460.1	0.95
Murphy belt	Amphibolite	CZam	949.8		24865.0	38.9	0.08
Inner Piedmont, etc	Amphibolite	CZma1			0.0	0.0	0.00
Charlotte/Milton belts	Mafic metavolcanic	CZmv			141016.4	220.3	0.45
Charlotte/Milton belts	Meta-gabbro and diorite	PzZg	1714.5		260059.5	406.3	0.83
Carolina State Belt	Meta-mafic rock	PzZm	8236.7		216302.3	338.0	0.69
Blue Ridge Belt	Meta-ultramafic	PzZu		272.5	21628.4	33.8	0.07
Blue Ridge Belt	Amphibolite	Ybam			1441.6	2.3	0.00
Blue Ridge Belt	Amphibolite	Yman			11637.0	18.2	0.04
Blue Ridge Belt	Amphibolite	Zaba		261.3	15952.0	24.9	0.05
Blue Ridge Belt	Amphibolite	Zata		5620.8	143310.5	223.9	0.46
Blue Ridge Belt	Greenstone	Zgmg			10074.1	15.7	0.03
Blue Ridge Belt	Amphibolite	ZYba			5493.5	8.6	0.02
Totals		**Acres**	10901.0	6154.6	1146223.7		
		Square miles	17.0	9.6		1791.0	
		Percent of state	0.03	0.02			3.7

its source water, or due to corrosion of asbestos cement pipe, or both, it may apply to the State for a waiver of the monitoring requirement in paragraph (b)(1) of §141.23. If the State grants the waiver, the system is not required to monitor" (emphasis added).

Section §141.23(5)(b)(3) permits the State to grant a waiver based on the consideration of the following factor (§141.23 (5)(b)(3)(i)): "*potential asbestos contamination of the water source . . .*" (emphasis added). Section §141.23(5)(b)(4) provides that the waiver remains in effect until completion of the three-year compliance period, *but systems that do not receive a waiver must monitor in compliance with §141.23(5)(b)(1)* (emphasis added).

Two other provisions apply. In the case where a public water supply system is "vulnerable to asbestos contamination due solely to source water" the system must monitor in accordance with section §141.23 (a) (Federal Register, 1991, p. 3579–3580). The other case is: "a system vulnerable to asbestos contamination due both to its source water supply and corrosion of asbestos cement pipe shall *take one sample at a tap* served by asbestos cement pipe and under conditions where the *asbestos contamination is most likely to occur*" (emphasis added) (Federal Register, 1991, §141.23 (b)(7), p. 3580).

Regulatory definition of asbestos

On June 8, 1992, the Occupational Safety and Health Administration (OSHA) lifted their Administrative Stay and ". . . amends the revised asbestos standards to remove nonasbestiform tremolite, anthophyllite and actinolite from their scope" (Federal Register, 1992, p. 24310). However EPA's decision did not address the issue of confused fiber definition and test procedure. Left unaddressed are what nonasbestiform minerals may be regulated that are not now subject to the asbestos standard. Such minerals include fibrous aluminum silicates (andalusite and sillimanite) and kyanite (a bladed aluminum silicate mineral).

The EPA's drinking water standards do not define asbestos. Discussion of the inorganic MCLSs was based on the "administration to rats of intermediate, (>1μ micrometer range) size chrysotile fibers." However, the EPA's "Drinking Water Criteria Document for Asbestos" (U.S. Environmental Protection Agency, April 1988) contains similar language to that used by OSHA for defining asbestos as discussed above.

REFERENCES CITED

Carpenter, R. H., and Reid, J. C., 1994, Asbestos monitoring and regulation in drinking water supplies: Geological Society of America Abstracts with Programs (Seattle), p. A-386.

Conrad, S. G., Wilson, W. F., Allen, E. P., and Wright, T. J., 1963, Anthophyllite asbestos in North Carolina: Raleigh, North Carolina Geological Survey Bulletin 77, 61 p.

Federal Register, Wednesday, January 30, 1991, Part II, Environmental Protection Agency, 40 CFR Parts 141, 142, and 143, National primary drinking water regulations, Final Rule, p. 3526–3597.

Federal Register, Monday, June 8, 1992, Occupational exposure to asbestos, tremolite, anthophyllite and actinolite, v. 57, No. 110, p. 24310–24331.

Lamarche, R. Y., 1981, Geology and genesis of the chrysotile asbestos deposits of northern Appalachia, *in* Riodon, P. H., ed., Geology of asbestos deposits: New York, New York, Society of Mining Engineers, p. 11–23.

Levy, B. S., Sigurdson, E., Mandel, J., Laudon, E., and Pearson, J., 1976, Investigation possible effects of asbestos in city water: Surveillance of gastrointestinal cancer incidence in Duluth, Minnesota: American Journal of Epidemiology, v. 103, no. 4, p. 362–368.

North Carolina Geological Survey, 1985, Geologic map of North Carolina: North Carolina Geological Survey, scale 1: 500,000, color.

North Carolina Geological Survey, 1988, Preliminary explanatory text for the 1985 Geologic Map of North Carolina: North Carolina Geological Survey, Contractual Report 88-1, November 4, 1988, 271 p. (unpublished).

Pratt, J. H., and Lewis, J. H., 1905, Volume I: Corundum and the peridotites of western North Carolina, North Carolina Geological Survey, 464 p.

Toft, P., Meek, M. E., Wigle, D. T., and Meranger, N. O., 1984, Asbestos in drinking water: Canadian Research Council, Critical Reviews in Environmental Control, v. 14, Issue 1, p. 151–97.

U.S. Environmental Protection Agency, April 1988 (March 1985), Drinking water criteria document for asbestos: Cincinnati, Ohio, U.S. Environmental Protection Agency, ECAO, 190 p.

Van Baalen, M. R., 1995, Chrysotile asbestos in public water systems: Hazardous or not?: Geological Society of America, Abstracts with Programs, v. 27, no. 6, p. A–233.

Virta, R. L., and Mann, E. L., 1994, Asbestos, *in* Carr, D. D., and 14 others, eds., Industrial minerals and rocks (sixth edition): Littleton, Colorado, Society for Mining, Metallurgy, and Exploration, Inc., p. 97–124.

MANUSCRIPT ACCEPTED BY THE SOCIETY JUNE 5, 1997

Printed in U.S.A.

Geological Society of America
Reviews in Engineering Geology, Volume XII
1998

Evaluating debris-flow hazards in Davis County, Utah: Engineering versus geological approaches

Jeffrey R. Keaton
AGRA Earth & Environmental, Inc., 3232 West Virginia Avenue, Phoenix, Arizona 85009-1502
Mike Lowe
Utah Geological Survey, 1594 West North Temple, Salt Lake City, Utah 84114-6100

ABSTRACT

Widespread debris-flow damage occurred in northern Utah intermittently between 1912 and the spring of 1983. The worst damage in 1983 was at the mouth of Rudd Creek, a canyon that previously had not generated significant debris flows in historical time. Floodlike damage extended well outside federally mapped flood-plain boundaries. Debris basins built in the 1930s were refurbished, and new basins, at a cost about $1.1 million each, were constructed at the mouths of some canyons that produced debris flows in 1983.

Engineering analyses, assuming that the 1983 Rudd Creek debris flow was the 100-year event, used observed characteristics (debris volume, depth distribution, time to peak discharge, speed of debris advance, and duration of discharge) to construct an inflow hydrograph for use with a finite-element grid network, alluvial-fan slope values for the Rudd Creek fan, and debris-flow fluid properties. The viscosity of the fluid was varied until the 1983 debris-flow characteristics on the Rudd Creek fan were obtained. Debris production rates normalized to drainage-basin area for Wasatch Front canyons were used to estimate 100-year debris-flow volumes from other canyons in Davis County. The finite-element grid, input hydrograph shape, and debris-flow fluid properties from Rudd Canyon were used with canyon-specific fan slopes to redefine the 100-year flood plains at the other canyons. Large urbanized areas were found to be within the newly defined flood plains, and nearly all debris basins were too small to protect against the predicted 100-year sediment discharges.

Studies of the structural fabric, hydrogeology, stream channels, and landslides within canyon watersheds, and the stratigraphy and geomorphology of alluvial fans, indicate major debris flows in Davis County are rare geological events. The majority of alluvial-fan building appears to have occurred during the early Holocene when much ice-age sediment was available in the Wasatch Range. The alluvial fans are small landforms and most historical debris-flow sediment came from stream channels. Debris production and accumulation in channels is a slow, intermittent process, and channels having historical sediment discharges cannot produce large flows again until the drainages have been recharged.

Approximately $12 million were spent in 1983 in Davis County to build or refurbish debris basins; fewer than approximately $50,000 were spent on a rapid, regional assessment of debris-flow hazards along the Wasatch Front in Davis and Weber Counties and parts of Salt Lake and Box Elder Counties. Had geologic studies to

Keaton, J. R., and Lowe, M., 1998, Evaluating debris-flow hazards in Davis County, Utah: Engineering versus geological approaches, *in* Welby, C. W., and Gowan, M. E., eds., A Paradox of Power: Voices of Warning and Reason in the Geosciences: Boulder, Colorado, Geological Society of America Reviews in Engineering Geology, v. XII.

understand the debris-flow processes been conducted before the debris basins were built, more emphasis would have been placed on canyons without historical debris flows, tempering the engineering approach that may have overestimated the 100-year-frequency debris-flow volumes.

INTRODUCTION

Debris flows, transitional flows, hyperconcentrated sediment flows (debris floods), and clear-water flooding form a continuum of sediment/water mixtures that present hazards to development on alluvial fans (Fig. 1; Wieczorek, 1986; Keaton et al., 1988a, b). Debris flows may be initiated by (1) landslides reaching flowing streams, or (2) erosion during cloudburst rainstorms. Once a debris flow is initiated, saturated stream-channel sediment may liquefy in response to the rapidly applied stress of an advancing debris-flow lobe and be incorporated into the flowing debris.

Debris flows and debris floods have occurred often in Davis County (Fig. 2) during historical time and have caused loss of life and significant damage to property. Debris-flow hazards in Davis County have been studied, using both engineering and geological approaches, since the early 1920s. Conclusions regarding the magnitude of debris-flow hazards reached using geological approaches are substantially different from those based on engineering hydrology and hydraulics.

GEOGRAPHIC AND GEOLOGIC SETTING

Davis County (Fig. 2) is in north-central Utah at the boundary between the Basin and Range Province, which includes the Great Salt Lake basin in the western portion of the county, and the Middle Rocky Mountains, which includes the Wasatch Range in the eastern portion of the county (Stokes, 1977). The Weber segment of the Wasatch fault zone runs along the foothills of the mountains, separating the physiographic provinces. Thurston Peak, elevation 2,959 m (9,707 ft), rises approximately 1,676 m (5,500 ft) above the level of the Great Salt Lake, which fluctuates around 1,280 m (4,200 ft) in elevation.

The Great Salt Lake basin is a structural trough filled with unconsolidated sediments of predominantly lacustrine and alluvial origin and semiconsolidated sedimentary and volcanic rocks that exceeds 3,000 m (9,850 ft) in thickness in Davis County (Mabey, 1992). The lacustrine sediments were deposited during periods when lakes occupied the Great Salt Lake basin, including Lake Bonneville between approximately 28,000 and 13,000 yr B.P. (Currey, 1990; Oviatt et al., 1992). The Bonneville shoreline, at an elevation of about 1,579 m (5,180 ft), marks the highest level reached by Lake Bonneville (about 15,000 yr B.P.; Currey and Oviatt, 1985). Alluvial processes in the basin dominate during interlacustrine periods, including approximately the past 13,000 years.

Bedrock in the Wasatch Range in Davis County is predominantly Precambrian Farmington Canyon Complex that consists of schist, gneiss, quartzite, and migmitite with some pegmatite

and amphibolite (Bryant, 1984, 1988). Other bedrock units that crop out in southeastern Davis County include the Cambrian Maxfield Limestone, Ophir Formation (shale and limestone), and Tintic Quartzite; the Devonian Stansbury Formation (sandstone and dolomite) and Pinyon Peak Limestone; the Mississippian Deseret and Gardison limestones; and Tertiary conglomerates (Bryant, 1984, 1988). These bedrock units have been folded and are cut by numerous thrust and normal faults (Bell, 1952). Areas of colluvium overlying the bedrock units are more common than bedrock outcrops and may exceed 9 m (30 ft) in thickness. Many debris slides have occurred in this colluvium (Pack, 1984, 1985). The canyons discussed in this paper have been eroded into bedrock of the Farmington Canyon Complex only.

Three types of canyons are present in the Wasatch Range: through-going canyons, full canyons, and half canyons. The only through-going canyon in Davis County is the Weber River canyon at the northeastern county boundary. Full canyons are those that extend from the crest of the Wasatch Range, which is the eastern county boundary. Half canyons are those that originate below the crest of the Wasatch Range. Table 1 contains selected data for canyons in Davis County.

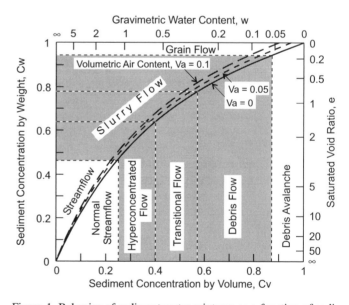

Figure 1. Behavior of sediment-water mixtures as a function of sediment concentration (modified from Wieczorek, 1986, p. 220; and Keaton, 1988, p. 17 and 73). Theoretical relationship between sedimentation concentration by weight and by volume are shown for sediment with a specific gravity of 2.65 and volumetric air (va) contents of 0, 0.05, and 0.10. Also shown are gravimetric water content and void ratio at saturation (air content = 0).

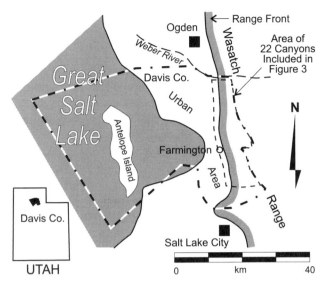

Figure 2. Location of selected features in Davis County, Utah.

TABLE 1. SELECTED DATA FROM 22 CANYONS IN DAVIS COUNTY*

Canyon	Size[†]	Basin Order	Basin Area (km²)	Basin Length (m)	Basin Relief (m)	Relief Ratio
Corbett	F	3	3.233	4,115	1,270	0.309
Hobbs	H	3	3.115	3,764	1,113	0.296
Lightning	H	2	0.547	1,920	689	0.359
Kays (Middle)	F	4	4.238	4,450	1,337	0.300
Kays (South)	F	4	4.491	4,450	1,392	0.313
Snow	H	3	2.022	3,719	1,244	0.334
Adams	F	4	5.485	4,907	1,435	0.292
Webb	F	5	6.465	4,877	1,375	0.282
Baer	F	4	8.502	5,304	1,435	0.271
Half	H	2	1.090	2,438	896	0.368
Shepard	F	3	5.958	4,892	1,370	0.280
Farmington	F	5	27.145	10,119	1,438	0.142
Rudd	H	3	1.781	3,307	1,146	0.347
Steed	F	4	6.706	5,029	1,435	0.285
Davis	F	4	4.283	4,968	1,414	0.285
Halfway	H	3	1.627	3,658	1,079	0.295
Ricks	F	4	6.341	5,395	1,451	0.269
Barnard	H	4	3.730	5,334	1,318	0.247
Parrish	F	4	5.452	5,883	1,342	0.228
Centerville	F	4	8.148	6,401	1,291	0.202
Buckland	H	3	2.436	4,511	843	0.187
Ward	F	5	11.302	6,126	1,221	0.199

*Modified from Keaton, 1988, 1995; basin order is by Strahler's method, 1952; relief ratio (nominal basin slope) is basin relief divided by basin length.
[†]F = full canyon; H = half canyon.

Davis County is a relatively small county with an area of about 1,635 km² (1,016 mi²) and a 1990 population of about 188,000. It is an area of increasing urbanization because of its proximity to Salt Lake City and Ogden (Fig. 2). About 57% of the county's area is the Great Salt Lake, and about 21% is state or federal land, leaving 22% available for urban development (Keaton, 1995). Little urban development in Davis County is located above the Bonneville shoreline because of local development ordinances and National Forest boundaries or within about 6 m (20 ft) of the level of Great Salt Lake because of shallow ground water. Thus, much of the urban development in Davis County is along a narrow strip at the mouths of Wasatch Range canyons. Alluvial-fan deposits overlying lake deposits at the mouths of these canyons are younger than approximately 15,000 years old.

HISTORICAL DEBRIS-FLOW AND DEBRIS-FLOOD EVENTS

Davis County residents periodically have been impacted by debris flows and debris floods since the first settlers arrived in 1847 in what is now Davis County. Most of the early development in Davis County was on mountain-front alluvial fans where water was more accessible and field stones (debris-flow boulders), commonly used for construction, were generally available.

The first reported alluvial-fan sedimentation event, in "1860 or 1861," was considered to be beneficial at the time by the local residents and "has become part of local legend" (Keate, 1991, p. 9). According to the legend, pioneers in Farmington wanted to build a new chapel from stone, but were unable to get the rock material out of a nearby canyon. The pioneers reportedly held prayer meetings to help them find a solution (Keate, 1991). "Shortly" after the prayer meetings a "flood" deposited a "large number of rocks" that were used to construct the chapel (Keate,

1991, p. 9). The description of this event illustrates the difficulty in categorizing some of the earlier alluvial-fan flooding and sedimentation events as either debris flows or debris floods. Keate (1991) concludes that the event in 1860 or 1861 probably was from Rudd Canyon; however, the flood histories of Farmington Canyon, a short distance to the north of Rudd Canyon, and Steed Canyon, a short distance to the south of Rudd Canyon, suggest that the event could have been from either of these canyons, which are still close enough to Farmington to have provided a source of rocks to construct the chapel.

A total of 78 alluvial-fan flooding and sedimentation events have been reported in Davis County since settlement in 1847 (Woolley, 1946; Butler and Marsell, 1972; Keaton, 1988), with 56 events having sufficient information to permit the volumes of discharged sediment to be estimated (Keaton, 1988). The earliest major historical event, probably a debris flow, was generated on July 23, 1878, from Farmington and Davis Canyons by a cloudburst rainstorm (Woolley, 1946; Keaton, 1988; Keate, 1991). Forty of the major alluvial-fan-flooding and sedimentation events were caused by cloudburst rainstorms whereas 16 were initiated by landslides caused by rapid snowmelt (Woolley, 1946; Croft, 1967; Butler and Marsell, 1972; Anderson et al., 1984; Lindskov, 1984; Keaton, 1988). The most severe and damaging sedimentation events occurred in response to cloudburst rainstorms in 1912, 1923, and 1930, and in response to landslides caused by rapid snowmelt in 1983 (Woolley, 1946; Keaton, 1995). The temporal distribution of flood events for each of 22 drainage basins comprising Keaton's (1988) study area is shown on Figure 3. Selected data for these canyons are presented in Table 1, whereas estimated volumes of historical sediment discharge from the 22 drainage basins are presented in Table 2.

Events of 1923

The damage caused by the flood and debris-flow events of August 12 and 13, 1923, contrasts sharply with the beneficial nature of the flood of 1860 or 1861. The debris flows, generated by erosion during a westward-moving cloudburst rainstorm that began on Sunday evening, August 12, issued from South Fork Kays, Baer, Farmington, Steed, Davis, and Ricks (Ford) Canyons (Woolley, 1946; Keaton, 1988; Keate, 1991; Fig. 3). The events from Farmington, Steed, Davis, and Ricks Canyons are discussed below.

Farmington Canyon. Seven people died, one due to a heart attack, in the August 12, 1923, Farmington Canyon event, the most disastrous flood in Utah history (Lowe et al., 1992). A loud roar, the sound of rushing water and large boulders clashing together, could be heard coming from Farmington Canyon before about 8 p.m.; the source of the sound reached the canyon mouth soon afterward, less than 15 minutes after rain began falling in town (Keate, 1991). Observers reported the flood water coming

out of Farmington Canyon to be about 9 m (30 ft) high (Keate, 1991) and 60 m (200 ft) wide. As the moving debris came into view, an unnamed eyewitness observed sparks created by boulders clashing together in the nose area of the debris flow (Croft, 1981).

The flood inundated many campers near the mouth of the canyon, causing most of the fatalities (Keate, 1991). Significant damage occurred to a number of homes, the Farmington Canyon road, an electrical power station, irrigation canals, crops, water systems, and telephone lines. The state highway at Farmington, about 900 m (3,000 ft) west of the canyon mouth, was covered with 6 m (20 ft) of debris for a distance of about 3.2 km (2 mi; Keate, 1991). Keaton et al. (1988b) estimated debris-flow volumes on the basis of damage descriptions or proportion to other canyons where flood events occurred in the same years. Croft (1967) provided information on total sediment delivery between 1923 and 1947. The total volume deposited by the 1923 debris-flow event from Farmington Canyon is estimated at 528,000 m³ (691,000 yd³; Keaton et al., 1988b).

Steed and Davis Canyons. Steed and Davis Canyons also produced debris flows as a result of the August 12, 1923, cloudburst rainstorm. Because of sparse development in this area in 1923, little damage occurred and few reports were made on the nature of the debris-flow events (Keate, 1991). One house damaged by the Davis Canyon debris flow is shown on Figure 4. Crops, irrigation systems, and telephone lines were also damaged. The deposits from the event blocked the highway, located about 600 m (2,000 ft) west of the mouth of Steed Canyon and about

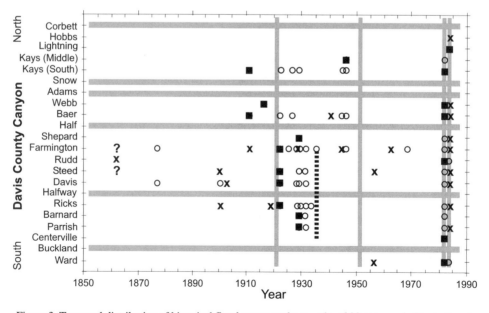

Figure 3. Temporal distribution of historical flood events at the mouths of 22 canyons in Davis County, Utah. Modified from Keaton (1988, 1995). Solid square symbols denote flood events with the largest estimated sediment volume. Open circle symbols denote flood events with estimated sediment volume. X symbols denote flood events with no estimated volumes. ? symbols at Farmington and Steed in 1860 or 1861 denote uncertainty in the report that a flood event occurred in Rudd Canyon. Horizontal shaded lines denote canyons without reported historical floods. Vertical shaded lines at 1922, 1952, 1983, and 1984 denote years with major snowmelt floods. Vertical line at 1935 from Farmington to Centerville denotes construction of contour trenches in these watersheds.

TABLE 2. SUMMARY OF HISTORIC FLOOD EVENTS FROM 22 CANYONS IN DAVIS COUNTY FROM 1847 TO 1995*

Canyon	Year	Estimated Volume (m³)	Normalized Volume† (m³/km²)	$\frac{V§}{V_o}$	$\frac{V**}{V_{max}}$	Canyon	Year	Estimated Volume (m³)	Normalized Volume† (m³/km²)	$\frac{V§}{V_o}$	$\frac{V**}{V_{max}}$
Corbett	None					Rudd	1860?	n.d.	n.d.	n.d.	n.d.
Hobbs	1984	n.d.					1983	68,000	38,181	1.0	1.0
Lightning	1984	9,000	16,453	1.0	1.0		1984	1,350	758	0.02	0.02
Kays (Middle)	1947	1,000	236	1.0	1.0	Steed	1860?	n.d.	n.d.	n.d.	n.d.
	1983	500	118	0.5	0.5		1901	n.d.	n.d.	n.d.	n.d.
Kays (South)	1912	51,000	11,356	1.0	1.0		1923	155,200	23,293	1.0	1.0
	1923	1,500	334	0.03	0.03		1930	53,000	7,903	0.34	0.34
	1927	1,200	267	0.02	0.02		1932	26,300	3,922	0.17	0.17
	1930	19,000	4,231	0.37	0.37		1957	n.d.	n.d.	n.d.	n.d.
	1945	1,000	223	0.02	0.02		1983	16,000	2,386	0.1	0.1
	1947	16,000	3,563	0.31	0.31		1984	n.d.	n.d.	n.d.	n.d.
	1983	500	111	0.01	0.01	Davis	1878	6,000	1,401	1.0	0.05
Snow	None						1901	16,000	3,736	2.67	0.14
Adams	None						1903	n.d.	n.d.	n.d.	n.d.
Webb	1917	2,500	387	1.0	1.0		1923	112,400	26,243	18.73	1.0
	1983	500	77	0.2	0.2		1929	12,000	2,802	2.0	0.11
	1984	n.d.	n.d.	n.d.	n.d.		1930	20,700	4,833	3.45	0.18
Baer	1912	51,000	5,999	1.0	1.0		1932	8,700	2,031	1.45	0.08
	1923	39,700	4,669	0.78	0.78		1983	500	117	0.08	0.00
	1927	12,000	1,411	0.24	0.24		1984	n.d.	n.d.	n.d.	n.d.
	1941	n.d.	n.d.	n.d.	n.d.	Halfway	None				
	1945	24,000	2,823	0.47	0.47	Ricks	1901	n.d.	n.d.	n.d.	n.d.
	1947	32,500	3,823	0.64	0.64		1923	72,000	11,355	1.0	0.72
	1983	2,400	282	0.05	0.05		1929	n.d.	n.d.	n.d.	n.d
	1984	n.d.	n.d.	n.d.	n.d.		1930	100,000	15,770	1.39	1.0
Half	None						1932	34,000	5,362	0.47	0.34
Shepard	1930	10,000	1,678	1.0	1.0		1934	22,000	3,469	0.31	0.22
	1983	5,000	839	0.5	0.5		1983	8,000	1,262	0.11	0.08
	1984	n.d.	n.d.	n.d.	n.d.		1984	n.d.	n.d.	n.d.	n.d.
Farmington	1860?	n.d.	n.d.	n.d.	n.d.	Barnard	1930	43,300	11,609	1.0	1.0
	1878	100,000	3,684	1.0	0.19		1932	21,600	5,791	0.5	0.5
	1912	n.d.	n.d.	n.d.	n.d.		1983	9,700	2,601	0.22	0.22
	1923	528,000	19,451	5.28	1.0	Parrish	1930	402,000	73,734	1.0	1.0
	1926	31,000	1,142	0.31	0.06		1932	33,000	6,053	0.08	0.08
	1929	40,000	1,474	0.4	0.08		1983	1,600	2,935	0.04	0.04
	1930	n.d.	n.d.	n.d.	n.d.		1984	n.d.	n.d.	n.d.	n.d.
	1931	61,700	2,273	0.62	0.12	Centerville	1983	2,000	245	1.0	1.0
	1932	29,400	1,083	0.29	0.06	Buckland	None				
	1936	23,100	851	0.23	0.04	Ward	1957	n.d.	n.d.	n.d.	n.d.
	1945	n.d.	n.d.	n.d.	n.d.		1983	15,500	1,371	1.0	1.0
	1947	10,000	368	0.1	0.02		1984	n.d.	n.d.	n.d.	n.d.
	1963	n.d.	n.d.	n.d.	n.d.						
	1969	16,000	589	0.16	0.03						
	1983	20,000	737	0.2	0.04						
	1984	n.d.	n.d.	n.d.	n.d.						

*Modified from Keaton, 1988.
†Drainage-basin area from Table 1.
§V_o is the volume of the earliest historic event in the canyon with an estimated volume.
**V_{max} is the volume of the largest historic event in the canyon.

300 m (1,000 ft) west of the mouth of Davis Canyon, for about two weeks (Keate, 1991). The total volume of debris deposited by the Steed Canyon event is estimated at 156,200 m³ (204,000 yd³); the total volume of debris deposited by the Davis Canyon event is estimated at 112,400 m³ (147,000 yd³; Keaton et al., 1988b).

Ricks (Ford) Canyon. The 1923 Ricks Creek debris flow, also generated by the August 12 cloudburst rainstorm, caused a great deal of property damage. Several homes were destroyed,

the highway was blocked at a location approximately 600 m (2,000 ft) west of the canyon mouth, and railroad tracks were buried at a location approximately 1,100 m (3,600 ft) west of the canyon mouth (Keate, 1991). Crops, irrigation systems, and telephone lines were also damaged. Two people were killed in an accident during cleanup of the debris (Keate, 1991), which is estimated to have had a total volume of about 72,000 m³ (94,000 yd³; Keaton et al., 1988b).

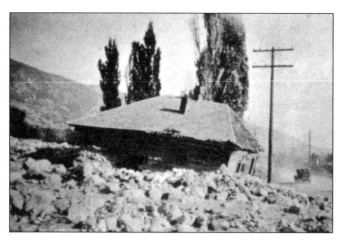

Figure 4. House damaged by the 1923 Davis Canyon debris flow (from Marston, 1958).

Observations and conclusions following the 1923 events

J. Cecil Alter, meteorologist with the Salt Lake Weather Bureau, surveyed the Farmington Canyon watershed following the debris-flow event (Keate, 1991). He believed that rainfall on slopes near the head of the canyon, denuded of vegetation by recent forest fires, produced the debris flow. He observed that the debris flow likely moved down the canyon in a series of "relays" (pulses) as the debris periodically formed dams that were subsequently breached (Keate, 1991, p. 28). He also noted that the stream channel had been "swept clean" and estimated that it would be "twenty five years before accumulated deposits could cause another flood" (Keate, 1991, p. 28).

The earliest scientific discussion of sedimentation events in Davis County was prepared by Pack (1923), who described the flowing debris and deposits from the 1923 events. He also noted that much debris and vegetation had been removed from the channel and channel margins, and, based on the size of the boulders in the flows (up to "hundreds of tons"), determined that "water was not the transporting agent" (Keate, 1991, p. 29).

Paul and Baker (1925) also discussed the floods of 1923, but focused more on the source of sediment in the mountains. They comment on the contribution of overgrazing and "an extensive burn" on steep slopes in Steed Canyon southeast of Farmington (Keaton, 1995, p. 187). They also note that Rudd Canyon, adjacent to the north side of Steed Canyon, was exposed to the same rainfall as Steed and Farmington Canyons; however, erosion from Rudd Canyon was insignificant because it was protected by vegetation (Paul and Baker, 1925).

Government response following events of 1923

Utah Governor Charles R. Mabey issued a proclamation on August 14, 1923, asking the people of Utah to give aid to Davis County residents impacted by the disaster (Keate, 1991). This resulted in both financial donations and citizen volunteers to aid

in the cleanup. In addition, 20 men from the 145th Field Artillery, Utah National Guard, were sent to Farmington to help carry out sanitary measures, and the Utah State Engineer's Office sent personnel to advise Farmington officials on the repair of water systems and clearing of highways (Keate, 1991).

Events of 1930

Four separate cloudburst-rainstorm events produced major alluvial-fan flooding and sedimentation in Davis County during the summer of 1930 (July 10, August 11, August 13, and September 4; Woolley, 1946). Sediment discharged from South Fork Kays, Shepard, Steed, Davis, Ricks (Ford), Barnard, and Parish Canyons caused damage at or beyond the canyon mouths (Fig. 3). The events from Steed and Davis Canyons, Ricks (Ford) Canyon, and Parrish Canyon are discussed below.

Steed and Davis Canyons. The first events from Steed and Davis Canyons occurred on July 10th. Crops were once again damaged. A number of structures and automobiles were severely damaged or destroyed (Keate, 1991). The state highway 600 m (2,000 ft) west of the mouth of Steed Canyon was blocked by debris 1.5 m (5 ft) thick for a distance of about 240 m (800 ft). The highway 300 m (1,000 ft) west of the mouth of Davis Canyon was blocked by 1.8 m (6 ft) of debris for a distance of about 180 m (600 ft; Keate, 1991).

Davis Canyon produced more flooding and sedimentation during cloudburst rainstorms on August 11 and 13, causing additional damage to homes and farmland. When the August 11 flood reached the highway west of the canyon mouth, rain had not yet fallen in town (Keate, 1991). Cannon (1931) estimated the weight of one of the boulders involved in one of the August events from Davis Canyon to be about 273,000 kg (300 tons).

Flooding and sedimentation from Steed and Davis Canyons occurred again on September 4, during another cloudburst rainstorm. Additional homes, crops, and farmland were damaged and the highway was again blocked by debris (Keate, 1991). The total volume of debris deposited from Steed Canyon by the four cloudburst rainstorms is estimated at 53,000 m³ (69,000 yd³); the total volume of debris deposited from Davis Canyon by the four storms is estimated at 20,700 m³ (27,000 yd³; Keaton et al., 1988b).

Ricks (Ford) Canyon. Alluvial-fan flooding and sedimentation from Ricks Creek occurred during the July 10 cloudburst storm. Homes, crops, irrigation systems, and farmland were damaged. Sediment blocked the Bamberger Interurban Railway tracks about 2.4 km (1.5 mi) west of the canyon mouth. Much of the sediment produced from the 1930 Ricks Creek event was eroded from sandy lake deposits below the canyon mouth. The post-1930 event Ricks Creek channel had been lowered 12 m (40 ft) by downcutting where it crossed Lake Bonneville sand and gravel deposits (Cannon, 1931), and an irrigation ditch crossing Ricks Creek had to be replaced with a pipe (Keate, 1991). Additional damage from Ricks Creek flooding and sedimentation occurred during the August 11 rainstorm (Keate, 1991). The total volume of debris deposited from Ricks Canyon by the four cloudburst rainstorms is estimated at 100,000 m³ (131,000 yd³; Keaton et al., 1988b).

Parrish Canyon. Most of the damage caused by the 1930 flooding and sedimentation events took place in Centerville. Parrish Canyon, which had not produced significant sediment during the 1923 cloudburst rainstorm, produced two debris flows, one debris flood, and a clear-water flood during the 1930 cloudburst rainstorms (Keate, 1991). The first debris flow, a result of the July 10 storm, killed at least 2,000 farm animals (mostly chickens), destroyed or damaged farm structures, crops, and automobiles, and deposited debris that blocked the highway in Centerville. The second debris flow, on August 11, caused additional damage including (1) destruction of the east wall of the eight-room Centerville School located about 600 m (2,000 ft) west of the mouth of Parrish Canyon, (2) damage or destruction of many homes and farm buildings, and (3) the death of farm animals. The August 13 storm produced a debris flood from Parrish Canyon, causing more damage to the already battered town of Centerville. The September 4 storm caused only clear-water flooding (Keate, 1991). The total volume of debris deposited from Parrish Canyon by the four cloudburst rainstorms is estimated at 402,000 m³ (526,000 yd³; Keaton et al., 1988b).

Observations and conclusions following the 1930 events

Total damages from the combined events of 1923 and 1930 were estimated at about $1 million, nearly one-fifth of the total assessed value of the property in that portion of Davis County (Bailey et al., 1947; Marston, 1958). Following the 1930 events, Bailey et al. (1947, p. 6) note that

the floods did more than physical damage to land and other property. For a time they caused severe economic shock and paralysis in the community. Interest and mortgages remained unpaid. Banks refused to extend credit. Many people wanted to sell and get out, but no one would buy the property in the flood zone. Real estate brokers refused even to list property for sale.

Some victims in the disaster area became more concerned with whether steps would be taken to prevent future disasters than repairing their damaged farms (Keate, 1991).

On September 9, 1930, Utah Governor George H. Dern appointed a Special Flood Commission to evaluate the extent and cause of the flooding problems in northern Utah (Keaton, 1995). This commission included geologist R. W. Bailey, forester C. L. Forsling, and ecologist R. J. Becraft, who deserve "much of the credit for correctly analyzing the flood causes" (Craddock, 1960). The report of the commission (Cannon, 1931) concluded that the causes of the 1930 flood damage were (1) uncommonly heavy rainfall, (2) steep topography and geological conditions conducive to sudden runoff and to a large quantity of flood debris, and (3) scant vegetation on portions of the watersheds of the canyons that flooded. This scantiness of vegetation, in some cases, was natural barrenness or semibarrenness of the land, but in many cases was caused by the depletion of the natural plant

growth by overgrazing, fire, and to a small extent over-cutting of timber (Cannon, 1931).

Members of the commission found the flood sources by following "the gutted channels to their origin on headwater slopes" (Craddock, 1960, p. 292). The source areas in each canyon showed evidence of plant-cover depletion, were scattered, and ranged in size from "less than one to only a few acres" (Bailey et al., 1947, p. 6). Soils were eroded from the poorly to unvegetated source areas, which covered only about 10% of the drainage basins, but no signs of runoff from adjacent vegetated areas were observed (Craddock, 1960). The channel fill below the source areas was washed out to depths of 21 m (70 ft), creating deep gorges the full length of the flooded canyons; the eroded channels contained long stretches of exposed bedrock (Bailey et al., 1947). No mention was made of the ratio of material contributed by channels to material contributed by drainage-basin slopes for the canyons that produced the 1930 events.

The commission (Cannon, 1931, p. 17) also compared the deposits of 1923 and 1930 in Davis County to the alluvial fans at the mouths of the canyons and noted that the floods of 1923 and 1930

mark a distinct increase from the normal rate of erosion and deposition of the thousands of years since Lake Bonneville receded to the present level of Great Salt Lake. In depth of cutting, in quantity of material and size of boulders carried, these floods far exceed the normal occurrence since the recession of Lake Bonneville. The post-Bonneville alluvial deposits are small, and the quantity of material brought down and added to them by the 1923 and 1930 floods is all out of proportion to the amount brought down through the thousands of years of post-Bonneville history. . . . If floods had occurred at intervals of one-half century for the 30,000 [sic] or more years since the recession of Lake Bonneville, the alluvial structures would be found extending far out into the lake.

Crawford and Thackwell (1931) observed prehistoric debris-flow deposits exposed in the eroded channel at the mouth of Ricks Creek. They acknowledged the importance placed by others on overgrazing and fire on sediment production and flooding, but argued that these factors had been "over-stressed and that the primary factors lie in other unbalanced conditions in nature, and that these other conditions are of sufficient importance to cause intermittent floods even if the contributing causes of over grazing [sic] and forest fires did not exist" (Crawford and Thackwell, 1931, p. 100). This warning would later prove to be prophetic.

Government response following events of 1930

Government response to the events of 1930 included constructing sediment catch basins (debris basins) at the mouths of some of the canyons that produced sediment, acquiring the watersheds into public ownership (U.S. Forest Service) and prohibiting grazing and burning, and creating contour trenches to promote infiltration and inhibit runoff. The contour trenches were constructed by the Civilian Conservation Corps (depression-era Work Projects Administration) beginning in 1934 in the upper parts of the watersheds from Farmington Canyon to Centerville Canyon (Bailey and Croft, 1937; Croft, 1967, 1981). The effectiveness of these contour trenches is indicated on Figure 3 by the small number of reported flood events between 1935 and 1982.

Events of 1983

During the last week of September 1982, nearly half of the 396-mm (15.6-in) average annual precipitation, over 178 mm (7 in), fell at Salt Lake City International Airport, helping make hydrologic year 1982 (October 1, 1981 to September 30, 1982) one of the wettest years in Salt Lake City history (Anderson et al., 1984; Kaliser and Slosson, 1988). The total precipitation for 1982 was 639 mm (25.2 in). The most important factor in the flooding of May and June 1983 was the heavy snowpack that persisted into late May and then melted rapidly. Under average conditions, snowpack peaks around April 1, then declines through April, May, and June. The snowpack conditions in the Davis County area for the first five months of 1983, compared to the 15-year average conditions, are shown on Figure 5. The 1983 snowpack continued to accumulate through the month of April, and was still 115% of average yearly maximum on June 1, even though rapid snow melting began on May 21 (Anderson et al., 1984).

Rapid and sustained melting of the record snowpack filled colluvial soils and even bedrock aquifers in the mountain watersheds (Mathewson et al., 1990) and resulted in hundreds of debris slides. The debris slides formed in colluvial soils that mobilized readily into debris flows because the average liquid-limit and plastic-limit moisture contents were within about 1 percent of each other (Keaton, 1988). As a slope movement began, the soil mass would dilate, creating negative pore-water pressures (Keaton, 1995). The abundant water from melting snow was sucked into the dilated soil mass, increasing the moisture content above the liquid limit, and the soil mass would mobilize into a debris flow. The sediments in stream channels also were saturated by water from the melting snow. Once the debris slide-generated debris flows reached the channels, the advancing debris imposed

a rapid load on the saturated channel sediments, causing an abrupt increase in pore-water pressure that liquefied the channel sediments (Keaton, 1995). The channel sediments were thus entrained into the debris flow.

Most of the canyons in Davis County produced landslide-generated debris floods (Wieczorek et al., 1983) during the 1983 snowmelt (Fig. 3). The worst damage in 1983 occurred at the mouth of Rudd Creek, a canyon that, except for the small suspected event in 1860 or 1861, had not generated significant debris earlier in historical time.

Rudd Canyon. A major debris flow issued from Rudd Canyon at about 6:30 p.m. on Memorial Day, May 30, and several smaller sedimentation events from the canyon occurred during the following eight days (Pierson, 1985; Keaton, 1988). The debris flow was initiated by a landslide (Fig. 6), which contributed approximately 12,230 to 15,290 m^3 (16,000 to 20,000 yd^3) of sediment and an unknown amount of water (Vandre, 1983). The 1983 landslide occurred in the lower portion of a much larger prehistoric landslide complex. Approximately 49,700 to 57,340 m^3 (65,000 to 75,000 yd^3) of sediment was deposited as a debris fan

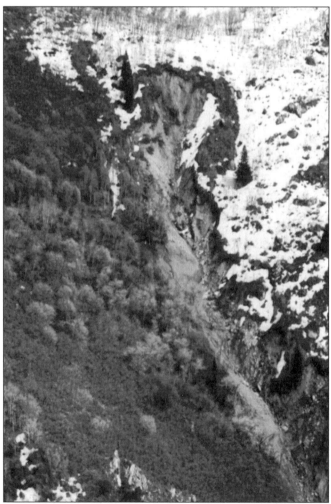

Figure 6. Rudd Canyon landslide shortly after 1983 debris-flow event.

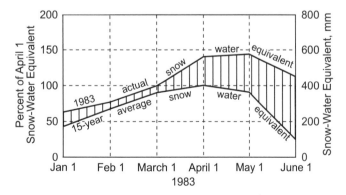

Figure 5. Snow-water equivalent for 1983 compared to a 15-year (1963–1977) average for all Wasatch Front snow course stations maintained by the U.S. Department of Agriculture Soil Conservation Service. Modified from Anderson et al. (1984) and Keaton (1995).

in Farmington and an additional 5,350 to 10,700 m³ (7,000 to 14,000 yd³) was deposited in a thin (<0.3-m, 1-ft, thick) veneer beyond the toe of the debris fan (Vandre, 1983). The initial pulse of sediment in Rudd Creek plugged the small channel of the creek near the head of the Rudd Canyon alluvial fan and diverted subsequent pulses to the south into a residential area. The first pulse of debris was reported to be a 6-m- (20-ft-) high wall as it came out of the canyon (Keate, 1991).

Five city blocks of residential development in Farmington were damaged by the initial debris flow, and a much larger area was damaged by subsequent flooding (Keate, 1991). Four or five homes were destroyed (Fig. 7a), and one home was pushed off its foundation (Fig. 7b) and carried by the flow approximately 30 m (100 ft; Keaton, 1995). A total of 35 homes were damaged, 15 severely (Lowe et al., 1989), as were some automobiles and the Weber Basin Conservancy District aqueduct (Keate, 1991). About 200 residents were forced from their homes. No one was killed, partly because the event occurred on a holiday weekend, but largely because residents could hear the "rumbling roar" of the debris flow coming down the canyon. Some residents, looking toward the noise, reported seeing trees "falling one after another like dominos" as the debris flow moved down canyon (Keate, 1991, p. 63).

Initial observations and conclusions following the 1983 events

Utah Geological and Mineral Survey, U.S. Geological Survey, and U.S.D.A. Forest Service personnel responding to the 1983 events determined that landslides mobilizing into debris flows in recently thawed colluvium near the snow line were the main cause of the flooding and sedimentation occurring on mountain-front alluvial fans in Davis County (Kaliser, 1983). Only those canyons with newly formed landslides generated significant debris, and eroded channels could be traced directly to the landslide scars (Wieczorek et al., 1983). The National Research Council Committee on Natural Disasters appointed a disaster reconnaissance team, consisting of a geotechnical engineer, an engineering geologist, an engineering hydrologist, and a social scientist, to document the research opportunities created by the 1983 events (Anderson et al., 1984). Two unique aspects of the late May and early June, 1983, Utah disaster were (1) its long duration (approximately two weeks), and (2) the Federal Emergency Management Agency (FEMA) already had established a disaster response center in Utah because of a landslide near Thistle, Utah, after President Reagan declared it a major disaster on April 30, 1983 (Anderson et al., 1984).

State and local officials became concerned about the effects that subsequent summer cloudburst rainstorms might have on the drainage basins in view of their now unstable conditions. Consequently, the state requested federal assistance with an evaluation of the potential hazard from subsequent cloudburst rainstorms in drainage basins where landslides occurred and partly detached landslide masses remained on the slopes. This hazard evaluation, funded by the FEMA and conducted by personnel from the U.S

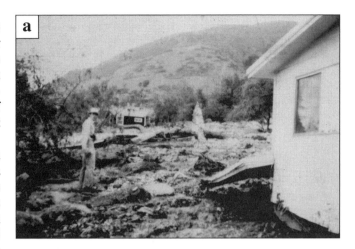

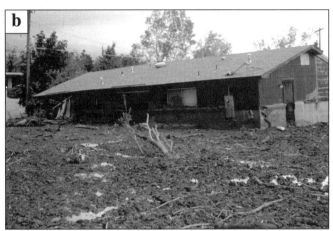

Figure 7. a. Houses at the mouth of Rudd Canyon destroyed by the 1983 debris-flow event. b. House on the Rudd Canyon alluvial fan that was pushed by the 1983 debris flow off its foundation a distance of approximately 30 m (100 ft).

Geological Survey and Los Angeles County Flood Control Department (Wieczorek et al., 1983), was based chiefly on features within the drainage basins, such as the volumes of partly detached landslides and on the likelihood that mobilized sediment would reach the canyon mouths. Wieczorek et al. (1983) also determined whether canyons were more likely to produce debris flows or debris floods. In general, the evaluation by Wieczorek et al. (1983) suggested a high to very high potential for significant volumes of sediment to reach canyon mouths in Davis County during cloudburst floods or rapid snowmelt events.

Wieczorek et al. (1983, p. 31) noted that 81 to 85% of the debris deposited at the mouth of Rudd Canyon was derived from the stream channel. However, their evaluation of short-term potential debris-flow volumes was based only on the largest detached landslide in each drainage basin (Wieczorek et al., 1983, 1989). Wieczorek et al. (1983) estimate of long-term debris production was determined by (1) replotting normalized debris-production/drainage-basin-area curves produced by the U.S.D.A. Forest Service in the 1950s for light, moderate, and severe flood events along the Wasatch Front; (2) comparing the curves to existing plots for debris production for Los Angeles County, California; and (3) adjusting the severe flood curve to match the debris produced by the 1983 Rudd Canyon event (Fig. 8). Wieczorek et al. (1983) assumed that those canyons rated as having a high relative potential for producing a debris-flow event would have debris-production potential in accordance with the severe curve. They assumed the canyons rated as having a high relative potential to produce debris floods would have debris-production potential in accordance with the moderate curve. Wieczorek et al. (1983, p. 19) also made general and canyon-specific recommendations for mitigation of debris-flow and debris-flood damage, principally construction of debris basins at canyon mouths to entrap debris and straightening and lining of stream channels to transport the remaining debris until it "can be deposited with minimal damage."

The hazard assessment by Wieczorek et al. (1983) was the only geologic study for subsequent government action along the Wasatch Front. This effort was initiated immediately following the May 31, 1983, debris flow from Rudd Canyon and was conducted with the aim of developing recommendations for hazard mitigation within a relatively short time (6 weeks) before the onset of summer cloudburst rainstorms. Although the cost of the FEMA-sponsored hazard assessment amounted to only about $50,000, the knowledge of debris-flow events, processes, and mitigation efforts brought to bear on the debris-flow problem in Utah represented millions of dollars and years of research by federal scientists and engineers who had been studying similar processes in southern and northern California (G. F. Wieczorek, written communication, 1996).

Initial government response following events of 1983

Based at least in part on the study by Wieczorek et al. (1983), Davis County and some cities began refurbishing debris basins constructed in the 1930s, or constructing new basins (Fig. 9) at a cost of about $12 million, or $1.1 million dollars each (Keaton, 1988). Some stream channels, primarily in Bountiful, were straightened and lined with concrete. Mitigation efforts focused primarily on those canyons that had produced historical debris flows or debris floods (Williams and Lowe, 1990). Davis County also established a system of remote weather stations, both in the mountains and along the mountain front, to measure precipitation, stream flow, soil-moisture conditions, landslide movement, and the level of water and debris in debris basins (Lowe et al., 1988).

Events of 1984

Heavy late-autumn rainfall, a near-record winter snowpack, and cool spring temperatures followed by sudden warming occurred again in the Wasatch Range of Davis County during the 1984 hydrologic year (Wieczorek et al., 1989). The soil mantle in the mountains of Davis County was saturated by the start of

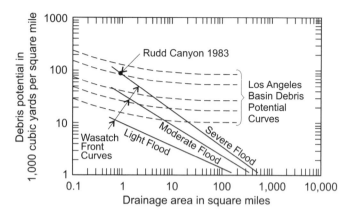

Figure 8. Graph showing potential for debris production (modified from Wieczorek et al., 1983).

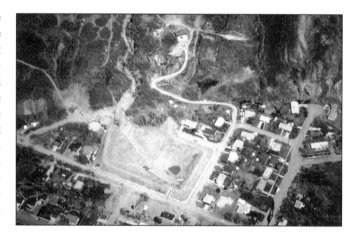

Figure 9. Debris basin constructed at the mouth of Rudd Canyon in the fall of 1983.

winter by late-autumn rains; at the end of September 1983 cumulative precipitation in upper Farmington Canyon was 161% of normal (Santi, 1988). On March 1, 1984, cumulative monthly precipitation was 160% of average (Wieczorek et al., 1989). Low temperatures during late winter and early spring prevented significant snowmelt and permitted retention of a deep snowpack (Santi, 1988). Moisture was added to the snowpack by additional rain and snow during the spring, and in early May snowpack water content was 203% of normal (U.S. Department of Agriculture, 1984). Beginning May 8, temperatures rose and stayed high, with the exception of May 16 and 17, and snowmelt generally continued once it began (Wieczorek et al., 1989). Colluvial soils and bedrock aquifers in the mountain watersheds were again filled, resulting in landsliding (debris slides; Mathewson and Keaton, 1986; Mathewson and Santi, 1987).

Once again, many Davis County canyons produced landslide-generated debris-flows and debris floods (Fig. 3). Debris volumes were smaller in 1984 for those canyons that had produced debris flows or debris floods in 1983, and most of the debris in these canyons was derived from the partly detached landslides created in 1983 (Wieczorek et al., 1989). For example, Rudd Canyon generated only 1,350 m³ (1,765 ft³) of debris in 1984 (Keaton, 1988). The worst damage in 1984 occurred at the mouth of Lightning Canyon, a canyon that, like Rudd Canyon in 1983, had not generated significant debris earlier in historical time (Table 2; Fig. 3). Only Lightning Canyon and Rudd Canyon produced debris flows that extended beyond canyon mouths in 1984 (Wieczorek et al., 1989); the debris basin that had been built at the mouth of Rudd Canyon in the fall of 1983 contained the debris discharged in 1984 and averted additional property damage (G. F. Wieczorek, written communication, 1996).

Lightning Canyon. A shallow, 1.5-m- (5-ft-) deep, 240-m³ (310-yd³) debris slide in the locally named Lightning Canyon mobilized and generated a debris flow on May 14, 1984 (Santi, 1988; Santi and Mathewson, 1988; Wieczorek et al., 1989; Mathewson et al., 1990). Large amounts of channel material were incorporated into the debris flow as it moved down a steep 2-km- (1.2-mi-) long stretch of canyon, ultimately depositing 9,000 m³ (11,800 yd³; Table 2) of debris in a residential subdivision and damaging five homes (Olson, 1985; Keaton, 1988; Santi, 1988; Santi and Mathewson, 1988; Wieczorek et al., 1989; Mathewson et al., 1990). Santi (1988) estimated that the debris flow reached velocities of 15.5 m/sec (19 ft/sec; 35 mi/hr) as it moved down the canyon.

Subsequent research following the 1983 and 1984 events

Considerable research into debris-flow hazards and processes in Davis County followed the events of 1983 and 1984. The U.S. Army Corps of Engineers (COE), at the request of the Federal Emergency Management Agency (FEMA), evaluated alluvial-fan flooding on the basis of conventional engineering hydrology/hydraulics (U.S. Army Corps of Engineers, 1984, 1988; Liou, 1989). Several Utah State University Department of Civil and Environmental Engineering graduate students studied the debris slides in the Wasatch Range of Davis County (Pack, 1984, 1985; Brooks, 1986; Jadkowski, 1987; Monteith et al., 1990). Texas A&M University Department of Geology graduate students conducted research on the geomorphology and stratigraphy of Davis County alluvial fans (Keaton, 1986a, b, 1988, 1989a, b; Keaton et al., 1987, 1988a, b; Keaton and Mathewson, 1987, 1988), the kinematics of debris-flow transport (Santi, 1988, 1989; Santi and Mathewson, 1988), the hydrogeology of the Wasatch Range in Davis County and its role in debris-flow initiation (Ala, 1989, 1990a, b; Ala and Mathewson, 1990; Mathewson, 1989; Mathewson and Keaton, 1986; Mathewson et al., 1990; Mathewson and Santi, 1987; Skelton, 1990, 1991), and watershed conditions (Coleman, 1990a; Eblin, 1990, 1991), including the influence of contour trenches on landslide-generated debris flows (Coleman, 1989, 1990b). The Davis County Planning and Flood Control Departments produced debris-flow hazard maps based on the boundaries of younger Holocene alluvial fans (Lowe, 1990, 1993; Lowe and Christenson, 1990), and studied stream-channel conditions in the mountains of Davis County (Williams et al., 1989; Williams and Lowe, 1990).

ENGINEERING VERSUS GEOLOGIC APPROACHES TO DEBRIS-FLOW HAZARDS

As a result of very costly floodlike damage in southern California in January 1969 (Campbell, 1975), damage resulting from "mudslides" was added to the National Flood Insurance Program (National Research Council, Advisory Board on the Built Environment, 1982). Damage from "landslides" was specifically excluded from the National Flood Insurance Program, and the term "mudslide" was intended to cover floodlike damage only.

Floodlike damage caused by the 1983 sedimentation events in Davis County occurred well outside flood-plain boundaries depicted on Flood Insurance Rate Maps prepared for the National Flood Insurance Program that is administered by the Federal Emergency Management Agency (FEMA). Consequently, the accuracy of the flood-plain maps was questioned and FEMA contracted with the U.S. Army Corps of Engineers (COE) to assess alluvial-fan flooding in central Davis County and produce new Flood Insurance Rate Maps that take into account debris-flow/flood hazards.

The evaluation of debris-flow hazards in Davis County requires an understanding of the amount of debris currently available for transport. Debris is derived from the drainage-basin slopes (overland erosion, landslides) and stream channels. The availability of debris also depends on the rate and process by which new sediment is produced by weathering of the bedrock materials. The nature and distribution of debris on alluvial-fan surfaces indicates the characteristics of the dominant processes of debris transport from the canyons (Keaton et al., 1988b).

The engineering hydrology and hydraulics approach used by the COE results in fundamentally different conclusions from the approach used by geologic researchers. These two approaches are described briefly in the following sections of this paper.

Engineering hydrology/hydraulics study

Modeling for flood-hazard delineation under the National Flood Insurance Program is based on a 100-year frequency. The most pronounced and severe damage from sedimentation events caused by the rapid snowmelt in the spring of 1983 occurred in Farmington. The COE examined records and discovered that a number of central Davis County drainages had produced debris-flow and flood damage between 1912 and 1983, and concluded that the 1983 Farmington damage represented a "100-year debris flow" in Rudd Creek (Anciaux, 1987, unpaginated).

The COE recognized that use of conventional hydrology/hydraulics would result in a very small estimated 100-year clear-water flood hydrograph in the 1.78-km² (0.69-mi²) Rudd Creek drainage basin, and very large bulking factors would be required to approximate the observed volume of discharged sediment-water slurry. A finite-element model with a moving front was developed for simulating transient debris-flow processes (Schamber, 1987). The model produced a modified dam-break hydrograph with compressed leading and trailing tails that was used to compute debris-flow thicknesses below the dam break. The observed characteristics of the 1983 debris-flow event from Rudd Creek, summarized by Anciaux (1987, unpaginated), were (1) volume of main event was 64,223 m³ (84,000 yd³), (2) debris-flow depths ranged from 3.6 m (12 ft) at the canyon mouth to 0.6 to 0.9 m (2 or 3 ft) at the front, (3) time to peak discharge was almost instantaneous (60 s or less), (4) the debris flow advance on the alluvial fan was "slower than a man could walk," and (5) the calculated length of the main event was approximately 4 to 5 min. Anciaux (1987, unpaginated) used these observed characteristics to construct an inflow hydrograph (Fig. 10) for use with Schamber's (1987) finite-element grid network (Fig. 11), alluvial-fan slope values for the Rudd Creek fan, and debris-flow fluid properties. The fluid properties, particularly the fluid viscosity, were varied until the thicknesses and distribution of debris observed in 1983 on the Rudd Creek fan were accurately modeled. The 100-year "mudflow" event from Rudd Creek was then defined in terms of the inflow hydrograph and the fluid properties. The dynamic viscosity that best modeled the sediment discharge was 1.27 kg-sec/m² (30 lb-sec/ft² or 0.127 poise; Anciaux, 1987).

The 100-year hydrograph and fluid viscosity defined for Rudd Creek was applied to other drainage basins in central Davis County, with the 100-year "mudflow" volume adjusted using the Wasatch Front curve for severe floods shown on Figure 8. The alluvial-fan slopes for the other canyons were used with the finite-element grid to compute debris-flow thicknesses on other selected Davis County alluvial fans (Anciaux, 1987).

The flood plains mapped by COE encompassed a large part of the urbanized areas in some communities. An example of the dramatic difference in mapped flood-plain boundaries is shown in Figure 12a and b for the Deuel Creek alluvial fan (Centerville Canyon). The Centerville Canyon drainage basin encompasses an area of 8.15 km² (3.15 mi²). Figure 12a is from the Flood Insurance Rate Map published in 1982 (Federal Emergency Management Agency, 1982) and shows that Zone A (the 100-year flood plain) was confined to the channel of Deuel Creek in the upper part of the Centerville Canyon alluvial fan. The street system is classified as Zone B (subject to flood depths less than 0.3 m, 1 ft, from the 100-year flood). Residential city blocks were classified as Zone C (area of minimal flooding).

Figure 12b is from the Flood Insurance Rate Map published in 1992 (Federal Emergency Management Agency, 1992) and shows that the current mapping of Zone A encompasses all or parts of 21 city blocks. Many other city blocks are classified as Zone X (subject to flood depths less than 0.3 m, 1 ft, from the 100-year flood).

The impact of the changes in alluvial-fan flood hazard mapping on the communities was two-fold: (1) extensive areas were suddenly within 100-year flood plain boundaries, and (2) many debris basins recently constructed to protect the communities

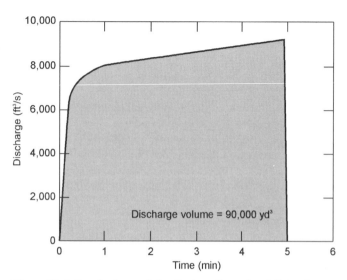

Figure 10. Inflow hydrograph for the two-dimensional finite-element model of the 1983 Rudd Creek debris flow (modified from Anciaux, 1987). The total volume of sediment discharged from Rudd Canyon in 1983 was 68,810 m³ (90,000 yd³); the initial event was the largest, with a volume of 64,220 m³ (84,000 yd³).

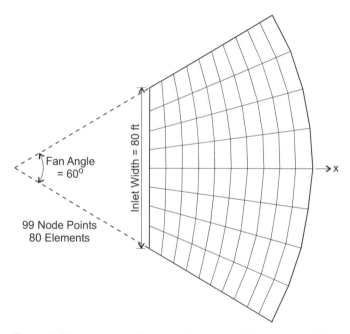

Figure 11. Finite-element grid network for the Rudd Creek fan (modified from Anciaux, 1987).

were suddenly deemed inadequate. Nearly all of the debris basins built and refurbished in response to the 1983 flood events were found to be significantly smaller than the volumes of predicted 100-year debris-flow flood events computed using the COE method (Table 3). The communities were faced with immediately devising and implementing flood-hazard mitigation measures to remain in compliance with provisions of the National Flood Insurance Program.

Geologic study of alluvial fans

Geologists who study the major sediment-discharge events of 1923 and 1930 noticed that the alluvial-fan landforms at the mouths of Wasatch Front canyons were too small to have been produced by frequent, major debris flows (Cannon, 1931). Keaton (1988) used the sediment sources and fan volumes to infer that the 1983 debris flows must have been rare geologic events.

The extensive contribution of stream-channel material to debris-flow volumes was noted by observers of the events of 1923 (J. C. Alter *in* Keate, 1991; Pack, 1923), 1930 (Craddock, 1960), 1983 (Wieczorek et al., 1983), and 1984 (Santi, 1988). Croft (1962) studied Baer Canyon, which produced debris flows in 1923 and 1927 (Fig. 3, Table 2), and estimated that 80 to 90% of the material deposited beyond the mouth of the canyon during these events came from channel erosion. He noted that "this material cut from the channels represents ages of accumulation" (Croft, 1967, p. 8). Because most of the sediment discharged into the central Davis County communities came from the stream channels, and because significant lengths of the stream channels have been substantially cleaned to bedrock, considerable time (more than 100 years) probably will be required for sediment to accumulate in the channels before the process can be repeated (Keaton, 1988; Williams and Lowe, 1990; Lowe et al., 1992). Therefore, geologic reasoning indicates that the 1983 event from Rudd Canyon cannot represent a 100-year frequency.

It is an oversimplification to suggest that debris flows remove all sediment from channels leaving only exposed bedrock (G. F. Wieczorek, written communication, 1996). Post-debris-flow observations typically reveal steep stretches of channels almost completely cleaned to bedrock, but some sediment remains in some stretches. In some channels with flatter gradients, deposition of debris-flow material predominates. In a few cases, debris flows deposit sediment and stop before reaching canyon mouths. Even in those channel reaches that are cleaned of sediment, small landslides from oversteepened side slopes in colluvial soils begin almost immediately to refill channels cleaned to bedrock. Nonetheless, the process of refilling a bedrock channel to its predebris flow volume of sediment would require a long period of time (G. F. Wieczorek, written communication, 1996).

The historical sediment accumulation rates on Davis County alluvial fans discussed above are relatively well constrained. Estimates of Holocene and late Pleistocene sediment accumulation rates are speculative and require some knowledge of the late Pleistocene history of Lake Bonneville. Lake Bonneville declined rapidly as evaporation greatly exceeded inflow during the period from approximately 14 ka to 11 ka (Currey and Oviatt, 1985). From approximately 11.5 ka to 10 ka, the lake rose to the Gilbert shoreline. Neilson and Wullstein (1985) used biogeography of gambel oak and scrub oak (*Quercus gambelii* and *Q. turbinella*) in Utah, Arizona, New Mexico, and Colorado to interpret that the northernmost populations of these species were established under a climate with greater summer precipitation than the current climate. They further suggest that the Holocene Hypsithermal Interval (Deevey and Flint, 1957) could have provided an expansion of the "Arizona Monsoon" that would have provided the summer precipitation, even if total annual precipitation had declined. Keaton (1988) recognized that the surface conditions in the Wasatch Range in the latest Pleistocene and early Holocene would have included substantial volumes of frost-shattered and solifluction rock debris created by the alpine glacial climate that existed when Lake Bonneville was at its highstand. Vigorous convective cloudburst storms associated with a summer "monsoon" climate beginning in the early Holocene, combined with easily eroded material in the steep mountain watersheds, would be expected to contribute much sediment to alluvial fans. Bull (1991) noted that plant fossils from packrat middens dated at 13 to 11 ka indicate that a plant-community transition in the deserts of the southwestern Basin and Range Province occurred just before a major aggradation event on piedmont slopes. Perhaps the climatic conditions responsible for the major aggradation event on the desert piedmont slopes also caused similar aggradation on the alluvial fans in Davis County. The apparent absence of major sedimentation events on alluvial fans in Davis County in the mid- to late Holocene may be explained on the basis of lack of available sediment in the mountain watersheds because it had been eroded during the earlier "monsoon" storms.

In a theoretical model of alluvial-fan deposition, Price (1976) recognized that the character of deposition on a fan is directly related to the volume of weathered material immediately available for erosion from the source basin. He used threshold values of weathered-layer thickness to predict responses on alluvial fans. For the same intensity of climatic event in the mountain drainage basin, Price (1976) reasoned that clear-water discharge would cause erosion on the fans if the weathered-layer thickness was small, no net erosion or deposition would occur on the fans if the weathered-layer thickness was moderate, and debris-flow deposition on the fans would result if the weathered-layer thickness was large. The source basins essentially were "cleaned out" after each storm of a certain magnitude or intensity; thus, large storms that occurred more frequently than weathered material could develop inhibited debris flows on the fans. Large storms that occurred less frequently than weathered material could develop promoted debris flows on the fans.

This concept is validated by the data in Figure 13 that show sediment-discharge volumes from Davis County canyons normalized on the basis of drainage-basin area for the years 1912, 1923, 1930, 1932, 1945, 1947, 1983, and 1984. The 39 values plotted in Figure 13 are listed in Table 2. Farmington Canyon (10 values in Table 2) is omitted from this plot because its drainage-basin area is more than twice the size of the next-largest basin (Ward Canyon). The volumes of seven sedimentation events from canyons other than Farmington that occurred in years other than those listed above are omitted from Figure 13.

Debris-production curves for severe, moderate, and light floods from Figure 8 are also shown on Figure 13. The equations

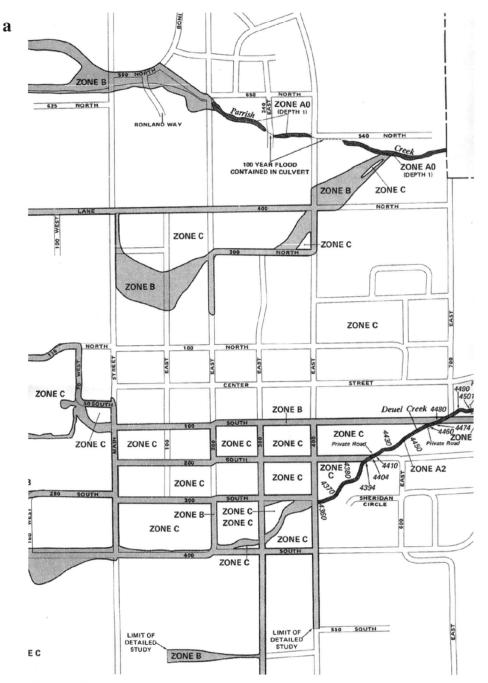

Figure 12 (this and facing page). a. "Flood Insurance Rate Map of Deuel Creek (Centerville Canyon)" published in 1982 (Federal Emergency Management Agency, 1982). b. "Flood Insurance Rate Map of Deuel Creek (Centerville Canyon)" revised in 1992 (Federal Emergency Management Agency, 1992).

for these reference curves are as follows:

$$V_s = 46024 \, Ad^{-0.685}$$
$$V_m = 17645 \, Ad^{-0.584}$$
$$V_l = 4282 \, Ad^{-0.427}$$

where V_s, V_m, and V_l are the normalized sediment volume or debris potential in m^3/km^2 for severe, moderate, and light floods, and Ad is the drainage-basin area in km^2. Normalized sediment volumes from historical Davis County events shown on Figure 13 are scattered above the severe-flood curve and below the light-flood curve.

The earliest historical sediment-discharge event with an esti-mated volume is the largest historical event from each canyon

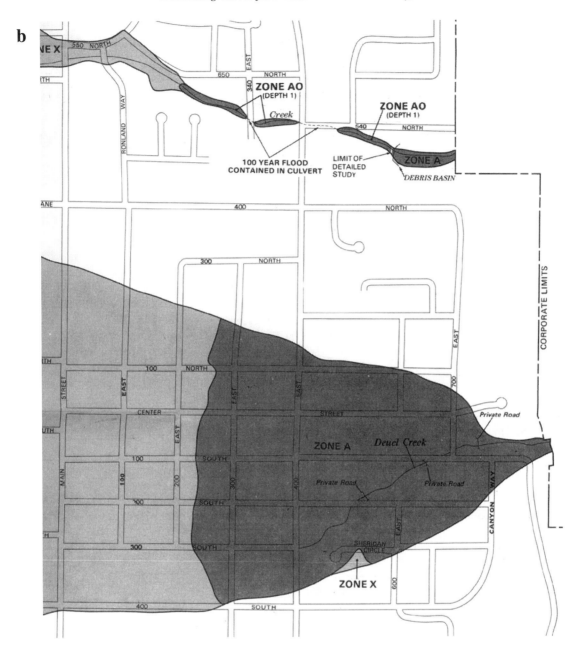

with the exceptions of Farmington, Ricks (Ford), and Davis Canyons (see Figs. 2 and 3, and Table 2). Trends in the normalized volume of the largest three events from each canyon except Farmington Canyon were evaluated by fitting a power function though that data plotted in Figure 14. The scattered data yield the following relationships:

$$V1 = 23067 \, Ad^{-0.946}; \quad n = 14; \quad r^2 = 0.138$$
$$V2 = 593 \, Ad^{0.753}; \quad n = 11; \quad r^2 = 0.031$$
$$V3 = 1718 \, Ad^{0.440}; \quad n = 7; \quad r^2 = 0.255$$

where V1, V2, and V3 are the sediment volumes in m^3/km^2 for the largest, second-largest, and third-largest sedimentation events, n is the number of values, and r^2 is the coefficient of determination. The scatter in the limited data and the low values of the coefficient of determination reveal that the trend lines are not reliable indicators of normalized debris potential. The significance of this observation is that the Davis County canyons historically have produced sediment in a way that does not follow a trend based on drainage-basin area. Therefore, using drainage-basin area to normalize the Rudd Canyon debris volume for estimating debris production from other canyons as used by COE is not supported by a trend in the historical data.

The concept that the earliest historical event in each canyon was also the largest historical event was tested by evaluating the ratio of each event volume to the volume of the earliest event. The

**TABLE 3. DEBRIS-BASIN CAPACITY, 100-YEAR DEBRIS-FLOW/FLOOD EVENT VOLUMES*,
VOLUME OF SEDIMENT WITH 10 PERCENT EXCEEDANCE PROBABILITY
IN A 50-YEAR TIME PERIOD†, AND ESTIMATED SEDIMENT YIELD
FOLLOWING A HIGH-INTENSITY BURN§ FOR SELECTED DAVIS COUNTY CANYONS**

Canyon	Debris-Basin Capacity (m³)	100-Year Event Sediment Volume* (m³)	10%-50-Year Sediment Volume† (m³)	High-Intensity Burn Sediment Volume§ (m³)
Shepard	24,200	85,000	180	4,990
Farmington	128,900	134,000	512,860	23,790
Rudd	35,200	64,000	90	1,530
Halfway (Lone Pine)	83,300	62,000	160	1,150
Ricks	30,600	86,000	3,160	4,540
Barnard	4,600	73,000	390	3,450
Parrish	30,600	83,000	320	3,700
Centerville (Deuel Creek)	3,400	92,000	25	7,320
Ward (Stone Creek)	185,000	115,000	40	10,610
Barton	252,000	107,000	n.d.	11,190
Mill	52,800	122,000	n.d.	20,150

*Modified from U.S. Army Corps of Engineers, 1988.
†Modified from Keaton, 1988, p. 226. An event with an exceedance probability of 10 percent in a period of 50 years has an average recurrence interval of approximately 475 years. Volumes were calculated as the average of binomial and extreme-value types of probability analyses associated with Holocene and historic periods of record.
§Modified from Evanstad and Rasely, 1995.

data in Table 2 were used to evaluate the 22 canyons in the study area. Six canyons have had no reported sedimentation events. One canyon (Hobbs) had only one event in 1984 for which a volume could not be estimated. Three other canyons have had only one historical sedimentation event. Six canyons have had two or three events for which estimated volumes are available; the ratios of the event volumes to the volume of the first event for these six canyons are plotted in Figure 15. It can be seen that the ratio of the second and third events is 0.5 or less in each case.

Six canyons have had four or more events for which estimated volumes are available. The ratios of the event volumes to the volume of the maximum event are plotted in Figure 16. The first historical event from three of these canyons was the largest historical event; the second historical event from two canyons (Farmington and Ricks) was the largest historical event, and the third historical event from one canyon (Davis) was the largest historical event. The ratios of historical event volumes to the volume of the first historical event for the three apparently anomalous canyons are plotted in Figure 17. We consider these historical events to be anomalous for reasons that are explained in the following paragraphs.

The earliest historical sedimentation event in Farmington Canyon for which an estimated volume is available occurred in 1878 (Fig. 3, Table 2). Only one other Davis County canyon (Davis) produced sediment in this year, indicating that the storm may have been localized. The second historical event in Farmington Canyon for which an estimated volume is available occurred in the disastrous year 1923, when six canyons produced sedimentation events. In Farmington Canyon, the third through

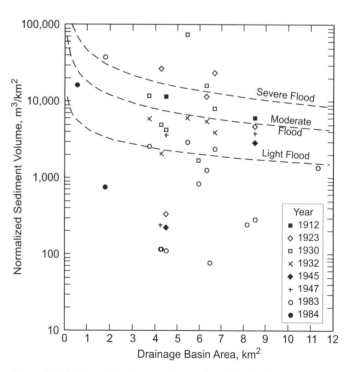

Figure 13. Sediment-discharge volumes from Davis County canyons (except Farmington Canyon) for eight selected years normalized on the basis of drainage-basin area. Based on data in Table 2. Curves for severe, moderate, and light floods are modified from Wieczorek et al. (1983) and are the same curves shown on Figure 8.

the tenth historical events all had volumes less than the volume of the earliest historical event (Fig. 17). Therefore, the earliest historical event probably was produced by a localized storm that was considerably smaller than the storm of 1923.

The earliest historical sedimentation event in Davis Canyon for which an estimated volume is available occurred in 1878; this was a relatively small event (Table 2) and probably was generated by a localized, relatively small storm. The second historical event in Davis County for which an estimated volume is available occurred in 1901. Two other canyons (Steed and Ricks) produced sediment in 1901, but no estimated volumes are available for either event, suggesting that the storm was relatively localized and centered on Davis Canyon. The third historical event in Davis Canyon for which an estimated volume is available occurred in 1923. Thus, Davis Canyon clearly had not been cleaned of available debris by the historical storms prior to 1923, and the volume of the third historical event was approximately 19 times larger than the volume of the earliest historical event.

The earliest historical sedimentation event on the Ricks Creek fan for which an estimated volume is available occurred in 1923. This event deposited a large volume of rocky debris on the fan, and appears to have cleaned colluvial deposits from the stream channel in the canyon and eroded through the previously deposited alluvial-fan deposits (Keaton, 1988). The second historical event for which an estimated volume is available occurred in 1930; the 1930 "event" actually represents four cloudbursts in the same year. The 1923 event not only cut down to erodible Lake Bonneville sand deposits on the alluvial fan at the mouth of the canyon, but also cleaned the canyon of most of the stream-channel

colluvium. Consequently, the flood events from the canyon mouth in 1930 were largely clear water which had considerable capacity to erode the exposed sandy Lake Bonneville sediments. The bulk of the sediment discharged into the community at the Ricks Creek fan in the 1930 events was sand (Keaton, 1988; Keate, 1991). Flood hazards typically are calculated on an annualized basis; therefore, it is appropriate to consider the four cloudburst events in 1930 as a single "event." Most of the volume of sediment from the second historical event (1930) probably actually came from erosion of the Lake Bonneville sand on which the late Pleistocene and early Holocene alluvial fan had been deposited, not from the mountain watershed. Therefore, the volume of sediment from this event is not directly comparable to volumes of historical events from other canyons. Furthermore, if only one cloudburst had occurred in 1930, the volume of sediment discharged into the community at Ricks Creek might have been less than the volume of the earliest historical event.

The explanation of the historical events from the three anomalous canyons indicates that the trend is reasonable for the earliest historical events from Davis County canyons to have the largest volumes. This trend supports the geologic interpretation that significant time is required for sediment to accumulate in canyon channels after it has been cleaned by either cloudburst rainstorms or rapid snowmelt. Because major debris flows were discharged from some Davis County canyons in historical time, future large-volume debris flows from these canyons should not be expected for a significant period of time, probably longer than 100 years, if the general condition of the watershed remains approximately the same or improves. Degradation of watershed conditions, because of factors such as fire, road building, or logging, could result in large-volume debris flows from canyons that produced major his-

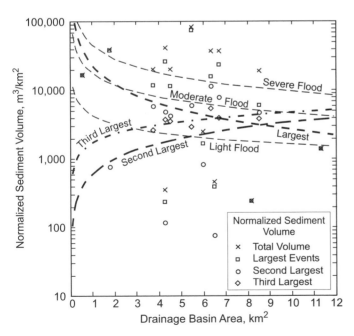

Figure 14. Normalized sediment-discharge volumes from the largest, second largest, and third largest historical flood events from Davis County canyons (except Farmington Canyon). Based on data in Table 2.

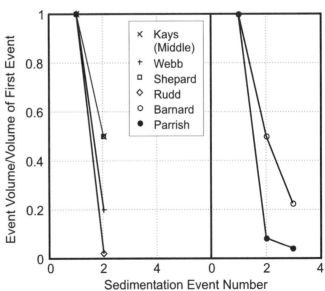

Figure 15. Ratio of flood-event volume to volume of the earliest historical event in Davis County canyons experiencing no more than three historical events. Based on data in Table 2.

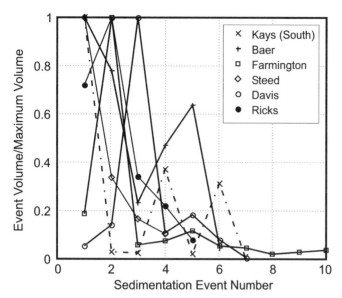

Figure 16. Ratio of flood-event volume to the volume of the largest historical event in Davis County canyons experiencing four or more historical events. Based on data in Table 2.

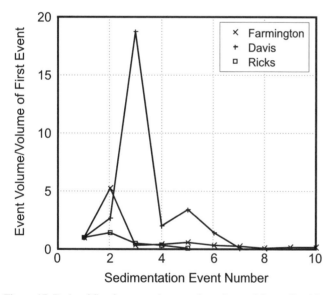

Figure 17. Ratio of flood-event volume to the volume of the earliest historical event in the three Davis County canyons from which the earliest historical event was not the largest historical event. Based on data in Table 2.

torical debris flows. However, the small sizes of the post-Lake Bonneville alluvial-fan landforms in Davis County indicate that debris flows were rare in prehistoric post–Lake Bonneville time, and the occurrence of major debris flows from some canyons in historical time indicates that debris flows from these canyons should be relatively rare in the near future. The phrase "relatively rare in the near future" in this context refers to an annual exceedance probability of 0.01 (the so-called "100-year" event).

The 1983 and 1984 debris flows were the only well-docu-

mented historical debris-flow events from Rudd Canyon, but exposures of alluvial-fan deposits on the upthrown side of the Wasatch fault scarp at the mouth of the canyon, and in a small borrow pit about 50 m (160 ft) north of the canyon, provide evidence for at least five prehistoric alluvial-fan sedimentation events from Rudd Canyon (Keaton, 1988). The volumes of the prehistoric Rudd Canyon sedimentation events, in order of decreasing size, are estimated on the basis of topography and distribution of exposures to have been on the order of 250,000, 146,000, 105,000, 94,000, and 64,000 m^3 (325,000, 190,000, 135,000, 120,000, and 80,000 yd^3), respectively (Keaton, 1988). The largest of these is inferred to have been the earliest post–Lake Bonneville sedimentation event.

Evidence of soil-profile development on the upper surfaces of buried prehistoric alluvial-fan deposits exposed at Rudd Creek could not be found, suggesting that the sedimentation events may have occurred over a relatively short period of time (Keaton, 1988). The soil developed at the ground surface on the oldest Ricks Canyon fan segments consists of an A-C profile, as described in Table 4 (Keaton, 1988). The degree of soil development observed by Keaton (1988) in test-pit exposures was uniform across the oldest post–Lake Bonneville fan and on fan deposits of clearly younger relative ages at both the Ricks Creek and Rudd Canyon fans. The uniformity of the soil and the absence of soil development on contacts separating deposits within the alluvial fan suggests that massive, rapid sedimentation was followed by an extensive period of landscape stability, during which the soil developed.

The 1983 and 1984 sedimentation events at Rudd Canyon did not exceed the capacity of the Rudd Creek channel above the fault scarp and, consequently, did not deposit significant amounts of sediment on the alluvial-fan above the fault; prehistoric sedimentation events with magnitudes similar to or smaller than the 1983 and 1984 events may have occurred at Rudd Creek, which have not yet been identified (Keaton et al., 1988b). Based on the geomorphology and stratigraphy of canyon-mouth alluvial fans, the recurrence intervals for debris flows of the magnitude of the 1983 event for Rudd Canyon range from 500 years (based on long-term erosion rates from the mountain block), to 1,000 years (over the past 10,000 years), to 3,700 years (based on the historical record; Keaton, 1988).

The stratigraphy and sedimentology of alluvial-fan sediments deposited from cloudburst discharge probably do not differ significantly from those deposited from rapid snowmelt discharge. The damaging intensities of historical cloudburst floods in Davis County had durations of 30 to 45 min, whereas rapid snowmelt floods had durations of days to weeks with diurnal fluctuations and individual sediment-discharge pulses of 30- to 45-min durations (Keaton, 1988). The frequency of cloudburst rainstorms can be estimated on the basis of rain-gauge data. The frequency of high-water-content snow pack can be estimated on the basis of snow course data. The frequency of sustained temperatures above freezing to cause rapid melting of record-breaking amounts of snow, such as existed in Utah in 1983 (Fig. 5) and 1984, can be estimated from temperature data. However, snowmelt floods require the pres-

**TABLE 4. DESCRIPTION OF SOIL FORMED ON
THE OLDEST SURFACE OF RICKS CREEK FAN**

Horizon	Depth (cm)	Description
A1	0 – 15	Very dark brown (10YR 2/2m) to very dark grayish brown (10YR 3/2m) silty coarse sand with gravel; very fine granular structure, friable; very slightly sticky; very slightly plastic; abundant fine roots; gradual smooth boundary.
A2	15 – 35	Very dark brown (10YR 2/2m) to very dark grayish brown (10YR 3/2m) gravely silty coarse sand; weak, fine granular structure; friable; nonsticky; nonplastic; few fine roots; gradual smooth boundary.
C2	35 – 70	Dark yellowish brown (10YR 3/4 to 4/4m) gravely silty coarse sand; massive; friable; nonsticky; nonplastic; few fine pores; gradual smooth boundary.
C3	70 – 100+	Dark yellowish brown (10YR 4/4m) to yellowish brown (10YR 5/6m) cobbly gravely silty sand; friable; nonsticky; nonplastic; few fine pores.

ence of both heavy snow pack and sustained warm temperatures to occur simultaneously, which together are relatively rare. Snowmelt floods also seem to be enhanced by antecedent soil moisture (Marsell, 1972). Snowmelt floods occurred along the Wasatch Front in 1922, 1952, 1983, and 1984 (Fig. 3). Only the snowmelt in 1983 created widespread landslides and debris flows.

Geologic study of stream channels

As a result of the 1983 and 1984 debris-flow and debris-flood events, Davis County formed a Flood Control Department and constructed debris basins below those canyons that had produced debris flows or debris floods during historical time. When Davis County received the COE's preliminary debris-flow potential analyses from FEMA, the county discovered the COE had calculated that most of the debris basins Davis County constructed as a result of the 1983/1984 events were inadequate to contain the 100-year debris-flow event (Table 3). Mayors and city engineers were concerned over the results of the COE's study and wanted to know why the newly constructed debris basins were inadequate when their sizes had been recommended by federally sponsored studies (Wieczorek et al., 1983) completed shortly or immediately after the events of 1983. To further complicate matters, geologic studies of alluvial fans at canyon mouths indicated that these same debris basins had been over-designed for the 100-year debris volumes or were constructed at the mouths of low-risk canyons (Keaton et al., 1988b).

To determine which set of conflicting volumetric estimates of potential debris flows was most accurate, the Davis County Planning and Flood Control Departments began a study of stream-

channel conditions (Williams et al., 1989; Williams and Lowe, 1990). Triggering mechanisms for alluvial-fan flooding and sedimentation events generally are either climatologically induced erosion or landsliding. Soil characteristics, topography, and vegetative conditions are important in determining the effects of these probabilistic events. The magnitude of the event, however, in terms of amount of debris produced is determined by the volume of debris produced by the triggering event and channel conditions. Davis County was aware that Wieczorek et al. (1983, p. 31) had estimated that 81 to 85% of the debris deposited at the mouth of Rudd Canyon was derived from the stream channel. Debris production and accumulation are slow, intermittent geologic processes. Our studies in Davis County suggest that a stream channel recently cleaned to bedrock usually cannot contribute the same volume of debris during subsequent events as it did during initial events until debris again accumulates in the channel. The potential for large debris-flow events is, therefore, deterministically controlled by channel conditions. Topographic profiles across selected stream channels (Fig. 18) were constructed and used to demonstrate current channel conditions and estimated rates of debris accumulation in channels since the 1930s.

Davis County research into the relationship of triggering events, channel conditions, and debris-flow magnitude produced some interesting results. Debris volumes produced during alluvial-fan sedimentation events in pristine drainages with perennial streams are largely a function of the length of the stream channel involved. Pristine canyons are those which have not had a historical or recent prehistoric debris-flow event that cleaned out debris in the channel bottom. Calculations based on debris volumes from historical events in which the contribution from the source areas (landslides or overland erosion) have been subtracted suggest that about 30 m^3 of debris per lineal m (12 yd^3 of debris per lineal ft) of channel may represent a characteristic maximum debris volume for first events from pristine Davis County canyons (Williams and Lowe, 1990). This relationship appears to apply to perennial streams for both the rainstorm-erosion-generated events of the 1920s and 1930s and the snowmelt-induced, landslide-generated events of 1983 and 1984 (Williams and Lowe, 1990).

The shape of profiles across the stream channels can be used to evaluate potential production from Davis County canyons

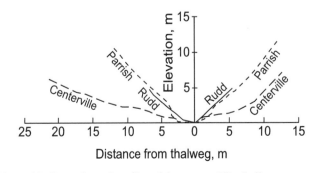

Figure 18. Cross-channel profiles of three central Davis County stream channels (from Lowe et al., 1992).

(Fig. 18). Rudd Canyon and Parrish Canyon have similar U-shaped channel profiles and side-channel slopes, in spite of the fact that the Parrish Canyon debris flows occurred more than 50 years prior to the Rudd Canyon debris flows. The Parrish Canyon channel is much deeper than the Rudd Canyon channel, perhaps because Parrish Canyon has a much larger drainage basin and flatter average channel gradient (Williams and Lowe, 1990). The Centerville Canyon cross-channel profile, however, has much gentler side slopes and a flat-bottomed shallow V-shape, indicating that the stream channel contains a large volume of material that could become incorporated into future debris flows (Williams and Lowe, 1990).

The amount of bedrock exposed in the channel bottoms of the three stream channels also varies significantly. Williams and Lowe (1990) estimate that the bottom of the Rudd Canyon channel is 50 to 70% bedrock. Although the Parrish Canyon debris flow occurred more than 50 years before the Rudd Canyon debris flow, Williams and Lowe (1990) estimate that 40–50% of the Parish Canyon stream channel is underlain by bedrock at shallow depths. Williams and Lowe (1990) estimate the amount of bedrock exposed in the Centerville Canyon stream channel to be 10% or less.

These observations lead to the conclusion that, for climatic conditions such as those experienced in central Davis County during the past 50 years, the rate of debris accumulation in stream channels is very low. Until the stream channels are reloaded with debris, drainages that have been cleaned out by recent debris flows will likely produce much smaller debris volumes than pristine, debris-choked canyons (Lowe et al., 1992).

Engineering versus geologic assumptions and conclusions

Engineering assumptions and conclusions. Five important engineering assumptions apparently were made by COE in the process of evaluating alluvial-fan flooding in Davis County after the damaging debris flows of 1983: (1) the sediment-discharge event at Rudd Canyon was the 100-year event, (2) sediment discharge can be modeled by an input hydrograph based on observed thicknesses and distribution of debris and duration of discharge, (3) the causative climatic process (cloudburst or snowmelt) is unimportant, (4) the supply of sediment (slopes or steam channels) is unimportant, and (5) the canyons in Davis County are sufficiently uniform in flood behavior that the observed sediment volume discharged from Rudd Canyon in 1983 can be used as the basis for debris-production curves to estimate 100-year sediment volumes from other canyons.

The number of damaging sedimentation events in central Davis County apparently was used by COE as the basis for making the judgment that the 1983 Rudd Canyon event was the 100-year event. The fact that Rudd Canyon apparently had not generated a significant sedimentation event in the 136-year history of Davis County apparently was unimportant in evaluating the frequency of sediment discharge.

The traditional engineering approach to flood-hazard analysis is the clear-water hydrograph. A reasonably direct method of using a hydrograph to model debris-flow discharge is to adjust its shape to produce the desired event volume. The alternative to the traditional hydrograph representing the 100-year debris-flow event is geologic interpretation of the volume and frequency of past sediment discharge events.

The engineering approach made no distinction between cloudburst processes, which had caused all sedimentation events in Davis County prior to 1983, and rapid snowmelt in the spring following rains that created high antecedent soil moisture the preceding fall as the causative climatic process. The annual frequencies of these two processes are distinct and cannot be combined readily. A conditional probability is required to model the likelihood of simultaneous heavy snow pack and temperatures for sustained melting. The frequency of occurrence of the climatic conditions in the Rudd Canyon drainage basin in 1983 are unknown, but probably much more rare than the so-called 100-year event.

The source and supply of sediment was not a factor in the COE model. However, observations and reports of historical sedimentation events in Davis County indicate that the source and availability of sediment could have been included in the model. The snowmelt events of 1983 began with slope movements which mobilized into debris flows that increased in volume as they traveled down channels by incorporating sediment from channel beds and banks. The cloudburst events of 1912, 1923, and 1930 began with erosion of overland flow on damaged watersheds and increased in volume as they traveled down channels by incorporating sediment from channel beds and banks. As mentioned above, those channels cleaned of sediment by an initial event yielded less sediment in subsequent events. Until sediment again accumulates in channels, large sediment discharges cannot recur. For the COE's engineering approach to modeling debris-flow processes to be reasonably valid, deterministic factors, such as the volume of debris in stream channels, must be used along with probabilistic modeling of climatological events.

Rudd Canyon is one of the smallest watersheds in central Davis County (Table 1) and had not produced a significant debris flow or debris flood in historical time prior to 1983 (Table 2). The shape of the debris-flow hydrograph determined for the 1983 event in this canyon appears to be unreasonable for a 100-year frequency for reasons discussed earlier in this paper. The assumption that the canyons are sufficiently uniform that the debris-production relationship determined for Rudd Canyon can be normalized and applied to canyons that are much larger also appears to be unreasonable (see Fig. 14).

Three important engineering conclusions following the COE analysis were clear to the Davis County Flood Control Department: (1) significant debris flows in Davis County should be expected to occur frequently, (2) most sediment catch basins built in 1983 have insufficient volumes to contain the newly defined 100-year sedimentation events, and (3) large urban areas are now located within the newly defined 100-year flood-plain boundaries.

Geologic findings and conclusions. Six important geologic factors were recognized by Keaton (1988, 1989a) during evaluation of alluvial-fan flooding hazards in Davis County: (1) each Davis County canyon has a unique history of sediment production and discharge; (2) prior to 1983, debris flows occurred two or more times during historical time from only 8 of 22 Davis County canyons; (3) the most severe debris flow in Davis County in 1983 occurred in a canyon that had not generated a significant event earlier in historical time; (4) debris flows in Davis County have been caused by both cloudburst and snowmelt processes; (5) stream channels in the Davis County canyons provided most of the sediment that caused damage in the communities; and (6) post–Lake Bonneville alluvial fans in Davis County are small landforms.

The COE concept that the 1983 discharge from Rudd Creek was a 100-year event apparently was based on historical sediment discharges from drainages in central Davis County other than Rudd Creek. The volume of sediment discharged during historical flood events appear to be unique for each canyon. Combining sediment-discharge histories from adjacent canyons should not be done in the same manner as combining data from regional precipitation gauges. The largest historical sediment discharge from Rudd Canyon occurred in 1983; therefore, the 1983 event must be at least the 136-year (1983–1847) event in that canyon.

The 1983 debris flows were triggered by landslides caused by high antecedent soil moisture, a heavy snow pack, an abnormally late rapid snowmelt, and an undrained bedrock aquifer (Mathewson et al., 1990). Geologic studies of the structural fabric (Ala, 1990a) and hydrogeology of the landslide source areas (Skelton, 1991) indicate these landslide-induced debris flows were infrequent events that certainly were rare in the historical time frame, and perhaps the first such large-volume event since the early to mid-Holocene. Most of the earlier historical debris flows were generated by overland erosion during cloudburst rainstorms on watersheds depleted of vegetative cover by overgrazing and burning. Geologic studies of alluvial fans at the mouths of central Davis County canyons (Keaton, 1988) indicate that (1) the majority of post–Lake Bonneville, prehistoric alluvial-fan building occurred rapidly, probably during the early Holocene when much frost-shattered and solifluction sediment in the Davis County canyons was available for transport; (2) apparently few major debris flows discharged significant volumes of sediment onto alluvial fans at canyon mouths between the early Holocene and the 1920s; and (3) if historical debris-flow events were representative of the long-term rate of sediment deposition on Davis County alluvial fans, the post–Lake Bonneville fans would be large, prominent landforms instead of the small features they actually are. The majority of sediment incorporated into debris flows triggered by either snowmelt-induced landslides or cloudburst rainstorms is derived from the stream channel. Geologic studies of central Davis County stream channels (Williams and Lowe, 1990) indicate that (1) debris production and accumulation in channels is a slow, intermittent process; (2) stream channels that have produced significant debris-flow events during historical time have not yet been recharged with sediment; (3) future debris flows

from drainages cleaned of sediment will likely be of less volume than initial historical events, until the drainages have been recharged with sediment; and (4) other factors (e.g., slope) being equal, the most likely channels to produce large debris flows in the near future are those that have not produced historical debris flows.

Four important geologic conclusions were made by Keaton (1988, 1989a) during evaluation of alluvial-fan flood hazards in Davis County: (1) debris flows in Davis County are rare geologic events; (2) a substantial amount of time is required for sediment to accumulate in channels that have been cleaned by previous sedimentation events; (3) most sediment catch basins will contain debris from the geologically defined 100-year event (Table 3); (4) other factors (e.g., slope) being equal, those canyons that have not had significant debris flows earlier in historical time have the greatest risk for future sedimentation events.

Subsequent government response to the new COE/FEMA maps

In 1991, based on the Davis County study of stream channels (Williams et al., 1989; Williams and Lowe, 1990), and augmented with the results of the study of central Davis County alluvial fans (Keaton, 1988; Keaton et al., 1988a, b), Davis County and Centerville City challenged the methods used by COE to construct the new FEMA flood maps for canyons above Centerville (Federal Emergency Management Agency, 1992). In 1992, Davis County and Farmington City challenged the new maps for canyons above Farmington. The third city for which new flood maps were prepared, Bountiful, did not challenge the maps because two of three debris basins in the city would have sufficient capacity to contain COE's calculated 100-year event volume. As a result of the challenges, the maps are currently being reviewed to determine if estimated sediment yield values from canyons with recently eroded channels are reasonable.

Beginning in 1994, FEMA sponsored a National Research Council Committee on Understanding Alluvial-Fan Flooding. This committee will study how to determine which areas are subject to alluvial-fan flooding, especially within the context of the National Flood Insurance Program. They may also study the methods available for quantifying the extent and probability of alluvial-fan flooding.

Changes that can dramatically affect the sediment production in drainage basins also need to be considered in preparing reasonable flood-hazard maps. Increasing urbanization results in increasing recreational pressure on the public land in the Wasatch Range, as it does elsewhere. Fire is a growing threat in the Wasatch-Cache National Forest. Sediment yield is known to increase following a fire (Branson et al., 1981, p. 135; Sidle et al., 1985, p. 77). Evanstad and Rasely (1995) systematically evaluated the sediment-yield potential for the canyons along the Wasatch Front under current management practices and immediately following a fire using a 1991 revision of an empirical sediment-yield model developed by the Pacific Southwest Inter-Agency Committee

(1968). The results of their evaluation provide needed information for debris-flow hazard management in Davis County. Evanstad and Rasely's (1995) estimates of sediment yield following a high-intensity burn in canyon drainage basins are presented for selected canyons in Table 3. These estimates are deterministic, and represent the sediment yield expected based on empirical factors, including climate, but not necessarily the 100-year precipitation. Although these estimates do not address the incorporation of channel material into debris flows, and even a channel cleaned to bedrock by a previous event will produce at least some additional debris, they estimate the contribution of material eroded from drainage-basin slopes. The estimates indicate that only the debris basin constructed near the mouth of Centerville Canyon (Deuel Creek) is inadequate to contain post-fire sediment yield from drainage-basin slopes (see Table 3).

CONCLUSIONS

In Davis County, approximately $12 million were spent to build or refurbish debris basins following the 1983 debris-flow events based on a 6-wk-long hazard assessment funded at less than $50,000. Geologic research to understand the debris-flow processes was conducted in Davis County after the debris basins were constructed. The new debris basins were constructed below those canyons that had partly detached landslides identified with potential for generating debris flows capable of reaching canyon mouths. Little emphasis was placed on construction of debris basins at the mouths of canyons that have not generated a damaging historical sedimentation event. Based on the geologic evaluation of the canyons in Davis County, these are potentially the most hazardous for future sedimentation events. Had detailed geologic studies of debris-flow processes been conducted prior to design and construction of the debris basins, more emphasis may have been placed on building debris basins at the mouths of canyons that have not produced historical debris flows instead of canyons that had produced debris flows during historical time.

Flood-plain-hazard evaluations are performed for FEMA on the basis of conventional engineering hydrology/hydraulics. The geologic approach to evaluating hazardous processes on the basis of evidence of past occurrences provides valuable information that should be included in the engineering analyses. A procedure does not yet exist that requires, let alone allows, geologic evidence and interpretations to be included in the FEMA approach to flood-plain-hazard evaluations.

The processes that led to historical debris-flow damage in Davis County consisted of rapid snowmelt in 1983 and 1984 and cloudburst rainstorms in all other years in which damaging debris flows occurred. Both of these climatological processes operate independently, and debris flows generated from them should be evaluated separately to estimate the 100-year event. Procedures for predicting the volume of the 100-year flood discharge from stream-flow gauges or precipitation records are well established. Procedures for predicting the 100-year snow-water equivalent are based on snow-course data; however, a conditional probability approach is required to predict temperatures for rapid melting given that the 100-year snowpack has accumulated. Additional conditional probabilities would be needed to include antecedent soil moisture and undrained bedrock aquifer conditions.

Geologic studies indicate that engineering approaches used by the COE to map "100-year flood-plain" boundaries in central Davis County overestimated 100-year-frequency debris-flow volume from Rudd Canyon, and therefore, also the 100-year volumes for many other canyons. Climatically controlled triggering events for alluvial-fan flooding and sedimentation can be probabilistically modeled. However, the volume of sediment produced during these events is, in part, determined by the amount of debris in stream channels and this factor must be incorporated into any model of potential debris-flow volumes. Two cities in central Davis County, Farmington and Centerville, have challenged the accuracy of the new FEMA flood-plain maps based on the COE flood volumes. Map revisions, which may not have been necessary if geologic data had been incorporated into the COE study, are currently under way.

The 6-week-long study funded by FEMA and conducted by personnel from the U.S. Geological Survey and Los Angeles County Flood Control District was a regional debris-flow hazard assessment of the area along the Wasatch Front from Salt Lake City to Willard. Geologic research to investigate debris-flow processes was not part of the scope of the hazard assessment. The understanding of debris-flow processes was greatly enhanced by subsequent studies supported by federal, state, county, and university sources. Much of what has been learned from these studies has significantly advanced the state of understanding of debris-flow processes in general, and along the Wasatch Front in particular, since 1983.

ACKNOWLEDGMENTS

This paper is based in part on research funded by the U.S. Geological Survey Landslide Hazards Reduction Program (Agreement No. 14-08-0001-A0507), sponsored by the Utah Geological Survey (Contract No. 88-0886), and administered through the Department of Civil and Environmental Engineering at Utah State University. Review comments by Gary E. Christenson, Gerald F. Wieczorek, Christopher C. Mathewson, and Kimm M. Harty improved the quality and clarity of this paper and are gratefully acknowledged.

REFERENCES CITED

Ala, S., 1989, The influence of bedrock on debris flows along the Wasatch Front, Utah: Association of Engineering Geologists 32nd Annual Meeting Abstracts and Program, Vail, Colorado, p. 48.

Ala, S., 1990a, Bedrock structure, lithology and ground water—influences on slope failure initiation in Davis County, Utah [M.S. thesis]: College Station, Texas A&M University, 236 p.; available as Utah Geological Survey Contract Report 95-4.

Ala, S., 1990b, Relationship between bedrock structural fabric and groundwater flow, Wasatch Front, Utah, in Robinson, L., ed., Proceedings, 26th Annual Symposium on Engineering Geology and Geotechnical Engineering:

Pocatello, Idaho, Idaho State University, p. 22-1–22-17.

Ala, S., and Mathewson, C. C., 1990, Structural control of ground-water induced debris flows, *in* Proceedings, International Symposium on the Hydraulics/Hydrology of Arid Lands (H²AL), July 30–August 3, 1990, San Diego, California: New York, American Society of Civil Engineers, p. 590–595.

Anciaux, A., 1987, Mud and debris flow case studies in Davis County, Utah, *in* Mud and debris flow workshop, Park City, Utah, September 10–11: Salt Lake City, Civil Engineering Department, University of Utah, and Federal Emergency Management Agency, unpaginated.

Anderson, L. R., Keaton, J. R., Saarinen, T. F., and Wells, W. G., II, 1984, The Utah landslides, debris flows, and floods of May and June, 1983: Washington, D.C., National Academy Press, 96 p.

Bailey, R. W., and Croft, A. R., 1937, Contour-trenches control floods and erosion on range land: Washington, D.C., U.S. Department of Agriculture Forestry Publication No. 4, 22 p.

Bailey, R. W., Craddock, G. W., and Croft, A. R., 1947, Watershed management for summer flood control, Utah: U.S. Department of Agriculture Miscellaneous Publication 639, 24 p.

Bell, G. L., 1952, Geology of the northern Farmington Mountains, *in* Marsell, R. E., ed., Geology of the Central Wasatch Mountains: Utah Geological Society Guidebook to the Geology of Utah, no. 9, p. 38–51.

Branson, F. A., Gifford, G. F., Renard, K. G., and Hadley, R. F., 1981, Rangeland hydrology: Dubuque, Iowa, Kendall/Hunt Publishing Company, Society for Range Management Range Science Series No. 1, 340 p.

Brooks, R. K., 1986, Instrumentation of the Steed Canyon landslide [M.S. thesis]: Logan, Utah, Utah State University, 183 p.

Bryant, B., 1984, Reconnaissance geologic map of the Precambrian Farmington Canyon Complex and surrounding rocks in the Wasatch Mountains between Ogden and Bountiful, Utah: U.S. Geological Survey Miscellaneous Investigation Series Map I-1447, scale 1:50,000, 1 sheet.

Bryant, B., 1988, Geology of the Farmington Canyon Complex, Wasatch Mountains, Utah: U.S. Geological Survey Professional Paper 1476, 54 p., scale 1:50,000, 1 sheet.

Bull, W. B., 1991, Geomorphic responses to climatic change: New York, Oxford University Press, 326 p.

Butler, E., and Marsell, R. E., 1972, Cloudburst floods in Utah, 1939–1969: Utah Division of Water Resources Cooperative Investigations Report No. 11, 103 p.

Campbell, R. H., 1975, Soil slips, debris flows and rainstorms in the Santa Monica Mountains and vicinity, southern California: U.S. Geological Survey Professional Paper 851, 51 p.

Cannon, S. Q., chairman, 1931, Torrential floods in northern Utah, 1930, report of Special Flood Commission: Utah Agricultural Experiment Station Circular 92, 51 p.

Coleman, K. W., 1989, Role of contour trenching in the alteration of hydrogeologic conditions of the Wasatch Front: Association of Engineering Geologists 32nd Annual Meeting Abstracts and Program, Vail, Colorado, p. 57.

Coleman, K. W., 1990a, Watershed conditions contributing to the 1983–1984 debris flows in the Wasatch Range, Davis County, Utah [M.S. thesis]: College Station, Texas A&M, University, 164 p., also available as Utah Geological Survey Contact Report 95-2.

Coleman, K. W., 1990b, The effect of contour trenching of hydrogeologic conditions of the Wasatch Front: Association of Engineering Geologists 33rd Annual Meeting Abstracts and Program, p. 100.

Craddock, G. W., 1960, Floods controlled on Davis County watersheds: Journal of Forestry, v. 58, no. 4, p. 291–293.

Crawford, A. L., and Thackwell, F. E., 1931, Some aspects of the mudflows north of Salt Lake City, Utah: Salt Lake City, Utah Academy of Sciences, v. 8, p. 97–105.

Croft, A. R., 1962, Some sedimentation phenomena along the Wasatch Mountain Front: Journal of Geophysical Research, v. 67, no. 4, p. 1511–1524.

Croft, A. R., 1967, Rainstorm debris floods—a problem in public welfare: University of Arizona Agricultural Experiment Station Report 248, 36 p.

Croft, A. R., 1981, History of development of the Davis County Experimental

Watershed: Ogden, Utah, U.S. Department of Agriculture Forest Service Special Publication, 42 p.

Currey, D. R., 1990, Quaternary paleolakes in the evolution of semidesert basins, with special emphasis on Lake Bonneville and the Great Basin, U.S.A.: Paleogeography, Paleoclimatology, Paleoecology, v. 76, p. 189–214.

Currey, D. R., and Oviatt, C. G., 1985, Durations, average rates, and probable causes of Lake Bonneville expansions, stillstands, and contractions during the last deep-lake cycle, 32,000 to 10,000 years ago, *in* Kay, P. A., and Diaz, H. F., eds., Problems of and Prospects for Predicting Great Salt Lake Levels, Conference Proceedings, Center for Public Affairs and Administration: Salt Lake City, University of Utah, p. 9–24.

Deevey, E. S., and Flint, R. F., 1957, Postglacial hypsithermal interval: Science, v. 125, p. 182–184.

Eblin, J. S., 1990, The influence of colluvial variations on the slope stability of three drainage basins along the Wasatch Front, Davis County, Utah: Association of Engineering Geologists, 33rd Annual Meeting, Abstracts and Program, Pittsburgh, Pennsylvania, p. 94–95.

Eblin, J. S., 1991, A probabilistic investigation of slope stability in the Wasatch Range, Davis County, Utah [M.S. thesis]: College Station, Texas A&M University, 98 p., also available as Utah Geological Survey Contract Report 95-3.

Evanstad, N. C., and Rasely, R. C., 1995, G.I.S. application in the northern Wasatch Front pre-fire hazard risk assessment, Davis and Weber Counties, Utah, *in* Lund W. R., ed., Environmental and engineering geology of the Wasatch Front region: Utah Geological Association Publication 24, p. 169–184.

Federal Emergency Management Agency, 1982, Flood insurance rate map, City of Centerville, Utah, Davis County: Federal Emergency Management Agency, Community-Panel No. 490040 0002 B, effective date March 1, Panel 2 of 3, scale 1:6,000.

Federal Emergency Management Agency, 1992, Flood insurance rate map, City of Centerville, Utah, Davis County: Federal Emergency Management Agency, Community-Panel No. 490040 0002 C, map revised February 19, Panel 2 of 3, scale 1:6,000.

Jadkowski, M. A., 1987, Multispectral remote sensing of landslide susceptibility areas [Ph.D. thesis]: Logan, Utah State University, 260 p.

Kaliser, B. N., 1983, Geologic hazards of 1983: Utah Geological and Mineral Survey, Survey Notes, v. 17, no. 2, p. 3–8, and 14.

Kaliser, B. N., and Slosson, J. E., 1988, Geologic consequences of the 1983 wet year in Utah: Utah Geological and Mineral Survey Miscellaneous Publication 88-3, 109 p.

Keate, N. S., 1991, Debris flows in southern Davis County, Utah [M.S. thesis]: Salt Lake City, University of Utah, 174 p.

Keaton, J. R., 1986a, Debris flow recurrence estimated from long-term erosion: Geological Society of America Abstracts with Program, v. 18, no. 6, p. 652.

Keaton, J. R., 1986b, Landslide inventory and preliminary hazard assessment, southeast Davis County, Utah: Association of Engineering Geologists, 29th Annual Meeting, Abstracts With Program, San Francisco, p. 59.

Keaton, J. R., 1988, A probabilistic model for hazards related to sedimentation processes on alluvial fans in Davis County, Utah [Ph.D. thesis]: College Station, Texas A&M University, 441 p.

Keaton, J. R., 1989a, Engineering versus geologic approach to evaluating debris flow hazards: Association of Engineering Geologists, 32nd Annual Meeting, Abstracts and Program, Vail, Colorado, p. 84.

Keaton, J. R., 1989b, A probabilistic model for sedimentation hazards on alluvial fans, *in* Watters, R. J., ed., Engineering geology and geotechnical engineering: Rotterdam, A. A., Balkema, p. 213–220.

Keaton, J. R., 1995, Dilemmas in regulating debris-flow hazards in Davis County, *in* Lund W. R., ed., Environmental and engineering geology of the Wasatch Front region: Utah Geological Association Publication 24, p. 185–192.

Keaton, J. R., and Lowe, M., 1993, Evaluation of debris-flow hazards in Davis County, Utah; engineering versus geological approaches: Geological Society of America Abstracts with Programs, v. 25, no. 6, p. A–3.

Keaton, J. R., and Mathewson, C. C., 1987, Proposed ideal alluvial fan stratig-raphy for risk assessment: Geological Society of America Abstracts with Program, v. 19, no. 7, p. 723.

Keaton, J. R., and Mathewson, C. C., 1988, Stratigraphy of alluvial fan flood deposits, *in* Abt, S. R., and Gessler, J., eds., Hydraulic engineering: Proceedings, 1988 National Conference of the Hydraulics Division of the American Society of Civil Engineers, Colorado Springs, Colorado, p. 149–154.

Keaton, J. R., Mathewson, C. C., and Anderson, L. R., 1987, Hazards and risks associated with alluvial fan processes in Davis County, Utah: Association of Engineering Geologists, 30th Annual Meeting, Abstracts with Program, Atlanta, Georgia, p. 42.

Keaton, J. R., Anderson, L. R., and Mathewson, C. C., 1988a, Assessing debris flow hazards on alluvial fans in Davis County, Utah, *in* Fragaszy, R. J., ed., Proceedings, Symposium on Engineering Geology and Soils Engi-neering, 24: Pullman, Washington State University, p. 89–108.

Keaton, J. R., Anderson, L. R., and Mathewson, C. C., 1988b, Assessing debris flow hazards on alluvial fans in Davis County, Utah: final report under U.S. Geological Survey Landslide Hazards Reduction Program Agree-ment No. 14-08-0001-A0507, Logan, Utah State University, Department of Civil and Environmental Engineering, 167 p., plus appendices, also available as Utah Geological Survey Contract Report 91–11.

Lindskov, K. L., 1984, Floods of May to June 1983 along the northern Wasatch Front, Salt Lake City to North Ogden, Utah: Utah Geological and Mineral Survey Water-Resources Bulletin 24, 11 p.

Liou, J., 1989, Mud flow and mudflow mapping in Davis County, Utah, *in* Pro-ceedings, 1988 Conference on Arid West Flood Plain Management Issues, Las Vegas, Nevada, October 19–21: Madison, Wisconsin, Association of Flood Plain Managers, p. 111–146.

Lowe, M., ed., 1990, Geologic hazards and land-use planning: background, explanation, and guidelines for development in Davis County in desig-nated geologic hazards special study areas: Utah Geological and Mineral Survey Open-File Report 198, 73 p.

Lowe, M., 1993, Debris-flow hazards—a guide for land-use planning, Davis County, Utah, *in* Gori, P. L., ed., Applications of research from the U.S. Geological Survey program, Assessment of regional earthquake hazards and risk along the Wasatch Front, Utah: U.S. Geological Survey Profes-sional Paper 1519, p. 143–150.

Lowe, M., Black, B. D., Harty, K. M., Keaton, J. R., Mulvey, W. E., Pashley, E. F., Jr., and Williams, S. R., 1992, Geologic hazards of the Ogden area, Utah, *in* Wilson, J. R., ed., Field guide to geologic excursions in Utah and adjacent areas of Nevada, Idaho, and Wyoming: Utah Geological Survey Miscellaneous Publication 92-3, p. 231–285.

Lowe, M., and Christenson, G. E., 1990, Geologic-hazards maps for land-use planning, Davis and Weber Counties, Utah: Geological Society of Amer-ica Abstracts with Programs, v. 22, no. 6, p. 37.

Lowe, M., Robison, R. M., Nelson, C. V., and Christenson, G. E., 1989, Slope-failure hazards in mountain front urban areas, Wasatch Front, Utah: Asso-ciation of Engineering Geologists, 32nd Annual Meeting, Abstracts and Program, Vail Colorado, p. 90–91.

Lowe, M., Williams, S. R., and Smith, S. W., 1988, The Davis County flood warn-ing and information system: Utah Geological and Mineral Survey Open-File Report 151, 15 p.

Mabey, D. R., 1992, Subsurface geology along the Wasatch Front, *in* Gori, P. L., and Hays, W. W., eds., Assessment of regional earthquake hazards and risk along the Wasatch Front, Utah: U.S. Geological Survey Professional Paper 1500-C, 16 p.

Marsell, R. E., 1972, Cloudburst and snowmelt floods, *in* Hilpert, L. S., ed., Envi-ronmental geology of the Wasatch Front, 1971: Utah Geological Associa-tion Publication 1, p. N1–N18.

Marston, R. B., 1958, The Davis County Experimental Watershed story: Ogden, Utah, unpublished Intermountain Forest and Range Experiment Station Guidebook, 37 p.

Mathewson, C. C., 1989, Hydrogeology and debris flows in the Farmington Can-yon Complex, Davis County, Utah: Association of Engineering Geolo-

gists, 32nd Annual Meeting, Abstracts and Program, Vail, Colorado, p. 93.

Mathewson, C. C., and Keaton, J. R., 1986, The role of bedrock groundwater in the initiation of debris flows: Association of Engineering Geologists 29th Annual Meeting, Abstracts and Program, p. 56

Mathewson, C. C., and Santi, P. M., 1987, Bedrock ground water: Source of sus-tained post-debris flow stream discharge, *in* McCalpin, J., ed., Proceed-ings, 23rd Annual Symposium on Engineering Geology and Soils Engineering: Logan, Utah, Utah State University Press, p. 253–265.

Mathewson, C. C., Keaton, J. R., and Santi, P. M., 1990, Role of bedrock ground water in the initiation of debris flows and sustained post-flow stream discharge: Association of Engineering Geologists Bulletin, v. 27, no. 1, p. 73–83.

Monteith, S., Anderson, L. R., and Keaton, J. R., 1990, Analysis of Steed Canyon landslide, *in* Robinson, L., ed., Proceedings, Annual Symposium on Engi-neering Geology and Geotechnical Engineering, 26th: Pocatello, Idaho, Idaho State University, p. 31-1–31-17.

National Research Council, Advisory Board on the Built Environment, 1982, Selecting a methodology for delineating mudslide hazard areas for the National Flood Insurance Program: National Academy Press, 23 p.

Neilson, R. P., and Wullstein, L. H., 1985, Comparative drought physiology and biogeography of *Quercus gambelii* and *Quercus turbinella*: The American Naturalist, v. 114, p. 259–271.

Olson, E. P., 1985, East Layton debris flow, Level 2 case study: Ogden, Utah, U.S. Department of Agriculture Forest Service, Intermountain Region Report, 20 p.

Oviatt, C. G., Currey, D. R., and Sack, D., 1992, Radiocarbon chronology of Lake Bonneville, eastern Great Basin, U.S.A.: Paleogeography, Paleoclimatol-ogy, Paleoecology, v. 99, p. 225–241.

Pacific Southwest Inter-Agency Committee, 1968, Report on factors affecting sediment yield in the Pacific southwest area and selection and evaluation of measures for reduction of erosion and sediment yield: Report of the Water Management Subcommittee, 10 p.

Pack, F. J., 1923, Torrential potential of desert waters: Pan American Geologist, v. 40, p. 349–356.

Pack, R. T., 1984, Debris flow initiation in Davis County, Utah, during the spring snowmelt period of 1983, *in* Proceedings, Annual Symposium on Engi-neering Geology and Soils Engineering, 21st, Moscow, Idaho, p. 59–77.

Pack, R. T., 1985, Multivariate analysis of relative landslide susceptibility in Davis County, Utah [Ph.D. thesis]: Logan, Utah, Utah State University, 233 p.

Paul, J. H., and Baker, F. S., 1925, The floods of 1923 in northern Utah: Univer-sity of Utah Bulletin, v. 15, no. 3, 20 p.

Pierson, T. C., 1985, Effects of slurry composition on debris flow dynamics, Rudd Canyon, Utah, *in* Bowles, D. S., ed., Delineation of landslide, flash flood, and debris flow hazards in Utah: Logan, Utah, Utah State University, Utah Water Research Laboratory Publication G-85/03, p. 132–152.

Price, W. E., 1976, A random-walk simulation model of alluvial-fan deposition, *in* Merriam, D. R., ed., Random processes in geology: New York, Springer-Verlag, p. 55–62.

Santi, P. M., 1988, The kinematics of debris flow transport down a canyon [M.S. thesis]: College Station, Texas A&M University, 85 p.

Santi, P. M., 1989, The kinematics of debris flow transport down a canyon: Bul-letin of the Association of Engineering Geologists, v. 26, no. 1 p. 5–9.

Santi, P. M., and Mathewson, C. C., 1988, What happens between the scar and the fan? The behavior of a debris flow in motion, *in* Fragaszy, R. J., ed., Pro-ceedings, Annual Symposium on Engineering Geology and Soils Engi-neering, 24th: Pullman, Washington State University, p. 73–88.

Schamber, D. R., 1987, One and two dimensional, transient simulations of mud-flows, *in* Mud and debris flow workshop, Park City, Utah, September 10–11: Salt Lake City, Civil Engineering Department, University of Utah, and Federal Emergency Management Agency, unpaginated.

Sidle, R. C., Pearce, A. J., and O'Loughlin, C. L., 1985, Hillslope stability and land use: American Geophysical Union Water Resources Monograph 11, 140 p.

Skelton, R. K., 1990, Investigation to determine the geological control of springs and seeps in the Farmington Canyon Complex, Davis County, Utah: Association of Engineering Geologists, 33rd Annual Meeting, Abstracts and Program, Pittsburgh, Pennsylvania, p. 100.

Skelton, R. K., 1991, Geological control of springs and seeps in the Farmington Canyon Complex, Davis County, Utah [M.S. thesis]: College Station, Texas A&M University, 98 p., also available as Utah Geological Survey Contract Report 95-1.

Stokes, W. L., 1977, Subdivisions of the major physiographic provinces in Utah: Utah Geology, v. 4, no. 1, p. 1–17.

Strahler, A. N., 1952, Hypsometric (area-altitude) analysis of erosional topography: Geological Society of America Bulletin, v. 63, p. 1117–1142.

U.S. Army Corps of Engineers, 1984, Wasatch Front and central Utah flood control study, Utah: U.S. Army Corps of Engineers, Sacramento District, 180 p.

U.S. Army Corps of Engineers, 1988, Mudflow modeling, one- and two-dimensional, Davis County, Utah: U.S. Army Corps of Engineers, Omaha District, 53 p.

U.S. Department of Agriculture, 1984, Water Supply Outlook for Utah, June, 1984: Salt Lake City, U.S. Soil Conservation Service, unpaginated.

Vandre, B. C., 1983, Geotechnical evaluation, Rudd Creek above Farmington: Ogden, Utah, U.S. Department of Agriculture, Forest Service, Intermountain Region, unpublished report, 11 p.

Wieczorek, G. F., 1986, Debris flows and hyperconcentrated streamflows, *in* Pro-

ceedings, Water Forum '86: World Water Issues in Evolution: New York, American Society of Civil Engineers, p. 219–226.

Wieczorek, G. F., Ellen, S., Lips, E. W., Cannon, S. H., and Short, D. N., 1983, Potential for debris flow and debris flood along the Wasatch Front between Salt Lake City and Willard, Utah, and measures for their mitigation: U.S. Geological Survey Open-File Report 83-635, 45 p.

Wieczorek, G. F., Lips, E. W., and Ellen, S. D., 1989, Debris flows and hyperconcentrated floods along the Wasatch Front, Utah, 1983 and 1984: Bulletin of the Association of Engineering Geologists, v. 26, no. 2, p. 191–208.

Williams, S. R., and Lowe, M., 1990, Process based debris-flow prediction method, *in* Proceedings, International Symposium on the Hydraulics/Hydrology of Arid Lands (H²AL), July 30–August 3, 1990, San Diego, California: New York, American Society of Civil Engineers, p. 66–71.

Williams, S. R., Lowe, M., and Smith, S. W., 1989, The discrete debris-mud flow risk analysis method, *in* Proceedings, 1988 Conference on Arid West Flood Plain Management Issues, October 19–21, 1988, Las Vegas, Nevada: Madison, Wisconsin, Association of Flood Plain Managers, p. 157–167.

Woolley, R. R., 1946, Cloudburst floods in Utah, 1850–1938: U.S. Geological Survey Water-Supply Paper 994, 128 p.

MANUSCRIPT ACCEPTED BY THE SOCIETY JUNE 5, 1997

Printed in U.S.A.

Geological Society of America
Reviews in Engineering Geology, Volume XII
1998

Preliminary assessment of the seismicity of the Malibu Coast Fault Zone, southern California, and related issues of philosophy and practice

Vincent S. Cronin and Keith A. Sverdrup
Department of Geosciences, University of Wisconsin-Milwaukee, Milwaukee, Wisconsin 53201

ABSTRACT

The Malibu Coast Fault Zone (MCFZ) is an east-west–trending fault system that marks the southern boundary of the western Transverse Ranges along the Santa Monica Mountains of southern California. Focal mechanism solutions for 107 earthquakes in the study area are mostly associated with thrusts or thrust-dominated oblique faults with a small left-lateral component of strike slip. The average azimuth of hanging-wall slip is 206°, which is approximately perpendicular to the trace of the San Andreas fault through the Transverse Ranges. Approximately 60% of the inferred slip vectors had azimuths between 180° and 240°. Six $M_L \geq 5$ earthquakes have been located along the MCFZ, most or all of which are attributed to the offshore Anacapa fault or to nonemergent structures to the south of the Anacapa fault. Hundreds of smaller earthquakes have been located in the vicinity of the MCFZ.

The MCFZ merges eastward with the active Potrero, Santa Monica, Hollywood, Raymond, and Cucamonga faults of the western and central Transverse Ranges. Offshore west of Sequit Point, the MCFZ merges with the active Santa Cruz Island and Santa Rosa Island faults. As part of the complex boundary zone between the Pacific and North American plates, the western Transverse Ranges is characterized by rates of uplift and crustal convergence that are comparable to the rates observed in the Himalayan Mountains, between the Indian and Eurasian plates. Documented Holocene slip, large gradients in topography and isostatic residual gravity, fault-related geomorphology, active uplift, distribution of micro- and macroearthquakes, and its position along a major structural/tectonic boundary are evidence that the MCFZ is an active fault zone.

The Malibu Coast fault of the MCFZ is an anastamosing zone of fault strands within a few kilometers of the Malibu coastline between longitudes 118.5° and 119°W. The Solstice and Winter Mesa strands of the Malibu Coast fault have been officially recognized as active faults under California's Alquist-Priolo Act. Rupture of the entire zoned length of the Solstice strand could have been generated by a M_L ~5.3 to 5.7 earthquake along the Malibu Coast fault: comparable in size to several historical earthquakes that have been attributed to the Anacapa fault. Although Holocene displacements have been officially recognized across only two strands of the Malibu Coast fault to date, we consider the Malibu Coast fault to be active and capable of producing a magnitude 6.5 to 7 earthquake.

Fault-zone studies involve scientific problems as well as problems of law and applied professional/scientific ethics. In addition to the basic ethics of science, a pri-

Cronin, V. S., and Sverdrup, K. A., 1998, Preliminary assessment of the seismicity of the Malibu Coast Fault Zone, southern California, and related issues of philosophy and practice, *in* Welby, C. W., and Gowan, M. E., eds., A Paradox of Power: Voices of Warning and Reason in the Geosciences: Boulder, Colorado, Geological Society of America Reviews in Engineering Geology, v. XII.

mary ethic in the engineering geosciences involves the legal and moral necessity to protect the public's safety. The incomplete nature of the geologic record and technical difficulties associated with dating Holocene geologic materials can make it difficult or impossible to establish the age of the most recent movement on a fault. The dilemma in fault-zone studies involves the potential conflict between the need to protect the safety of the public and the need to protect the property and wealth of the public by not mistakenly zoning fossil faults as active. The resolution of this dilemma must come through the evolution of public policy and professional practice concerning the assessment of fault-zone hazards. The formal reintroduction of the category *potentially active*, to characterize faults whose most recent displacement is ambiguous but that are likely to be active, might provide a useful intermediate category between *active* and *inactive* faults.

INTRODUCTION

This paper has two general purposes: (1) to review a spectrum of published data concerning the activity of the Malibu Coast Fault Zone (MCFZ) and offer a preliminary assessment of its Holocene activity, and (2) to engage in a brief discussion of issues related to the identification of significant seismogenic faults in populated areas. Discussions of issues that involve applied ethics in the engineering geosciences literature are as important as discussions of technical issues. We emphasize from the outset that we are not directly, obliquely, or tacitly questioning the ethics or scientific competency of any individuals, groups, companies, or governmental entities involved in fault-zone studies, particularly along the MCFZ. Where scientific interpretations are challenged in this paper, it is in the spirit of normal scientific discourse.

The study area for this paper lies within a geographic box between latitudes 33°55′–34°10′N and longitudes 118°30′–119°5′W (Figs. 1 and 2). The MCFZ includes the family of subparallel, east-west–trending faults adjacent to the Malibu coastline within the study area, many of which have been active during the Quaternary (Fig. 2). The MCFZ includes the Potrero fault, the various strands of the Malibu Coast fault (e.g., Puerco Canyon fault, Ramirez thrust, Escondido thrust, Point Dume fault, Latigo fault, Solstice fault, Paradise Cove fault), the Anacapa fault ("Dume fault" of Junger, 1976), Fault Z, and several unnamed offshore faults interpreted from marine geophysical data (see references in Table 1).

The Malibu Coast fault is mapped from Sequit Point along the Malibu coastline to a point between Carbon Canyon and Las Flores Canyon, where the fault trace extends offshore toward the Santa Monica coastline (Fig. 2). Nomenclature for the various strands of the Malibu Coast fault is not yet consistent. For example, the Solstice fault and Puerco Canyon fault (Treiman, 1994) are coincident with the southern strand of the Malibu Coast fault, as mapped by Dibblee (1993). The northern strand of the Malibu Coast fault (Dibblee, 1993; Dibblee and Ehrenspeck, 1993) is sometimes called the *main* branch—a term that is imprecise and potentially misleading. If, for example, a fault strand known as the *main* branch has not been active in the Quaternary, one might reasonably assume that the entire fault lacks Quaternary dis-

placement. In the case of the Malibu Coast fault, two strands that are south of the main or northern strand of the fault have been officially recognized as active during the Holocene (Division of Mines and Geology, 1995a, b). We prefer to use the term *Malibu Coast fault* to include the structurally interrelated fault strands that have been active during the Quaternary and that are located within ~3 km of the Malibu coastline between longitudes 118.5° and 119°W.

The subaerially exposed strands of the Malibu Coast fault are typically marked by gouge/breccia zones ranging in width from less than a meter to tens of meters. The gouge/breccia within the faults is typical of low-temperature deformation in the upper crust. Strands of the Malibu Coast fault generally dip toward the north at 30° to 70° and show evidence of reverse oblique slip, typically with a left-lateral strike-slip component. Field observations concerning Quaternary or Holocene activity along the Malibu Coast fault have recently been compiled by Treiman (1994).

The Malibu Coast fault is a fundamental boundary separating terranes with near-surface lithologies that appear to be quite different from one another and that were first juxtaposed through major rotations and horizontal translations in the late middle Miocene (Campbell, 1990; Campbell and Yerkes, 1976; Hornafius et al., 1986). The crystalline basement complex of the block north of the Malibu Coast fault is inferred to consist of Mesozoic igneous and metamorphic units similar to those exposed east of the study area in the Santa Monica Mountains. The basement complex is covered by marine and nonmarine strata of Late Cretaceous to middle Miocene age, which are locally interbedded or overlain by basaltic-andesitic volcanic rocks of middle Miocene age. The cover sequence of the northern block is locally mantled by Pleistocene marine terraces and other Quaternary deposits. South of the Malibu Coast fault are Miocene marine formations atop the Catalina schist (Campbell et al., 1966; Keller and Prothero, 1987). Total vertical displacement across the Malibu Coast fault has not been determined and may be indeterminate due to the differences in formations across the fault. Vertical separation of middle Miocene units to the east along the Santa Monica fault is approximately 2.1 km (Wright, 1991). The total amount of left-lateral slip along the Santa Monica/Hollywood–Malibu Coast

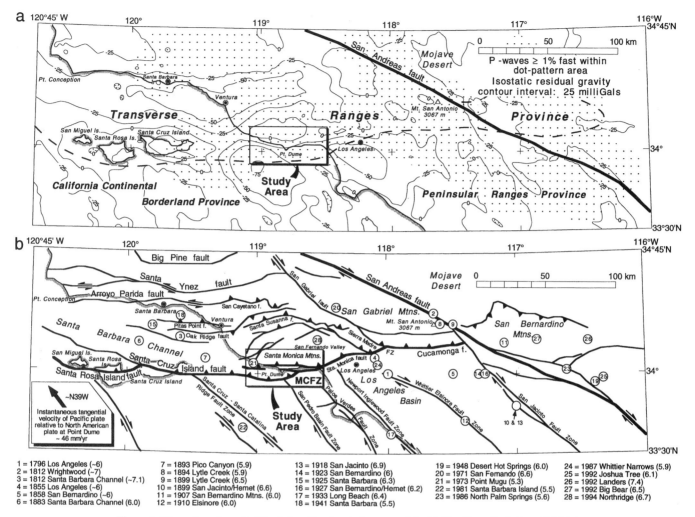

Figure 1. Maps of southern California locating the study area and the Malibu Coast Fault Zone (MCFZ). a, Location of physiographic provinces, contoured isostatic residual gravity (Roberts et al., 1990), and dot-patterned area within which *P*-wave velocities are 1–3% faster than normal (Humphreys and Clayton, 1990; Humphreys and Hager, 1990). Dashed curve is the approximate boundary of the Transverse Ranges Province. b, Location of selected major faults (Jennings, 1994; Wallace, 1990) and earthquake epicenters (Real et al., 1978; Hileman et al., 1973; Ellsworth, 1990; Hutton and Jones, 1993; Glen Reagor of NEIC, written communication, 1996). Epicenters for the numbered earthquakes listed at bottom are shown on map b. The Santa Cruz Island fault, MCFZ, Santa Monica fault, and Cucamonga fault are along the southern boundary of the Transverse Ranges Province. Inset box shows the present-day instantaneous tangential velocity of the Pacific plate relative to the North American plate, determined for Point Dume based on plate-motion data from NUVEL-1a (DeMets et al., 1994).

fault trend is estimated to be as much as 60 to 90 km (Lamar, 1961; Yeats, 1968; Colburn, 1973; Sage, 1973; Campbell and Yerkes, 1976; Link et al., 1984; Hornafius et al., 1986; Yerkes and Lee, 1987).

Late Cenozoic setting

The MCFZ is a fundamental physiographic boundary forming the southern edge of the Transverse Ranges Province and separating it from the California Continental Borderland Province to the southwest and the Peninsular Ranges Province to the south-

east (e.g., Jahns, 1954). The California Continental Borderland and Peninsular Ranges are part of a compound terrane of continental crust that extends from the southern edge of the Transverse Ranges south to the tip of the Baja California Peninsula. The MCFZ is also a fundamental structural-tectonic boundary. The surface traces of the northwest-trending strike-slip faults of southern California terminate along the north-dipping thrust faults at the southern edge of the Transverse Ranges (Fig. 1b). Only the San Andreas fault among these northwest-trending strike-slip faults passes through the Transverse Ranges (Hutton et al., 1991).

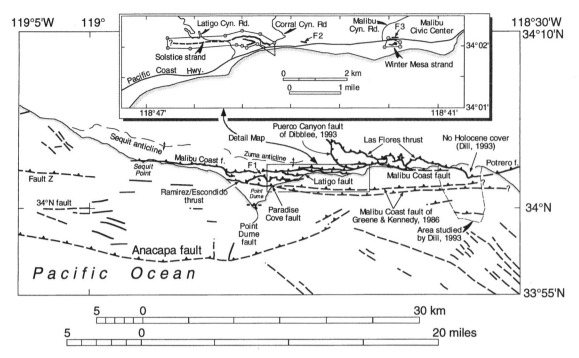

Figure 2. Map of principal faults in study area, after Dibblee (1992, 1993), Dibblee and Ehrenspeck (1990, 1993), Yerkes and Lee (1979b), Greene and Kennedy (1986), Yerkes and Campbell (1980), and Dill (1993). Inset detail map shows boundaries of Alquist-Priolo Special Studies Zones surrounding the Solstice and Winter Park strands of the Malibu Coast fault (Division of Mines and Geology, 1995a, b).

As the Baja California terrane has moved with the Pacific plate toward the northwest in the last ~4–5 million years, it has rotated clockwise relative to the North American plate, opening the Gulf of California in its wake and converging with other lithospheric elements to the north (e.g., Atwater, 1970; Bohannon and Parsons, 1995). The principal areas of convergence during the Quaternary are generally inferred to be along the Transverse Ranges and across the restraining bend in the San Andreas fault south of the "big bend" in its trace at ~35°N latitude (Hill and Dibblee, 1953; Hill, 1981; Wallace, 1990). The trend of the San Andreas fault along the restraining bend through the Transverse Ranges is ~25° anticlockwise from the direction in which the Pacific plate is currently moving relative to the North American plate: ~46 mm/yr toward N39°W, as computed for the coordinates of Point Dume using plate-motion data from NUVEL-1a (inset, Fig. 1b; DeMets et al., 1994).

The nature of the convergence in the Transverse Ranges and across the restraining bend of the San Andreas fault in southern California is still problematic. The western and central Transverse Ranges have been inferred to be a crustal flake/terrane/microplate that is in motion relative to both the Pacific and North American plates (Yeats, 1981). Weldon and Humphreys (1986) infer that this terrane is translating parallel to the trend of the San Andreas fault along the restraining bend, toward ~N60–65°W. The direction of maximum horizontal stress trends toward the north-northeast throughout the western Transverse Ranges and Santa Monica Bay (Hauksson and Saldivar, 1989; Zoback et al.,

1990). The average slip azimuth for earthquakes in the western and central Transverse Ranges is approximately perpendicular to the trace of the San Andreas fault along the restraining bend through the Transverse Ranges (Jackson and Molnar, 1990).

A regional detachment is inferred to exist in the mid- to lower crust beneath southern California, based on focal mechanism solutions and the inferred kinematics of the upper crust (e.g., Anderson, 1971; Hadley and Kanamori, 1978; Sibson, 1983; Crouch et al., 1984; Webb and Kanamori, 1985; Weldon and Humphreys, 1986; Davis et al., 1989). Hearn and Clayton (1986a, b) developed a velocity model for the upper crust based on backprojection tomography using Pg arrivals and a second tomographic model for the lower crust based on Pn arrivals. The results for the upper crust differed significantly from those for the lower crust, from which they inferred that the upper crust is decoupled from the lower crust in southern California. Yeats (1981) speculated that a regional detachment exists beneath the Transverse Ranges that rises to the surface along two major subparallel thrust zones with concurrent Holocene activity: the Santa Cruz Island–MCFZ–Santa Monica–Raymond–Cucamonga fault zone and, to the north, the Red Mountain–San Cayetano–Santa Susanna–Sierra Madre–Cucamonga fault zone. Davis et al. (1989) named these two subparallel zones the Santa Ynez–San Gabriel zone and the Santa Monica zone. Hauksson (1990) has associated the Santa Monica zone with the Elysian Park fold and thrust belt of Davis et al. (1989).

Motion of the Transverse Ranges terrane has a significant

TABLE 1. ACTIVITY ASSESSMENT AND REFERENCES FOR FAULTS WITHIN OR ADJACENT TO THE MALIBU COAST FAULT ZONE

Fault	Status	Sources
Santa Rosa Island fault	Active	Kew, 1927; Hileman et al., 1973; Junger, 1976, 1979; Yerkes and Lee, 1979b; Ziony and Yerkes, 1985; Vedder et al., 1987.
Santa Cruz Island fault	Active	Junger, 1976, 1979; Patterson, 1979; Yerkes and Lee, 1979a, b; Ziony and Yerkes, 1985; Vedder et al., 1986; Ziony and Jones, 1989; Pinter and Sorlien, 1991.
Anacapa (Dume) fault	Active	Vedder et al., 1974; Junger, 1976; Junger and Wagner, 1977; Lee et al., 1979; Yerkes and Lee, 1979a, b; Greene and Kennedy, 1986.
Fault Z	Active	Yerkes and Lee, 1979b; Lee at el., 1979.
Malibu Coast fault	Active/potentially active	Yerkes and Wentworth, 1965; Campbell et al., 1970; Campbell and Yerkes, 1976; Yerkes and Campbell, 1980; Clark et al., 1984; Greene and Kennedy, 1986; Ziony and Yerkes, 1985; Vedder et al., 1986; Ziony and Jones, 1989; Dibblee and Ehrenspeck, 1990, 1993; Wright, 1991; Drumm, 1992; Dibblee, 1992, 1993; Treiman, 1994.
–Escondido strand	Potentially active	Campbell, et al., 1966; Dibblee and Ehrenspeck, 1993; Treiman, 1994.
–Las Flores strand	Potentially active	Yerkes and Campbell, 1980; Dibblee, 1992, 1993.
–Latigo strand	Potentially active	Yerkes and Campbell, 1980; Dibblee, 1993; Dibblee and Ehrenspeck, 1993; Treiman, 1994.
–Paradise Cove strand	Potentially active	Dibblee and Ehrenspeck, 1993; Treiman, 1994.
–Point Dume strand	Potentially active	Treiman, 1994.
–Puerco Canyon strand	Potentially active	Yerkes and Wentworth, 1965; Campbell et al., 1970; Yerkes et al., 1971; Birkeland, 1972; Yerkes and Campbell, 1980; Dibblee, 1993; Treiman, 1994.
–Solstice strand	Active	Cleveland and Troxel, 1965; Campbell et al., 1970; Birkeland, 1972; Yerkes and Campbell, 1980; Dibblee, 1993; Traiman, 1994.
–Winter Mesa strand	Active	Yerkes and Campbell, 1980; Rzonca et al., 1991; Dibblee, 1993; Treiman, 1994.
–Ramirez strand	Potentially active	Dibblee and Ehrenspeck, 1993; Treiman, 1994.
Potrero fault	Active/potentially active	Hill, 1979; McGill, 1981, 1982, 1989; McGill et al., 1987; Wright, 1991; Dibblee, 1992.
Santa Monica fault	Active/potentially active	Buika and Teng, 1979; Hill, 1979; Hill et al., 1979; McGill, 1981, 1982; Crook et al., 1983; Clark et al., 1984; Ziony and Yerkes, 1985; Real, 1987; Ziony and Jones, 1989; Wright, 1991; Dibblee, 1991a, b, 1992; Crook and Proctor, 1992.
Hollywood fault	Active	Hill et al., 1979; Weber, 1980; Crook et al., 1983; Wesnousky, 1986; Real, 1987; Dibblee, 1991a, b; Wright, 1991; Crook and Proctor, 1992.

After Jennings, 1994 and Ziony and Yerkes, 1985.

rotational component. Hornafius et al. (1986) infer a 78° ± 11° clockwise rotation of the Santa Monica Mountains since the early Miocene based on paleomagnetic data and 60 km of left-lateral slip along the Santa Monica/Hollywood–Malibu Coast fault trend. Northern Santa Cruz Island is inferred to have rotated by approximately the same amount (76° ± 9°) concurrently, so it is thought to be part of the same element of rigidly rotating and translating upper crust (Hornafius et al., 1986). Jackson and Molnar (1990) interpreted present-day rotation rates of 6°/Ma clockwise for the western Transverse Ranges, based on very long baseline interferometry (VLBI) experiments conducted over a five-year period in the 1980s. Feigl et al. (1993) described comparable angular velocities for the western Transverse Ranges, based on a larger dataset including VLBI and global positioning system observations made between 1984 and 1992. Jackson and

Molnar (1990; after Lamb, 1987) suggest that the observed rotation and faulting in the western Transverse Ranges can be viewed as being similar to the rotation of essentially rigid blocks riding atop a viscous substratum that is homogeneously deforming across a wide boundary zone between two rigid plates. As applied to the Transverse Ranges, the modeled boundary zone between the Pacific and North American plates is ≥100 km wide.

The Transverse Ranges Province has several distinctive seismic attributes in comparison with surrounding provinces. The deepest earthquakes in southern California occur within the Transverse Ranges, with depths to ~30 km (Humphreys and Hager, 1990; Ziony and Jones, 1989; Bryant and Jones, 1992). These deep crustal earthquakes occur in areas of rapid crustal convergence (Weldon and Humphreys, 1986). Another distinctive feature is called the *Transverse Ranges velocity anomaly*: a volume of crust and upper mantle within/beneath the Transverse Ranges characterized by *P*-wave velocities that are 1–3% faster than average (Hadley and Kanamori, 1977, 1978; Raikes and Hadley, 1979; Raikes, 1980; Walck and Minster, 1982; Humphreys et al., 1984; Humphreys and Clayton, 1988, 1990; Humphreys and Hager, 1990). Perhaps not coincidentally, the deep crustal earthquakes occur within the Transverse Ranges velocity anomaly (Humphreys and Hager, 1990). A tomographic inversion on teleseismic *P*-wave delays indicates that the Transverse Ranges velocity anomaly is nearly vertical, approximately 200 km wide, and extends in depth to approximately 250 km (Humphreys et al., 1984; Humphreys and Clayton, 1988, 1990). The anomaly has been interpreted as resulting from upper-mantle lithosphere sinking vertically into the sublithospheric mantle (e.g., Bird and Rosenstock, 1984; Humphreys and Hager, 1990; cf. Griggs, 1939). If the rate at which the lithosphere sinks is approximately the same as the local rate at which the Pacific plate moves horizontally relative to the North American plate (~46 mm/yr; DeMets et al., 1994), then it would take ~5 million years for the slab(s) to reach a depth of 250 km, which is approximately the same time that Baja California and the parts of coastal California west of the San Andreas fault have been moving with the Pacific plate (Atwater, 1970).

The areal extent of the upper 30 km of this velocity anomaly is indicated by the dot-patterned area in Figure 1a (Humphreys and Clayton, 1990). It is significant to note that this velocity anomaly extends across the San Andreas fault. Although the Transverse Ranges velocity anomaly does not correlate well with surface topography or gravity anomalies, it is a further indication that the fault zones that mark the sharp southern edge of the Transverse Ranges are significant, active, crustal boundary structures.

ALQUIST-PRIOLO ACT

The Alquist-Priolo Earthquake Fault Zoning Act was developed in the immediate aftermath of the 1971 San Fernando earthquake (M_L 6.6) and was signed into law December 22, 1972, as part of California's Public Resources Code, sections 2621–2630 (Hart, 1994). Through 10 revisions to date, the purpose of the Alquist-Priolo Act is to "prohibit the location of most structures for human occupancy across the traces of active faults" and to facilitate "seismic retrofitting to strengthen buildings, including historical buildings, against ground shaking" (section 2621.5[a]).

Although the Alquist-Priolo Act mentions ground-shaking hazards, it is effectively limited to the identification and avoidance of ground-rupture hazards. As experience in the 1987 Whittier Narrows earthquake (M_L 5.9), 1989 Loma Prieta earthquake (M_L 7.1), and 1994 Northridge earthquake (M_L 6.7) clearly attests, ground shaking can cause loss of life and many billions of dollars in damage at significant distances from the epicenter without any ground rupture along the causative fault plane (see Yeats et al., 1981). Mitigation of ground-shaking hazards must be accomplished regionally, through the strengthening of building codes in seismically active areas.

The implementation of the Alquist-Priolo Act is "pursuant to the policies and criteria established and adopted by the (State Mining and Geology) Board" (section 2621.5[c]). It is the responsibility of the State Geologist to delineate "appropriately wide earthquake fault zones to encompass all potentially and recently active traces of the San Andreas, Calaveras, Hayward, and San Jacinto faults, and such other faults, or segments thereof, as the State Geologist determines to be sufficiently active and well-defined as to constitute a potential hazard to structures from surface faulting or fault creep" (section 2622[a]). The State Geologist utilizes fault-zone maps and written characterizations by geoscientists registered in the State of California, as well as studies by geoscientists of the Division of Mines and Geology, to evaluate the activity of fault zones.

The policies and criteria of the State Mining and Geology Board with respect to the Alquist-Priolo Act are established in the California Code of Regulations, Title 14, Division 2, sections 3600–3603. This chapter specifies that an active fault is one "that has had surface displacement within Holocene time (about the last 11,000 years)" (section 3601[a]). Also specified in this chapter is the prohibition against placing a structure across the trace of an active fault, or within 50 feet (~15 m) of the trace of an active fault (section 3603[a]).

The operational definitions used in the implementation of the Alquist-Priolo Act are noteworthy. "A *fault* is defined as a fracture or zone of closely associated fractures along which rocks on one side have been displaced with respect to those on the other side... A fault is distinguished from those fractures or shears caused by landsliding or other gravity-induced surficial failures" (Hart, 1994, p. 3). By this definition, a mode I extensional fracture or joint without shear displacement could be classified as a fault. The phrase "potentially and recently active traces" currently has no operational definition, although a potentially active fault was originally understood to mean a fault that had demonstrable movement during the Quaternary Period, within the last 1.6 million years.

Earthquake fault zones are currently established based on the operational definitions associated with the phrase "sufficiently active and well-defined" (Alquist-Priolo Act, section 2622[a]).

Sufficiently active. A fault is deemed sufficiently active if there is evidence of Holocene surface displacement along one or more of its segments or branches. Holocene surface displacement may be directly observable or inferred; it need not be present everywhere along a fault to qualify that fault for zoning.

Well-defined. A fault is considered well-defined if its trace is clearly detectable by a trained geologist as a physical feature at or just below the ground surface. The fault may be identified by direct observation or by indirect methods (e.g., geomorphic evidence...). The critical consideration is that the fault, or some part of it, can be located in the field with sufficient precision and confidence to indicate that the required site-specific investigations would meet with some success (Hart, 1994, p. 5).

Hence, there are effectively two classes of faults under the Alquist-Priolo Act: sufficiently active and well-defined faults with demonstrable Holocene displacement histories, and all other faults.

Hart (1994) lists guidelines for evaluating the hazard of surface fault rupture, which are derived largely from other published guidelines (Division of Mines and Geology, 1975a, b, 1982, 1986a–c; also see Slosson, 1984; Larson and Slosson, 1992). An evaluation of the historic record of earthquakes is not currently a requirement or significant suggestion in the development of fault evaluation studies under the Alquist-Priolo Act, which is somewhat curious given that it is explicitly called an *earthquake* fault zoning act that calls for the compilation and publication of maps of *earthquake* fault zones. Jennings (1994, p. 17) notes that "the Nuclear Regulatory Commission . . . defines a capable fault, in part, on macroseismicity instrumentally determined with records of sufficient precision to demonstrate a direct relationship with the fault." Aligned seismicity using both macro- and microearthquakes ($M_L \leq 3$) is used as an indicator of fault activity on the *Fault Activity Map of California and Adjacent Areas* (Jennings, 1994).

INDICATORS OF HOLOCENE ACTIVITY

Primary indicators of Holocene fault activity include instrumentally recorded earthquakes that can be associated with specific faults or fault zones, and offset markers that are datable as Holocene. Secondary indicators include a wide variety of data that tend to indicate fault activity, including fault-related geomorphology such as scarps or offset drainages, linear gradient anomalies in topographic or structural surfaces, linear gradient anomalies in gravity or magnetic potential fields, evidence of differential uplift provided by leveling surveys or mineral cooling ages, linear ground-water anomalies, and linear trends of hydrocarbon seeps. General criteria for identifying active faults are amply discussed elsewhere, and will not be repeated here (e.g., Taylor and Cluff, 1973; Allen, 1975; Slemmons, 1977; Wallace, 1977; Hatheway and Leighton, 1979; Bonilla, 1982; Ziony and Yerkes, 1985; Slemmons and dePolo, 1992; Hart, 1994; Keller and Pinter, 1996). The secondary indicators discussed below are not intended to be a comprehensive review of the topic with respect to the MCFZ. Analysis of the structural geomorphology of the MCFZ and a compilation of the many observations made by consulting geologists along the MCFZ have not been included in this paper. Some of these data are included by Treiman (1994) in the most current fault evaluation report concerning the Malibu Coast fault.

Primary indicators

Documented Holocene activity along MCFZ. Holocene or Quaternary activity has been documented by California's Division of Mines and Geology for several elements of the MCFZ exposed subaerially along the Malibu coastline (Treiman, 1994). The Solstice and Winter Mesa strands of the Malibu Coast fault have documented Holocene displacement and have been identified as Earthquake Fault Zones under California's Alquist-Priolo Earthquake Fault Zoning Act (inset map, Fig. 2; Hart, 1994; Divi-

sion of Mines and Geology, 1995a, b; Rzonca et al., 1991). As defined in the Alquist-Priolo Act, the boundaries of the "official Earthquake Fault Zone are established about 500 ft away from major active faults and about 200 to 300 ft away from well-defined minor faults" with some exceptions where faults are locally complex or are not vertical (Hart 1994: p. 5 and 7). The fault traces used to determine the boundaries are shown on the official maps of the Earthquake Fault Zones published by the California Division of Mines and Geology.

Dill (1993) imaged an area that was devoid of Holocene sedimentary cover offshore of Topanga and Will Rogers Beaches, which may indicate Holocene tectonic uplift along the Malibu Coast fault (Fig. 2). The southern boundary of this anomalous sea floor is along the inferred offshore trend of the Malibu Coast fault and coincides to the east with the Potrero fault. Green et al. (1975) mapped a parallel pair of offshore strands of the Malibu Coast fault and inferred Holocene activity along them. The inferred Holocene age and the location of these faults have been questioned by Treiman (1994).

The offshore Anacapa fault is seismically active (e.g., "Santa Monica fault" of Ellsworth et al., 1973; Stierman and Ellsworth, 1976; Yerkes and Lee, 1979a). Holocene activity has also been indicated for most of the fault elements of the southern boundary of the western and central Transverse Ranges (Table 1), including the Santa Cruz Island fault (Pinter and Sorlien, 1991) and the Hollywood/Santa Monica faults (Hill et al., 1979; Real, 1987; Crook and Proctor, 1992; James Dolan, written communication, 1995), which are immediately adjacent to the MCFZ to the west and east, respectively.

MCFZ seismicity. A history of instrumentally recorded earthquakes is a strong indicator of fault activity. A database was compiled including 638 earthquakes reported to have occurred within the MCFZ study area through 1995 (Fig. 3; Appendix 1). The nucleus of the earthquake database was provided by Dr. Glen Reagor of the U.S. Geological Survey's National Earthquake Information Center (NEIC), whose data were supplied by the California Division of Mines and Geology (CDMG; Real et al., 1978; Toppozada et al., 1984; Seismological Laboratory of the California Institute of Technology, Seismological Stations of the University of California-Berkeley), the Geological Society of America's Decade of North American Geology Project (DNAG; Engdahl and Rinehart, 1988, 1991), Stover and Coffman (1993), and NEIC's Preliminary Determination of Epicenter files (PDE and PDE-W, which are weekly updates to PDE files). These data were augmented with other published data and, for the most recent two earthquakes, by data posted by Dr. L. K. Hutton of the Caltech Seismological Laboratory via Internet/World Wide Web (newsgroup ca. earthquakes; Caltech seismology home pages http://scec.gps.caltech.edu or http://www.gps.caltech.edu/seismo/seismo.page.html). NEIC data are now available (as of December 1997) via the World Wide Web at http://www.NEIC.cr.usgs.gov/neis/epic/epic.html. Another useful path to earthquake data on the web is available at http://www.geophys.washington.edu/seismosurfing.html.

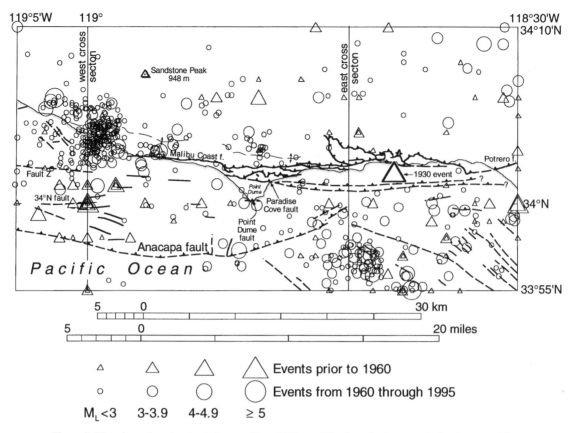

Figure 3. Historic earthquakes in study area. Since 1960, proliferation of seismographs has improved the detection and location of earthquakes; pre-1960 earthquakes are indicated by triangles. Corresponding data and sources are listed in Appendix 1.

The earliest reported earthquake within the study area occurred in 1827 and is estimated to have had a magnitude of 5.5 (Toppozada et al., 1981). Sixty-two percent of the earthquakes listed in Appendix 1 occurred in the 1970s and most were associated with the 1973 Point Mugu (M_L 5.3, as revised by Hutton and Jones, 1993) and 1979 Malibu (M_L 5.2) earthquakes. More than 80% of the earthquakes have occurred since 1960. Rather than necessarily indicating an increase in seismicity during recent decades, this increase in reported earthquakes is probably due in large part to the expansion in the number of seismographs installed in southern California and the consequent decrease in the threshold of detection for small earthquakes. Six of the reported earthquakes had magnitudes ≥5 (events 1, 11, 12, 181, 492, and 600), and 154 had magnitudes ≥3. Hypocenter depths range from 19.2 km to less than 1 km, with 26 events reported with depths of <2 km.

Focal mechanism solutions were compiled for 107 events (Fig. 4a–c, Appendix 1). More than one focal mechanism solution has been published for several of the earthquakes (events 176, 181, 259, 273, 325, 492, 495, and 547). Where published focal mechanism solutions did not include the inferred orientation of the slip vector (i.e., the direction that the hanging wall moved relative to the foot wall), the fault plane and slip vector

were inferred based upon the orientation of mapped faults in the area. Nodal plane orientations for the earthquakes analyzed by Stierman and Ellsworth (1976) were estimated using the published focal mechanism diagrams and unpublished data provided by Donald Stierman and William Ellsworth (written communication, 1995, 1996).

Of the focal mechanism solutions compiled in this study, approximately 70% are associated with either the 1973 Point Mugu or 1979 Malibu earthquake sequences (Fig. 4b, c). The dip of fault planes inferred from the focal mechanisms range from 0 to 90°, averaging 51°. Almost 70% of the inferred fault planes dip between 30° and 60°, generally toward the north quadrant. Most of the focal mechanism solutions indicate thrust or thrust-dominated oblique faults, typically with left-lateral strike-slip components. Webb and Kanamori (1985) interpreted six of the focal mechanism solutions as indicating slip on low-angle detachments (events 176, 261, 273, 325, 495, and 547). The average azimuth of hanging-wall slip vectors inferred from the focal mechanism solutions is 206°, which is approximately perpendicular to the trend of the San Andreas fault through the Transverse Ranges. Just over 60% of the slip azimuths are between 180° and 240° (see inset rose diagram, Fig. 4a).

The relocated 1930 Santa Monica earthquake (M_L 5.2) has

been attributed to the eastern end of the Anacapa fault or the western end of the Santa Monica fault (Hauksson and Saldivar, 1986). (As a matter of common usage, use of the term *Santa Monica fault* is generally restricted to the area east of longitude 118°30'; to the west, this fault is considered one of the strands of the Malibu Coast fault; (cf. Dibblee 1991a, b, 1992.) The relocated epicenter of the 1930 Santa Monica earthquake lies between the offshore trace of the Malibu Coast fault inferred by Dibblee (1992) and the offshore trace of the Malibu Coast fault inferred by Greene and Kennedy (1986; Figs. 2 and 3). If the 1930 Santa Monica earthquake occurred at a depth of 15 km as reported (Gutenberg et al., 1932; Hauksson and Saldivar, 1986), it is more likely to have occurred on either the Anacapa fault or another, structurally lower, fault surface (Fig. 5).

The 1973 Point Mugu earthquake was interpreted to have occurred along the Anacapa fault, with a slip surface dipping ~36 to 44°N (Ellsworth et al., 1973; Stierman and Ellsworth, 1976; Lee et al., 1979). The local magnitude of the Point Mugu earthquake was initially reported to be 5.9 to 6.0 (Ellsworth et al., 1973; Stierman and Ellsworth, 1976; Lee et al., 1979). Hutton and Jones (1993) reevaluated the local magnitudes of earthquakes that occurred in southern California since 1932 that had reported magnitudes of ≥4.8. The local magnitude of the Point Mugu earthquake was adjusted to 5.3 as a result of that reevaluation. Several of the more shallow aftershocks of the Point Mugu earthquake clustered along Fault Z, which is interpreted to dip 41°N (Fig. 5; Lee et al., 1979). Fault Z may be the western offshore extension of the Escondido/Ramirez thrust, Paradise Cove fault, or Point Dume fault that are exposed at Point. Dume (Fig. 2).

The 1979 Malibu earthquake (M_L 5.2) has been associated with the eastern end of the Anacapa fault (Hauksson and Saldivar, 1986). However, the Anacapa fault as it is typically mapped (e.g., Yerkes and Lee, 1979b; Greene and Kennedy, 1986) is above the reported hypocenter (Fig. 5), so the 1979 Malibu earthquake may have occurred along a nonemergent fault below the Anacapa fault, perhaps along a propagating thrust or within a duplex. Hauksson (1990, 1992) has suggested that thrust earthquakes south of the Malibu coastline may be associated with a westward extension of the Elysian Park fold-and-thrust belt (Davis et al., 1989).

Other selected indicators

Slip and convergence rates. Yeats (1981) estimated a convergence rate of 18 mm/yr across the central and western Transverse Ranges. He subsequently estimated the convergence across the Ventura basin within the western Transverse Ranges at 23 mm/yr during the past 200,000 years (Yeats, 1983), which compares favorably with the slightly smaller convergence-rate estimate of 17 ± 4 mm/yr by Rockwell (1983, cited in Weldon and Humphreys, 1986). Taking the average of the convergence rates reported by Yeats (1983) and Rockwell (1983), Weldon and Humphreys (1986) used a convergence rate of 20 mm/yr across the western Transverse Ranges. Namson and Davis (1988) sug-

gest that the shortening of the western Transverse Ranges began during the late Pliocene, 2 to 3 million years ago, and has averaged 17.6 to 26.5 mm/yr since then for the area north of the Santa Monica Mountains. Bryant and Jones (1992) argue that the rapid shortening of the Ventura basin is not characteristic of the western Transverse Ranges as a whole, but rather that high rates of shortening are confined to a small region that is marked by anomalously thick crust, deep-crustal earthquakes to 30 km, and low heat flow. Dolan et al. (1995) estimate the current rate of shortening in the western Transverse Ranges to be ~10 mm/yr, based on geodetic measurements made between 1984 and 1992 (Donnellan et al., 1993a, b; Feigl et al., 1993). For comparison, the convergence rate across the Himalaya between India and Tibet is thought to be 18 ± 7 mm/yr (Molnar et al., 1987).

Clark et al. (1984) estimated the long-term minimum slip rate on the Malibu Coast fault to be 0.04 mm/yr, with an estimated maximum of 0.09 mm/yr. The estimated maximum slip rate seems inconsistent with the Quaternary uplift rates of ~0.3 to 0.4 mm/yr along the Malibu coastline (Birkeland, 1972; Lajoie et al., 1979), discussed more fully in the next section. The estimated maximum slip rate for the Malibu Coast fault is much less than the 0.27 to 0.39 mm/yr estimated slip rate for the Santa Monica fault immediately to the east, or the 0.2 to >0.56 mm/yr vertical component of slip for the Santa Cruz Island fault immediately to the west (Clark et al., 1984). Part of this apparent discrepancy may be accommodated by slip on the Anacapa fault or on other offshore or nonemergent structures such as blind thrusts or duplexes. Dolan et al. (1995) suggest a slip rate of 1 to 1.5 mm/yr along the Malibu Coast fault, primarily as strike-slip displacement, and 4 mm/yr across a hypothetical nonemergent structure that they call the Santa Monica Mountains thrust.

Uplift. Three prominent marine terraces that are exposed subaerially along the Malibu coastline have been termed the Dume terrace, Corral terrace, and the Malibu terrace, listed in order of increasing age and increasing elevation (Davis, 1933; Yerkes and Wentworth, 1965; Birkeland, 1972). Currently, the ages of the Dume, Corral, and Malibu terraces are thought to be 124,000 yr, 210,000 yr, and 320,000 yr, respectively (Lajoie, written communication, 1996; Lajoie et al., 1979; Treiman, 1994; cf. Szabo and Rosholt, 1969). The maximum elevations of the Dume, Corral, and Malibu terraces along the Malibu coastline west of Topanga Canyon (longitude ~118.58°W) are 40 m, 58 m, and 97 m, respectively (Birkeland, 1972). All three terraces increase in elevation from west to east along the Malibu coastline, at rates of ~0.3 m/km for the Dume terrace, ~0.8 m/km for the Corral terrace, and ~1.3 m/km for the Malibu terrace. Birkeland (1972) inferred that most of the differential uplift is younger than the Dume terrace based upon what he considered the parallel geometry of the Dume and Corral terraces; however, this supposed parallelism is not strongly supported by existing elevation data for these terraces (Yerkes and Wentworth, 1965; Lajoie, written communication, 1996).

Birkeland (1972; Yerkes and Wentworth, 1965) noted three

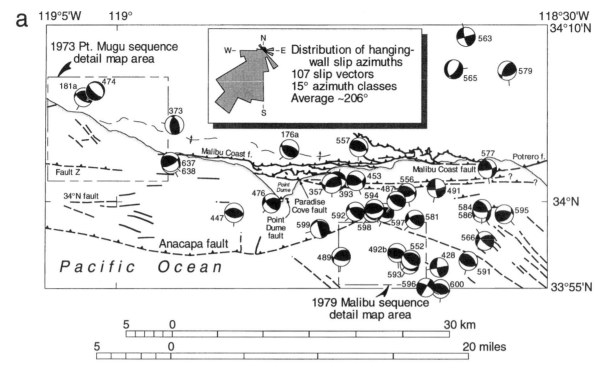

Figure 4 (on this and facing page). Focal mechanism solutions along the Malibu Coast Fault Zone. Focal mechanism solutions shown as lower hemisphere projections with compressional quadrants in black and the direction of hanging-wall slip indicated by the short line extending out from the edge of the projection. Adjacent number corresponds to the event number in Appendix 1, where sources and corresponding data are listed. a, Focal mechanism solutions for the entire study area, with the locations of the detail maps for the Point Mugu and Malibu earthquake sequences bounded by dashed lines. Inset box includes rose diagram of 107 hanging-wall slip directions derived from the focal mechanism solutions. b, Focal mechanism solutions associated with the 1973 Point Mugu earthquake, including two different solutions for the main earthquake. Inset map clarifies the positions and focal mechanisms of several tightly clustered aftershocks. c, Focal mechanism solutions associated with the 1979 Malibu earthquake, including two different solutions for the main earthquake. Inset box shows solution for the main earthquake by Hauksson (1990), which is obscured on the main map.

sites where Quaternary deposits are displaced vertically along a strand of the Malibu Coast fault (sites F1, F2, and F3 on Fig. 2). At site F1, just north of Point Dume, minimum vertical separation of "pre-Malibu nonmarine deposits" is 4 m (Birkeland, 1972, p. 441). Site F2 is located between the official Earthquake Fault Zone boundaries around the Solstice strand and Winter Mesa strands of the Malibu Coast fault (Division of Mines and Geology, 1995a, b). At site F2, vertical separation of the Corral terrace is 5.2 m across a strand of the Malibu Coast fault (Puerco Canyon fault of Treiman, 1994). Site F3 is located just north of the official Earthquake Fault Zone boundary around the Winter Mesa strand of the Malibu Coast fault (Division of Mines and Geology, 1995b). At site F3, vertical separation of the Corral terrace is 14 m across two fault strands. The north sides are uplifted relative to the south sides at sites F1 and F2, but the south side is up at F3.

After compensation for the effects of global variations in late Quaternary sea level, the altitudes of the marine terraces indicate that the Malibu coastline has been rising during the late Quaternary. When the Dume terrace was formed 124,000 years ago, sea level was ~6 m above current sea level (Lajoie et al., 1979, after Shackleton and Opdyke, 1973), so the average uplift rate over that time interval has been 0.27 mm/yr. As adjusted to reflect more recent dating of the Dume and Corral terraces, Birkeland's (1972) inferred uplift rate along the Malibu coastline is ~0.2–0.4 mm/yr. Yerkes and Lee (1979a, p. 34) refer to a ~105,000-yr marine terrace (the 124,000-yr Dume terrace?) thrust "more than 15 m over upper Miocene strata at one locality near Malibu Canyon" by the Malibu Coast fault, suggesting an uplift rate of ~0.1 mm/yr. Johnson (1932, in Hill, 1979) illustrated a marine terrace, inferred to be the Dume terrace by Lajoie (written communication, 1996), vertically offset by 47 m along the Potrero Canyon fault. Lajoie et al. (1979) estimated the long-term uplift rate of the Dume terrace to be 0.2 mm/yr south of the Malibu Coast fault and 0.6 mm/yr north of the fault, requiring 0.4 mm/yr of vertical displacement along the fault.

For comparison, the apparent uplift rates in the northwest Himalaya of Pakistan, as measured using fission-track and $^{40}Ar/^{39}Ar$ cooling ages, range from 0.2 to 0.9 mm/yr (Zeitler, 1985). Late Cenozoic uplift rates in the northwest Himalaya are

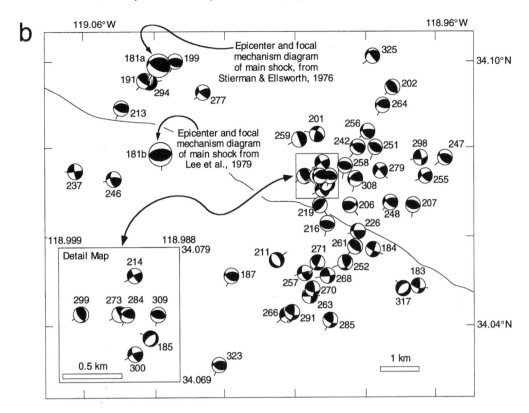

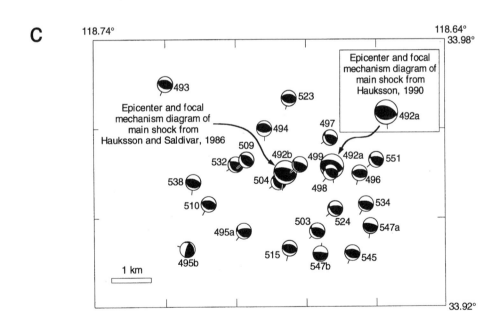

similar to the Quaternary uplift rates estimated along the Malibu coastline. The uplift rate for the massif that culminates in Nanga Parbat (8,126 m) is estimated to be ~5 mm/yr (Zeitler, 1985), a rate that is comparable to the 4 to 10 mm/yr uplift rate estimated by Lajoie et al. (1979) for parts of the western Transverse Ranges. On Santa Cruz Island, along trend to the west of

the MCFZ, an uplift rate of 2.1 mm/yr can be inferred from the 25-m vertical displacement of a fluvial terrace that formed 11,780 ± 100 years ago across the Santa Cruz Island fault (Pinter and Sorlien, 1991).

Castle et al. (1977) measured changes in surface elevation associated with the 1973 Point Mugu earthquake. The region

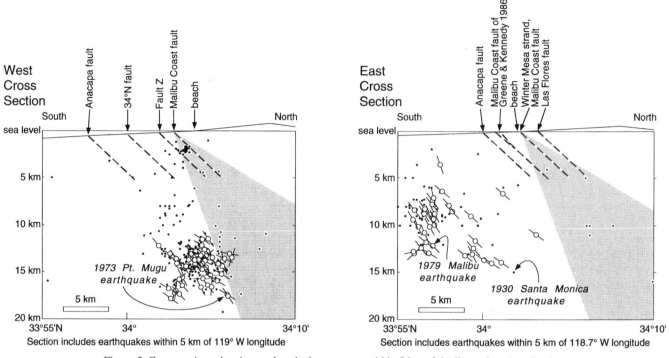

Figure 5. Cross sections showing earthquake hypocenters within 5 km of the lines of section. Section-line locations are shown on Figure 3. Hypocenters were projected due east/west to the line of cross section without change in reported depth. Open circles depict hypocenters of earthquakes for which focal mechanism solutions have been determined. The lines through the open circles indicate the apparent plunge of the interpreted slip vector in the plane of the cross section. Hypothetical fault orientations, based on the mapped surface trace of major faults that intersect the line of section, are dashed. Gray region extending from the surface trace of the Malibu Coast fault is bounded by lines dipping 30° and 60°, within which the actual Malibu Coast fault is likely to be located. Corresponding data and sources are listed in Appendix 1.

north of the Anacapa fault, called the "Santa Monica fault" in Castle et al. (1977), rose by 30 to 40 mm between 1960 and 1968, subsided by a similar amount between 1968 and 1971, and rose back to nearly its 1968 elevation between 1971 and 1973, for a total uplift along the Malibu coastline of 20 to 30 mm relative to the 1960 datum. It is unclear whether the uplift between 1971 and 1973 surveys was preseismic or coseismic with the 1973 Point Mugu earthquake sequence. Coincident with this episode of uplift in the Santa Monica Mountains was a subsidence of as much as 200 mm in the Oxnard Plain, ~5 to 10 km northwest of the epicenter of the 1973 Point Mugu main shock (Castle et al., 1977).

Topographic gradient. Along the south face of the Santa Monica Mountains at Malibu, from Sandstone Peak (elevation 948 m; Fig. 3) across the MCFZ to the floor of the Santa Monica basin between the San Pedro basin fault zone and the Santa Cruz–Santa Catalina Ridge fault zone (~2,550 m below sea level; Fig. 1), the average topographic gradient is ~80 m/km. In the San Gabriel Mountains from San Antonio Peak (3,067 m; Fig. 1) to the active Cucamonga fault (~600 m; Morton and Matti, 1987), the average topographic gradient is ~170 m/km. The topographic gradient along the south slope of the San Gabriel Mountains is

approximately twice as steep as the topographic gradient of the south slope of the Santa Monica Mountains. The difference in topographic gradient may be due in part to the differing erosional characteristics of the two mountain ranges resulting from different lithologies exposed at the surface. The exposed core of the San Gabriel Mountains includes Precambrian-Mesozoic metamorphic and intrusive igneous rock units, whereas the surficial lithologies of the Santa Monica Mountains are Cretaceous-Quaternary sedimentary units and Miocene volcanics (Jennings and Strand, 1969; Dibblee, 1992, 1993; Dibblee and Ehrenspeck, 1990, 1993).

Gravity gradient. Isostatic residual gravity tends to reflect mass anomalies in the mid- to upper crust, correlating better with surface geology than Bouguer or free-air gravity (Jachens and Griscom, 1985; Simpson et al., 1986; Jachens et al., 1989; Griscom and Jachens, 1990). The isostatic regional gravity field is caused by masses that isostatically compensate the surface topography. When the isostatic *regional* gravity field is subtracted from the Bouguer gravity field, the remainder is the isostatic *residual* gravity field (Jachens et al., 1989). Faults that juxtapose rock of different physical properties generally coincide with steep gradients in the isostatic residual gravity field.

The range in isostatic residual gravity from the crest of the Santa Monica Mountains (+5 to +10 mGal) across the MCFZ to the regional gravity low in the Santa Monica basin (–75 mGal) is ~80–90 mGal (Fig. 1a; Roberts et al., 1990). The average isostatic residual gravity gradient across the MCFZ on the south slope of the Santa Monica Mountains is ~4.5 mGal/km, which contrasts with the 1 mGal/km gradient along the topographically steeper south slope of the San Gabriel Mountains across the active Cucamonga fault. The trend of the –25 mGal contour along the Malibu coastline parallels the surface trace of the Malibu Coast and Santa Monica faults.

Crustal thickness and crustal roots. The crustal thickness in the study area ranges from ~25 km in the southwest corner of the area to ~30–35 km along the axis of the Santa Monica Mountains (Mooney and Braile, 1989; Mooney and Weaver, 1989; Bryant and Jones, 1992). The average crustal thickness in southern California is 29 km (Hearn, 1984; Bryant and Jones, 1992). Bryant and Jones (1992) have inferred an anomalous crustal thickness of ~41 km in an east-trending oval centered on the Ventura basin, between the Santa Monica Mountains and the Santa Ynez Mountains. The crustal structure in this area is complex (e.g., Keller and Prothero, 1987). In general, surface topography as significant as the Transverse Ranges is isostatically compensated by a thick lower-crustal root zone. The eastern Transverse Ranges (San Bernardino Mountains, Fig. 1) have a small crustal root of 2–3 km thickness, while the central and western Transverse Ranges are generally considered to be essentially rootless (Hearn, 1984; Hearn and Clayton, 1986a, b; Mooney and Weaver, 1989).

The lack of a significant crustal root under the Transverse Ranges is an indicator of the youth and vigorous structural evolution of this province. In the kinematic model of Weldon and Humphreys (1986) the upper crust of the western and central Transverse Ranges is inferred to move essentially parallel to the San Andreas fault along a trajectory that is oblique to the motion of the Pacific plate relative to the North American plate. Hence, the western and central Transverse Ranges are thought to be moving with respect to the upper-mantle lithosphere beneath them, which would inhibit the development of a lower-crustal root. Sheffels and McNutt (1986) have developed an alternative explanation, based on a series of simple one-dimensional models of Bouguer gravity anomalies in the Transverse Ranges. They infer that the western Transverse Ranges are supported north of the Ventura basin by the flexural rigidity of a slab of upper-mantle lithosphere, modeled to be ≥40 km thick, on which they rest (cf. Lyon-Caen and Molnar, 1983). South of Ventura basin, the western Transverse Ranges are inferred to be supported by a thin (~5–15 km), northward-subducting, elastic slab of upper-mantle lithosphere as it bends downward and is resorbed into the upper mantle in the area of anomalously fast P-wave velocities (gray area in Fig. 1a; Humphreys et al., 1984; Humphreys and Clayton, 1990; Humphreys and Hager, 1990).

Thrust sequencing. Models for the evolution of thin-skinned thrust belts often incorporate the idea that older thrust faults rotate into steeper, mechanically disadvantageous orientations as newer faults develop below them, progressively farther from the axis of the mountain range. The term "out-of-sequence thrust," used to describe an active or reactivated thrust in the middle of a thrust system, illustrates the tendency to think that the usual sequence involves progressively younger faults with increasing distance from the axis of the mountain range. While this order of faulting is observed in many simple mountain belts as well as in many computational and physical models of thrust systems, it is not the only sequence possible in a compressional orogen. The critical Coulomb wedge model (Davis et al., 1983; Dahlen, 1984; Dahlen et al., 1984), in which the entire thrust system is simultaneously at the point of failure, is an example of an alternative thrust-belt model in which fault displacement is not assumed to be limited to the basal/frontal structure.

The aftershocks associated with both the 1973 Point Mugu earthquake and the 1979 Malibu earthquake are distributed within a volume of crust 5–10 km wide on either side of the inferred main fault plane (Fig. 5; Stierman and Ellsworth, 1976; Yerkes and Lee, 1979a, b; Hauksson and Saldivar, 1986). From the width of this distribution it is inferred that elastic strain was released along more than one fault surface during these sequences. Yerkes and Lee (1979a, b) located the 1973 Point Mugu earthquake along the Anacapa fault, but ascribed many of the more shallow aftershocks to Fault Z, which is parallel to and just above the Anacapa fault. The concurrent seismic activity along the Anacapa fault and Fault Z is inferred to reflect displacement within an active imbricate fan of subparallel thrust faults that reach the surface from a common detachment at depth (Boyer and Elliott, 1982). A similar distribution of seismicity has been described within an imbricate fan associated with the 1978 Tabas-e-Golshan, Iran, earthquake (Berberian, 1982). While the youngest, most outboard thrust in an imbricate fan is likely to be the most seismically active, compressive stress transmitted across the entire thrust system may excite activity along any favorably oriented thrust.

The simplification that the only thrust that is likely to be active is the one farthest from the axis of the mountain range does not apply to the Transverse Ranges where Holocene deformation is distributed across several active structures. The Anacapa fault may be the most active element of the MCFZ; however, it is not the only fault element with Holocene activity.

SEISMOLOGY

Event size–rupture length relationships

It would be useful to be able to relate the length of fault rupture and amount of slip to the size of the earthquake that generated the displacement (e.g., Ellsworth, 1990; Bonilla et al., 1984). Unfortunately, the relationships among these characteristics are not simple and vary from one locality to another.

The size of an earthquake is typically measured in one of two ways: either by the magnitude of the event or by its seismic moment. Earthquake magnitude is a relative measurement. The concept of magnitude is complicated by the fact that there are many different magnitude scales. Various scales have been devised to allow independent measurements from body and surface waves, and to measure the relative size of events that vary by depth, energy released, and geographic location. Commonly used magnitude scales include the local or Richter magnitude (M_L), *P*-wave or body-wave magnitude (m_b), and surface-wave magnitude (M_S). (It should be noted that the abbreviations used above for the various magnitude scales are those most commonly in use, but these abbreviations are not used consistently by all authors.) M_L and m_b are typically used for small- to intermediate-size events, or deep events, and are based on measurements of body waves. M_S is usually a better measure for large events that are shallow enough to generate strong surface waves. The following empirical relationships have been developed between these magnitudes:

$$m_b = 2.5 + (0.63\ M_S)$$
$$M_S = (1.59\ m_b) - 3.97$$
$$m_b = 1.7 + (0.8\ M_L) - (0.01\ M_L^2)$$

The seismic moment (M_o) is a direct measure of the amount of energy radiated by an earthquake. M_o has been described as "perhaps the most fundamental parameter we can use to measure the strength of an earthquake caused by fault slip" (Aki and Richards, 1980). M_o is the product of the area of fault slip in cm^2 (A), the average fault slip in cm (S), and the shear modulus of the faulted material in dyne/cm^2 (μ):

$$M_o = \mu AS$$

(Bullen and Bolt, 1985). Measured values of M_o range from about 10^{12} dyne-cm for microearthquakes to about 10^{30} dyne-cm for the largest earthquakes (e.g., 1960 Chilean and 1964 Anchorage earthquakes).

In general, M_S, M_L, and m_b are strongly dependent on wave period. This is a problem because each of these magnitude scales will saturate at the upper end when the dimensions of the rupture surface exceed the wavelength of the seismic waves used in the calculation. In addition, while the results of the magnitude calculations might be quite similar when they are based on records from stations that are relatively close to one another, significant variations in calculated magnitude can arise from the changes in wave amplitude and frequency that are related to distance, azimuth, and instrument response. A more uniform magnitude scale that does not have the same saturation problem, the moment magnitude (M_W) scale, was proposed by Kanamori (1977). This scale provides more stable estimates of magnitude, or the energy released by an event, and is related to M_o by:

$$M_W = [(2/3)\log_{10}(M_o)] - 10.7$$

(Hanks and Kanamori, 1979). In practice, however, it is generally sufficient for engineering purposes to consider M_L, M_S, M_W,

and m_b to be roughly equivalent to one another for moderate size, shallow-focus events that cause damage at the surface (Bullen and Bolt, 1985, p. 377).

The relationship between magnitude and surface rupture length (L) has been investigated by Evernden et al. (1981) and Wells and Coppersmith (1994). Evernden et al. (1981) developed the following empirical relationship between local magnitude and surface rupture length:

$$M_L = [3.2667 + \log_{10}(L)]/0.711$$

Wells and Coppersmith (1994) used 244 historical earthquakes to develop empirical relationships between moment magnitude, surface rupture length, rupture width, rupture area, and surface displacement. They used a subset of 80 events to develop the following formula relating M_W to surface rupture length:

$$M_W = [1.16\ \log_{10}(L)] + 5.08$$

To the extent that these relationships are approximately valid, the entire 3.2-km-long segment of the Solstice fault that has been zoned as active (inset, Fig. 2) could have ruptured in a magnitude 5.3 to 5.7 earthquake. This magnitude is at least as great as the largest recorded earthquakes attributed to the Anacapa fault: 1930 Santa Monica earthquake (M_L 5.2), 1973 Point Mugu earthquake (M_L 5.3), and 1979 Malibu earthquake (M_L 5.2). Half of the Solstice strand could rupture in a magnitude 4.9 to 5.3 earthquake. The entire 0.25-km length of the zoned Winter Mesa strand of the Malibu Coast fault could have ruptured in a magnitude 3.7 to 4.4 earthquake.

Given the uncertainty in any computed magnitude or seismic moment, estimated rupture lengths based on these measures should be made with caution.

Maximum credible earthquake

Greensfelder (1972, 1973) assigned a maximum probable earthquake magnitude of 7.5 to the Malibu Coast fault, based on Bonilla's (1970) data on fault rupture length, in creating maps of maximum credible ground acceleration for California earthquakes (see description and reproduction of Greensfelder's map in Kockleman, 1985, p. 454–455). W. H. K. Lee and W. L. Ellsworth concluded, after reviewing the earthquake history of the Santa Barbara Channel region from 1800 through 1973, "that the maximum credible earthquake for engineering design purposes is an event of magnitude 7.5 occurring anywhere in the Santa Barbara Channel region" (Lee et al., 1979, p. 3). Ziony and Yerkes (1985, after Wesson et al., 1974) concluded that reasonable maximum earthquake magnitudes to be expected along the Santa Cruz Island–Anacapa–Santa Monica–Hollywood-Raymond fault system is M 7.5. For other late Quaternary reverse faults in the Transverse Ranges, Ziony and Yerkes (1985) suggested a design magnitude of 6.5 to 7 for noncritical structures. Mualchin and Jones (1992) assigned a maximum magnitude of 7.5 to the Malibu Coast–Santa Monica–Raymond fault system to estimate peak accelerations for the design purposes of the California Department of Transportation. Dolan et al. (1995) estimated moment magnitudes of between 6.9 and 7.3 for modeled earthquakes along faults of the MCFZ, with recurrence intervals ranging from 740 to >3,000 years.

Evernden et al. (1981, p. 50) chose the Malibu Coast fault as an example in their model to estimate the replacement value of constructed works damaged by earthquakes in California. In a hypothetical M 6.7 earthquake along the Malibu Coast fault, they predicted 31 km of surface rupture resulting in $760 million in damage in 1981 dollars—more than half as much as a repeat of the 1857 Fort Tejon earthquake (M 8.1) along the San Andreas fault.

PROFESSIONAL PRACTICE, MORAL PHILOSOPHY, AND FAULT-ZONE STUDIES

The investigation of potentially active faults seems to involve not only scientific problems, but also problems of law and applied professional/scientific ethics. There is a moral dimension to the work of engineering geoscientists, comparable to the moral dimensions of science and engineering in general (e.g., Martin and Schinzinger, 1989), because the work product of an engineering geoscientist affects the public's safety, property, and welfare.

An ethic is a moral principle or value that most, if not all, prudent individuals would accept and strive to follow. Ethical theories are developed to assist people in the resolution of moral dilemmas, in which two or more moral obligations, duties, rights, goods, or ideals conflict with one another. For example, an ethical conventionalist might assert that his/her moral and professional obligations are fulfilled when the requirements of applicable laws and customs are met. A utilitarian would choose the action that would result in the greatest benefit for the most people, or causes the least suffering (e.g., Quinton, 1988). Immanuel Kant (1785, 1788) advocated basing moral decisions on categorically imperative duties like "tell the truth" that are universally applicable and reflect an individual's autonomous commitment to morality. Act as if, by your actions, you are establishing universal law. It is clearly beyond the scope of this paper to provide a primer on ethical theory (e.g., Harman, 1977; Martin and Schinzinger, 1989); however, the personal study of ethics serves to prepare an individual to act rationally in accordance with definable moral principles when confronted with a moral dilemma.

A scientist seeks knowledge through the use of valid and reproducible methodology to collect and analyze relevant available data and to make a defensible interpretation. Implicit in this statement of what a scientist does is a fundamental scientific ethic: seek the truth and tell the truth (e.g., Bronowski, 1965, 1978; Woodford, 1956). As Einstein put it (Mackay, 1991), "Most people say that it is the intellect which makes a great scientist. They are wrong: it is the character."

In addition to the basic ethics of science, a primary ethic in the engineering geosciences involves the legal and moral neces-

sity to protect the public's safety. Interpretations made by a geoscientist who follows a safety-based professional ethic should be the same regardless of whether the individual has a personal, professional, or financial stake in the outcome (cf. Rawls, 1971; Martin and Schinzinger, 1989). We assert that professional ethics in the engineering geosciences are based primarily on the underlying ethics of science and the necessity to protect human safety and secondarily on the protection of property.

One of the central purposes of engineering geoscience is to identify and characterize geologic conditions that represent a potential hazard to the public. The principal client of engineering geoscientists in fulfilling this purpose is the public. In California as in many other jurisdictions, the public through its government has established registration laws comparable to those that apply to other professionals whose work affects the public's safety and welfare, so there is a reasonable expectation that engineering geoscientists will use their knowledge and technical skills in the public interest.

Engineering geoscientists are at the base of the organizational pyramid in protecting the public from geologic hazards. Engineers and architects cannot design to mitigate hazards that they do not know exist. Similarly, public officials cannot make informed policy decisions concerning hazards that they do not understand or know exist. Ideally, there is an orderly flow through the process of hazard identification and risk management, which can be generalized as follows: (1) the geologic hazard is recognized; (2) the hazard is characterized using appropriate scientific methods; (3) the risk posed by the investigated hazard is assessed and described; (4) the risk associated with the hazard is evaluated by an informed public authority; (5) conditions that are unacceptably hazardous are mitigated, or the area is zoned to avoid the hazardous conditions; (6) hazardous conditions that are not considered to be unacceptibly dangerous are routinely monitored against the possibility of future adverse developments; and (7) data concerning the hazards are maintained within the public record. If the geoscientist fails in his/her responsibilities within this process, for whatever reason, the system is rendered inoperable.

Cost of seismic safety

Geoscientists fear being held liable, based on the legal theory of inverse condemnation, for the loss of resale value for properties adjacent to faults for which they are able to demonstrate Holocene activity. Allen (1976) mentioned a threatened lawsuit by the City of Los Angeles against seismologist James Whitcomb and his employer the California Institute of Technology for allegedly lowering property values in the San Fernando Valley through the public discussion of earthquake predictions. Most individuals fear the financial consequences of being sued for whatever reason, even if the case has no merit. Although such financial and legal concerns may be valid criteria for an individual geoscientist or company to use in deciding whether to become involved in fault-zone studies, they are not valid criteria to use in the scientific process of assessing fault activity. Faults are active or inactive without regard to the economic value of the ground that they traverse.

What is the cost of designing a structure for seismic safety? The shear walls, lateral bracing, shock-mounting of utilities, and other relatively minor adjustments to the design of a house would increase its cost by an estimated 1–2% for a structure valued at $300,000 to $600,000 (Larson and Slosson, 1992). Relative to the value of people and property that are exposed to risk in a structure that is not designed for seismic safety, this amount is a very small premium to pay in new-building construction or in retrofitting existing buildings. This minimal additional cost is probably even less of a burden in Malibu, where the median income is substantially above the national average.

The more costly aspect of seismic safety involves the mandated setbacks from the trace of an active fault that may render some lots unusable. The property is unusable for its intended purpose because of a natural condition of the property, not because of the geoscientist who observed and characterized that condition. A qualified geoscientist who locates and characterizes an active fault on a property, using sound scientific methods and meeting the standards of care as well as the standards imposed by law, should not be in a position of being held liable for the loss of real or potential property value. If geoscientists have reason to fear adverse legal action in response to their competent and necessary scientific work, then society through its legal system has made it impossible for geoscientists to function in the public interest.

Uncertainty and hazard assessment

Evaluating fault activity. When a Holocene earthquake produces coseismic surface rupture along a recognizable fault, it would appear that there is little room for uncertainty about whether the fault is seismically active. However, there may be some uncertainty in the interpretation even in this case. (1) The most obvious interpretation is that the slipped fault patch propagated outward from the hypocenter of the main shock until it intersected the ground surface, where it was manifested as surface rupture. That is, the surface displacement is along the same fault that generated the earthquake. (2) The coseismic surface rupture may have occurred along a fault other than the one that generated the earthquake, due to a kinematic adjustment or a secondary earthquake. (3) The fault that displayed coseismic surface rupture may be the slip surface of a landslide that moved during or after the earthquake; however, the earthquake focus was along another fault. While there may be several possible causes, the effect is still the same: coseismic surface rupture.

Ground-surface ruptures caused by landslides are specifically excluded from the zoning restrictions of the Alquist-Priolo Act (Hart, 1994) because landslide hazards can generally be mitigated whereas fault-rupture hazards can only be avoided. However, it is not always obvious whether a particular fault offset is related to the motion of a landslide or a crustal-scale fault. A landslide slip surface is a fault by common definition: a surface along which there is shear displacement. Landslide slip surfaces are marked by the same fault-zone structures and gouge/breccia found along any other fault in the shallow crust. Most of a landslide slip surface is a normal fault; however, the segment of the slip surface along the toe or base of a landslide is commonly a thrust fault. Some landslides in coastal southern California are hundreds of feet thick and have surface areas of many square kilometers. Some landslides slip on preexisting fault surfaces that are favorably oriented to facilitate slope instability. Coseismic landsliding associated with the 1989 Loma Prieta earthquake was observed in the Santa Cruz Mountains, where it caused significant property damage.

In the absence of instrumentally recorded earthquakes or historical accounts of surface rupture, it can be difficult to demonstrate the age of the most recent movement along a fault. Sometimes there is no datable material along the fault with which to evaluate the Holocene activity of the fault. The orientation of the net-slip vector may coincide with the plane of a datable horizon. Fault strands known to have slipped during the 1992 Landers earthquake (M_L 7.4) could not be recognized in some trenches cut across an unambiguous ground-surface trace, in spite of competent and diligent efforts to identify the fault trace in the trench exposure (James Slosson, oral communication, 1995; Murbach, 1994).

Some of the many difficulties encountered in interpreting fault activity from field data can be appreciated by considering a few scenarios based on the cross section in Figure 6a.

a. Unit A is Holocene, but elsewhere along the fault unit A does not appear to be displaced. Any future slip along the fault would probably cause the fault to propagate.

b. Unit A is Holocene, but elsewhere along the fault there are no Holocene units that cross the fault trace.

c. Unit A is Holocene, but the fault trace projects into urbanized areas in both directions. Pre-development geological reports for the urbanized areas are insufficient to evaluate possible Holocene slip along the fault in those areas.

d. Unit A is pre-Holocene, but a Holocene unit is cut by the fault elsewhere along the fault trace.

e. Unit A is pre-Holocene, no Holocene units exist along the trace of the fault, and there is no record of observed surface rupture along the fault.

f. Unit A is pre-Holocene, no Holocene units exist along the trace of the fault, and there is no record of observed surface rupture along the fault; however, there are geomorphic or geodetic indicators of structural activity across the fault.

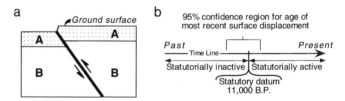

Figure 6. Dilemmas posed by legal definitions of fault activity. a, Fault exposure in a trench wall or outcrop. Unit A is younger than unit B. b, Error region for absolute age straddles a legally defined datum that separates *active* from *inactive* categories of fault.

g. Unit A is pre-Holocene, no Holocene units exist along the trace of the fault, and there is no record of observed surface rupture along the fault; however, a set of microearthquakes appears to coincide with the fault surface.

h. Unit A is pre-Holocene, no Holocene units exist along the trace of the fault, and there is no record of observed surface rupture along the fault; however, this fault surface is parallel to an adjacent fault surface on which there is demonstrable Holocene activity. Are two parallel faults in the same stress environment equally likely to experience future slip?

i. The statistical uncertainty in the absolute age of unit A makes it impossible to tell with certainty whether the unit is younger or older than the datum that statutorily differentiates active faults from inactive or potentially active faults (Fig. 6b).

In response to issues like these, there are two end-member approaches. Approach 1 is that a fault is to be considered *inactive* unless Holocene activity can be proven. Approach 2 is that a fault is to be considered *active* unless Holocene activity can be disproven. (In current practice, the only effective designations for a fault are *active* and *inactive*. This binary system will persist until the designation of a fault as *potentially active* results either in legally mandated restrictions on development or in legally mandated notification of potential fault activity included on real estate documents.)

Under approach 1, scenarios a through c would result in the fault being designated active, but the official Earthquake Fault Zone might include only the part of the fault that cuts a datable Holocene unit. Scenarios d through i would probably not result in an active designation for the fault shown in Figure 6a. Under approach 2, scenarios a through i might all result in the fault being designated active.

The problem with following approach 1 is that the hazard posed by at least some seismogenic faults will be discounted by labeling them inactive or just *potentially* active. The risk in approach 1 is borne by the individuals whose lives and property would be affected by coseismic surface rupture along the fault. These individuals do not generally have adequate knowledge or understanding of the risk they face, and so they cannot give their informed consent to the risk. These individuals rely on their public officials and the relevant technical professionals to recognize and manage the risk associated with geologic hazards on their behalf. In our opinion, approach 1 does not adequately protect the safety of the public.

Approach 2 would be effective in protecting the public from many potential fault-rupture hazards; however, it would also cause at least some faults that are actually fossil, inactive faults to be designated active. The inaccurate designation of a fault as active would result in the unnecessary imposition of setbacks from fault traces for new construction. Unnecessary setbacks make it needlessly expensive to develop some properties, and would make it impossible to develop other properties.

The dilemma. A classic moral/professional dilemma is presented by the problem of evaluating the Holocene activity of a fault given the incomplete nature of the geologic record as well as the technical limits on dating Holocene materials. In this dilemma the need to protect the safety of the public is potentially in conflict with the need not to waste the property/wealth of the public. Clearly, a balance needs to be struck between approaches 1 and 2 so that fault-rupture hazards are effectively identified and avoided with a minimum of collateral loss of usable property. Similar balances are prevalent in law and public policy as, for example, in the restrictions for hillside development in the Uniform Building Code (e.g., Scullin, 1983). Certain natural slope conditions, like high slope angles developed on weak materials or "daylighted" beds or joints that dip toward the slope face, are generally recognized as increasing the probability of future slope instability. Not every slope with adverse natural characteristics will fail during the useful life span of the adjacent structures, but development is still constrained by code when these conditions are present because of the reasonable expectation that these conditions will compromise the integrity of structures and the safety of their occupants.

The positive evolution of effective and appropriate public policy and professional practice concerning the assessment of fault-zone hazards requires an open and comprehensive dialog involving all of the stake-holders in the process: geoscience professionals, public servants, and the public. What can responsible geoscientists do to assess the hazard potential of potentially active faults and faults whose displacement history in the Quaternary is ambiguous? What can public officials do to expand statutory definitions and protections to include the hazards posed by potentially active faults? How can the public be better educated about seismic hazards, so that they can play a more effective role in enhancing their own seismic safety and in forming public policy?

Given a professional ethic that places the highest value on the protection of human life and safety, we prefer that public officials and geoscientists choose approach 2 as the starting point in the evolution of public policy and professional practice concerning the assessment of fault-zone hazards. The formal reintroduction of the category *potentially active* might provide a useful intermediate category between *active* and *inactive* faults to characterize faults that are likely to be active but whose most recent displacement is not unambiguously dated. The utility of designating a fault "potentially active" is contingent upon the legal effect of such a designation, which we feel should include clear notification on real estate documents associated with properties along the fault. The public cannot make an informed decision in evaluating the risk associated with a potentially active fault on a given property if they are not notified of the fault's existence and activity status.

IS THE MALIBU COAST FAULT ACTIVE?

Yerkes et al. (1987, p. 169) stated:

The intensity and relative youth of regional deformation in the Transverse Ranges have been emphasized in comparative or qualitative terms for more than 30 years. Gilluly's advocacy is both long standing (1949, 1962, 1979) and emphatic (1979, p. 475): 'there is no escape from the fact that this orogeny is active and active at a rate comparable to that of the formation of any mountain chain we know about.'

Recent seismicity and documented Holocene displacements within the MCFZ demonstrate conclusively that it is an active fault zone. The range of ancillary evidence described herein is uniformly supportive of that conclusion. Holocene slip is typically oblique: primarily reverse, with a minor left-lateral component. The average azimuth of hanging-wall slip relative to the foot wall is ~206°. The active emergent faults of the MCFZ appear to be a set of east-west–trending, north-dipping faults that are interpreted to constitute an imbricate, locally anastamosing thrust fan rising from a common detachment zone in the lower crust. The Anacapa fault appears to be the most active fault within the MCFZ although there may be other active, perhaps nonemergent, structures below and to the south of the Anacapa fault. Reliable published data on the position and characteristics of offshore faults are still sparse. Concurrent Holocene deformation has been observed or documented on many structures throughout the width of the western Transverse Ranges, so there is little reason to assume that deformation within the MCFZ is currently limited to the Anacapa fault and other offshore faults.

It has been shown that elements of the MCFZ are active, and that at least some strands of the Malibu Coast fault are active. The principal ambiguity involves the assessment of activity for the many individual strands of the MCFZ exposed along the Malibu coastline. While not all fault surfaces within the MCFZ may display unambiguous evidence of Holocene displacement, we feel that any favorably oriented fault surface within the MCFZ should be considered potentially active unless it can be shown conclusively to be otherwise.

We concur with Ziony and Yerkes (1985) that the Malibu Coast fault should be considered active and capable of producing a magnitude 6.5 to 7 earthquake. We feel that structures to be occupied by humans along the Malibu coastline should be built, or retrofitted, to withstand a magnitude 7 earthquake along the MCFZ, regardless of the proximity of the structure to an active fault strand. We also feel that critical facilities along the MCFZ should be built to withstand a magnitude 7.5 earthquake, as suggested by Mualchin and Jones (1992).

Identifying a fault and assessing the associated earthquake hazard is a matter of science and is governed by the methodology and ethics of science. Once compelling scientific evidence has been acquired that a fault zone is active, engineering geoscientists have a professional and moral obligation to act in an appropriate manner to inform and protect the public. An informed public can rationally assess the level of risk that it is willing to assume and can take steps, individually and collectively through its government, to protect itself from earthquake hazards.

ACKNOWLEDGMENTS

We thank Bob Dill, Jim Dolan, Bill Ellsworth, Leslie Ewing, Kate Hutton, Ken Lajoie, Lalliana Mualchin, Glen Reagor, Jim Slosson, Don Stierman, Robert Yerkes, and anonymous reviewers for providing data or constructive ideas to this paper. This paper could not have been written without the publications, basic science, and observational data contributed by the geoscientists of the U.S. Geological Survey and the California Division of Mines and Geology. We also thank Charles Welby for organizing this volume, and for his patience, encouragement, and many helpful comments with respect to this paper.

APPENDIX 1. DATA FOR EARTHQUAKES REPORTED FROM LATITUDE 33°55' TO 34°10'N AND FROM LONGITUDE 118°30' TO 119°5'W ALONG THE MALIBU COAST FAULT ZONE

EQ Ref. No.	Year	Date Mo	Da	Hypocenter/Epicenter Lat (°N)	Long (°W)	Location Depth (km)	Mag	Reported Arrivals	Focal Mechanism Soln Dip Azim	Dip Angle	Slip Azim	Source
1	1827	9	24	34	119		5.5					Toppozada et al., 1981
2	1911	5	10	34.1	118.8		4					CDMG via NEIC, 1995
3	1912	12	14	34	119		4					CDMG via NEIC, 1995
4	1914	11	8	34	118.5		4.5					CDMG via NEIC, 1995
5	1918	3	6	34	118.5		4					CDMG via NEIC, 1995
6	1918	3	8	34	118.5		4					CDMG via NEIC, 1995
7	1918	11	19	34	118.5		4					CDMG via NEIC, 1995
8	1920	6	22	34	118.5		4.9					USHIS via NEIC, 1995
9	1920	6	22	34	118.5		4.9					CDMG via NEIC, 1995
10	1920	6	23	34	118.5		4					CDMG via NEIC, 1995
11	1927	8	4	34	118.5		5					CDMG via NEIC, 1995
12	1930	8	31	34.03	118.643	15	5.2					Hauksson and Saldivar, 1986
13	1932	12	3	34	118.667		3					CDMG via NEIC, 1995
14	1934	1	14	33.967	118.583		2					CDMG via NEIC, 1995
15	1934	2	12	33.95	118.633		2.5					CDMG via NEIC, 1995
16	1934	3	10	33.95	118.633		3.5					CDMG via NEIC, 1995
17	1934	8	6	34.117	118.75		2.5					CDMG via NEIC, 1995
18	1934	8	6	34.117	118.75		2					CDMG via NEIC, 1995
19	1934	8	6	34.117	118.75		2					CDMG via NEIC, 1995
20	1934	8	6	33.95	118.633		2					CDMG via NEIC, 1995
21	1934	8	20	33.95	118.633		2.5					CDMG via NEIC, 1995
22	1935	5	13	33.95	118.633		2					CDMG via NEIC, 1995
23	1935	7	23	34.017	118.583		2.5					CDMG via NEIC, 1995
24	1936	2	5	34.117	118.75		2					CDMG via NEIC, 1995
25	1936	2	7	33.95	118.633		2					CDMG via NEIC, 1995
26	1936	3	7	34.117	118.75		2.5					CDMG via NEIC, 1995
27	1936	3	27	34.05	118.917		3					CDMG via NEIC, 1995
28	1936	4	18	34.117	118.75		2					CDMG via NEIC, 1995
29	1936	5	17	34.117	118.75		2					CDMG via NEIC, 1995
30	1936	5	22	34.117	118.75		2.5					CDMG via NEIC, 1995
31	1936	5	24	34.117	118.75		2.5					CDMG via NEIC, 1995
32	1936	6	3	34.117	118.75		2					CDMG via NEIC, 1995
33	1936	7	5	33.95	118.633		2					CDMG via NEIC, 1995
34	1936	8	14	33.95	118.633		2					CDMG via NEIC, 1995
35	1936	9	17	33.95	118.633		2					CDMG via NEIC, 1995
36	1936	10	8	34	118.533		3					CDMG via NEIC, 1995
37	1936	12	10	34.1	118.7		2					CDMG via NEIC, 1995
38	1937	5	11	33.95	118.633		2.5					CDMG via NEIC, 1995
39	1937	5	12	33.95	118.633		2.5					CDMG via NEIC, 1995
40	1937	5	24	33.95	118.633		2.5					CDMG via NEIC, 1995
41	1937	7	6	33.95	118.633		3					CDMG via NEIC, 1995
42	1937	11	7	33.95	118.633		2					CDMG via NEIC, 1995
43	1938	1	16	33.95	118.633		2.5					CDMG via NEIC, 1995
44	1938	5	24	34.117	118.75		2.5					CDMG via NEIC, 1995
45	1939	8	28	33.95	118.633		3.5					CDMG via NEIC, 1995
46	1940	8	16	33.95	118.633		3					CDMG via NEIC, 1995
47	1940	9	5	34.117	118.75		2.5					CDMG via NEIC, 1995
48	1940	10	16	33.95	118.583		2.5					CDMG via NEIC, 1995
49	1941	4	12	33.95	118.633		2.5					CDMG via NEIC, 1995
50	1941	7	13	34.1	118.85		3					CDMG via NEIC, 1995
51	1941	7	16	33.95	118.633		2.5					CDMG via NEIC, 1995
52	1942	10	9	34	118.717		3					CDMG via NEIC, 1995
53	1945	7	24	34	118.55		2.5					CDMG via NEIC, 1995
54	1945	12	19	34.1	118.683		2.7					CDMG via NEIC, 1995
55	1946	2	4	33.917	119		2.8					CDMG via NEIC, 1995
56	1946	4	27	34.017	119.017		3.1					CDMG via NEIC, 1995
57	1946	9	7	34.1	118.55		2.5					CDMG via NEIC, 1995
58	1947	6	30	33.983	118.9		2.4					CDMG via NEIC, 1995
59	1947	7	23	33.917	119		3.6					CDMG via NEIC, 1995
60	1947	7	27	34.117	118.8		2.8					CDMG via NEIC, 1995
61	1947	12	6	33.917	118.6		2.7					CDMG via NEIC, 1995
62	1948	4	16	34	118.933		3.3					CDMG via NEIC, 1995
63	1948	4	16	34.017	118.967		4.7					CDMG via NEIC, 1995
64	1948	4	17	34.017	118.967		2.9					CDMG via NEIC, 1995
65	1948	4	17	34.017	118.967		3.5					CDMG via NEIC, 1995

EQ Ref. No.	Year	Date Mo	Da	Hypocenter/Epicenter Location Lat (°N)	Long (°W)	Depth (km)	Mag	Reported Arrivals	Focal Mechanism Soln Dip Azim	Dip Angle	Slip Azim	Source
66	1948	4	17	34.017	118.967		2.7					CDMG via NEIC, 1995
67	1948	9	30	33.967	119		3.3					CDMG via NEIC, 1995
68	1948	9	30	33.967	119.033		3.1					CDMG via NEIC, 1995
69	1948	9	30	33.967	119.017		2.8					CDMG via NEIC, 1995
70	1948	10	4	34.017	119		3.8					CDMG via NEIC, 1995
71	1948	11	30	34	118.833		2.5					CDMG via NEIC, 1995
72	1949	2	9	33.933	118.65		3					CDMG via NEIC, 1995
73	1949	3	13	34	119		2.7					CDMG via NEIC, 1995
74	1949	4	23	34.05	118.8		2.9					CDMG via NEIC, 1995
75	1949	5	11	34.067	119.05		2.8					CDMG via NEIC, 1995
76	1949	6	28	34.067	119.033		2.7					CDMG via NEIC, 1995
77	1949	7	1	34.1	118.5		2.5					CDMG via NEIC, 1995
78	1949	9	23	33.967	118.95		3.2					CDMG via NEIC, 1995
79	1949	11	10	34.1	118.517		3					CDMG via NEIC, 1995
80	1949	11	16	33.983	118.533		2.4					CDMG via NEIC, 1995
81	1949	12	3	33.983	118.55		2.2					CDMG via NEIC, 1995
82	1949	12	10	34.05	118.5		3.2					CDMG via NEIC, 1995
83	1950	1	16	34.083	118.983		2.8					CDMG via NEIC, 1995
84	1950	10	9	33.917	118.717		2.7					CDMG via NEIC, 1995
85	1950	11	8	34.067	118.683		3.1					CDMG via NEIC, 1995
86	1950	11	8	34.067	118.717		2.6					CDMG via NEIC, 1995
87	1950	11	9	34.067	118.683		2.6					CDMG via NEIC, 1995
88	1951	3	6	34.017	119		2.9					CDMG via NEIC, 1995
89	1951	4	13	33.983	118.6		3.4					CDMG via NEIC, 1995
90	1951	4	25	34.166	118.733	16	3.2					DNAG via NEIC, 1995
91	1951	7	11	34	118.867		3.4					CDMG via NEIC, 1995
92	1951	10	21	34.133	118.567		2.2					CDMG via NEIC, 1995
93	1951	12	24	34	119.083		2.4					CDMG via NEIC, 1995
94	1952	2	12	34	119		3.2					CDMG via NEIC, 1995
95	1952	4	26	33.917	118.567		2.3					CDMG via NEIC, 1995
96	1952	11	18	34.1	118.5		2.5					CDMG via NEIC, 1995
97	1953	1	6	34	119.017		3.4					CDMG via NEIC, 1995
98	1953	9	7	34.083	118.5		2.1					CDMG via NEIC, 1995
99	1953	12	31	33.95	118.733		2.4					CDMG via NEIC, 1995
100	1954	1	22	33.95	118.75		2.3					CDMG via NEIC, 1995
101	1954	1	22	33.95	118.75		2.7					CDMG via NEIC, 1995
102	1954	7	24	34.166	118.65	16	3.2					DNAG via NEIC, 1995
103	1954	12	20	33.967	118.733		2.5					CDMG via NEIC, 1995
104	1955	5	29	33.99	119.058	17	4.1					CDMG via NEIC, 1995
105	1955	12	5	34.067	118.583		2.3					CDMG via NEIC, 1995
106	1955	12	13	34.033	119.05		2.8					CDMG via NEIC, 1995
107	1956	7	29	33.967	118.983		2.8					CDMG via NEIC, 1995
108	1956	10	22	33.967	118.5		2.3					CDMG via NEIC, 1995
109	1957	2	13	33.983	118.517		2.3					CDMG via NEIC, 1995
110	1957	4	26	34.1	118.867		2.7					CDMG via NEIC, 1995
111	1957	8	6	33.917	118.633		3.3					CDMG via NEIC, 1995
112	1957	8	6	33.917	118.633		2.9					CDMG via NEIC, 1995
113	1957	11	30	33.967	118.583		3.6					CDMG via NEIC, 1995
114	1958	5	19	34.05	119		3.1					CDMG via NEIC, 1995
115	1958	8	17	34.083	118.5		2					CDMG via NEIC, 1995
116	1958	12	15	33.917	118.667		2.6					CDMG via NEIC, 1995
117	1959	1	7	34.017	119.033		3					CDMG via NEIC, 1995
118	1959	3	29	34.033	118.5		2.7					CDMG via NEIC, 1995
119	1959	12	31	34.05	118.667		2.2					CDMG via NEIC, 1995
120	1960	1	29	34.083	118.633		2.3					CDMG via NEIC, 1995
121	1960	6	27	34	118.817		3.1					CDMG via NEIC, 1995
122	1960	12	26	34.133	118.633		2.6					CDMG via NEIC, 1995
123	1961	10	2	34.101	118.719	10	2.7					CDMG via NEIC, 1995
124	1961	11	13	34.018	118.849	13	3.8					CDMG via NEIC, 1995
125	1961	12	28	34.14	119.071	13	2.3					CDMG via NEIC, 1995
126	1962	1	16	34.166	119.083	13	3					DNAG via NEIC, 1995
127	1962	2	4	34.043	118.755		2.9					CDMG via NEIC, 1995
128	1962	2	6	34.1	118.73	5	3.1					CDMG via NEIC, 1995
129	1962	2	6	34.01	118.751	12	2.9					CDMG via NEIC, 1995
130	1962	3	19	34.069	118.896	15	3					CDMG via NEIC, 1995
131	1962	9	14	34.151	118.685		2.1					CDMG via NEIC, 1995
132	1962	12	9	34.007	118.59	14	2.7					CDMG via NEIC, 1995
133	1963	5	26	33.961	118.727	12	3.4					CDMG via NEIC, 1995
134	1963	8	27	34.139	119.019		2.6					CDMG via NEIC, 1995

EQ Ref. No.	Year	Date Mo	Da	Hypocenter/Epicenter Location Lat (°N)	Long (°W)	Depth (km)	Mag	Reported Arrivals	Focal Mechanism Soln Dip Azim	Dip Angle	Slip Azim	Source
135	1965	4	6	34.101	118.913	10	2.5					CDMG via NEIC, 1995
136	1965	5	2	33.989	118.575	10	2.7					CDMG via NEIC, 1995
137	1965	6	25	34.08	119.013	1	2.6					CDMG via NEIC, 1995
138	1965	10	5	33.919	118.651	10	2.8					CDMG via NEIC, 1995
139	1965	10	6	34	118.6	0	3.7					DNAG via NEIC, 1995
140	1965	10	6	34	118.6	0	3.7					DNAG via NEIC, 1995
141	1965	11	10	34.076	118.581	4	3					CDMG via NEIC, 1995
142	1965	12	9	34.104	118.688	11	2.7					CDMG via NEIC, 1995
143	1965	12	26	33.922	118.958	16	2.8					CDMG via NEIC, 1995
144	1966	9	4	33.938	118.525	10	2.7					CDMG via NEIC, 1995
145	1966	9	12	33.958	118.559	13	3.4					CDMG via NEIC, 1995
146	1966	9	12	33.993	118.562	5	3.2					CDMG via NEIC, 1995
147	1966	9	26	34.147	118.859	1	2					CDMG via NEIC, 1995
148	1966	10	1	33.959	118.803		2.3					CDMG via NEIC, 1995
149	1966	10	19	33.936	118.519		2.1					CDMG via NEIC, 1995
150	1966	12	20	33.961	118.842	10	3.3					CDMG via NEIC, 1995
151	1966	12	26	33.993	118.597	10	3.6					CDMG via NEIC, 1995
152	1966	12	27	33.958	118.63	0	2.9					CDMG via NEIC, 1995
153	1967	4	2	33.966	118.638	10	2.6					CDMG via NEIC, 1995
154	1968	3	13	33.96	118.531	13	2.5					CDMG via NEIC, 1995
155	1968	5	21	34.067	118.811	5	3.1					CDMG via NEIC, 1995
156	1968	6	6	33.98	118.688	10	2.7					CDMG via NEIC, 1995
157	1968	8	13	34.036	118.999	10	2.8					CDMG via NEIC, 1995
158	1969	6	22	33.924	118.72	9	3.6					CDMG via NEIC, 1995
159	1969	6	22	33.941	118.744		2.8					CDMG via NEIC, 1995
160	1970	3	7	33.942	118.825	5.3	2.7	9				Lee et al., 1979 (#10)
161	1970	3	29	34.06	118.987	8	1.9	5				Lee et al., 1979 (#16)
162	1970	7	1	34.037	118.85	0.5	1.8	6				Lee et al., 1979 (#36)
163	1970	11	22	34.132	119.033	12.6	1.9	5				Lee et al., 1979 (#50)
164	1971	2	9	34.166	118.516	7	3.7					DNAG via NEIC, 1995
165	1971	4	1	34.116	118.67		2.8					CDMG via NEIC, 1995
166	1971	4	15	34.15	118.54	8	4.2					Lee et al., 1979 (#79)
167	1971	4	15	34.15	118.518	9.1	3.2					Lee et al., 1979 (#80)
168	1971	11	16	34.102	118.832	3.2	2.1	6				Lee et al., 1979 (#130)
169	1971	11	23	34.063	118.827	0.5	2.1	6				Lee et al., 1979 (#131)
170	1971	12	18	34.117	118.818	3.4	2.1	8				Lee et al., 1979 (#134)
171	1972	1	13	34.052	118.792	6.1	2.1	7				Lee et al., 1979 (#140)
172	1972	1	15	34.113	118.832	0.5	2.1	7				Lee et al., 1979 (#141)
173	1972	1	20	34.102	118.837	1.8	2.2	8				Lee et al., 1979 (#147)
174	1972	3	2	34.013	118.563	3.5	1.9	7				Lee et al., 1979 (#153)
175	1972	4	27	34.07	118.982	12.8	3.1	11				Lee et al., 1979 (#163)
176a	1972	7	14	34.05	118.797	6.6	2.7	10	17	70	226	Lee et al., 1979 (#172)
176b	1972	7	14	34.05	118.797	6.6	2.7	10	227	22.8	17	Webb and Kanamori, 1985 (#60)
177	1972	11	9	34.053	118.795	5.1	2.5	11				Lee et al., 1979 (#184)
178	1972	12	22	34.003	118.548	8	2.6	8				Lee et al., 1979 (#189)
179	1973	2	8	33.982	118.703	6.6	2.8	16				Lee et al., 1979 (#194)
180	1973	2	14	34.09	119.053	14	2.2	6				Lee et al., 1979 (#195)
181a	1973	2	21	34.099	119.039	17.4	6	9	350	36	212	Stierman and Ellsworth, 1976 (#1)
181b	1973	2	21	34.078	119.038	12.2	5.9	16	356	44	167	Lee et al., 1979 (#197)
181c	1973	2	21	34.065	119.035	8	5.9		350	36	211	Hill et al., 1990 (#59)
181d	1973	2	21	34.099	119.039	17	6.0		339	49	181	Bent and Helmberger, 1991
181e	1973	2	21	34.065	119.035		5.3					Hutton and Jones, 1993
182	1973	2	21	34.061	118.967	15.4	2.9	8				Stierman and Ellsworth, 1976 (#2)
183	1973	2	21	34.049	118.965	14.1	4.1	10	209	62	108	Stierman and Ellsworth, 1976 (#3)
184	1973	2	21	34.057	118.978	14.6	3.8	9	207	78	116	Stierman and Ellsworth, 1976 (#4)
185	1973	2	21	34.072	118.991	12.7	2.1	9	327	64	290	Stierman and Ellsworth, 1976 (#5)
186	1973	2	21	34.066	118.992	14.5	2	8				Stierman and Ellsworth, 1976 (#6)
187	1973	2	21	34.051	119.018	17.3	2.9	9	354	50	214	Stierman and Ellsworth, 1976 (#7)
188	1973	2	21	34.079	118.983	12.6	2.9	7				Stierman and Ellsworth, 1976 (#8)
189	1973	2	21	34.098	119.003	15	2.1	8				Stierman and Ellsworth, 1976 (#9)
190	1973	2	21	34.107	119.005	11.4	2.5	8				Stierman and Ellsworth, 1976 (#10)
191	1973	2	21	34.096	119.043	13.6	4.2	10	87	30	217	Stierman and Ellsworth, 1976 (#11)
192	1973	2	21	34.095	118.972	14.2	2.3	9				Stierman and Ellsworth, 1976 (#12)
193	1973	2	21	34.066	118.97	14.6	2.9	9				Stierman and Ellsworth, 1976 (#13)
194	1973	2	21	34.099	118.986	14.8	2.1	7				Stierman and Ellsworth, 1976 (#14)
195	1973	2	21	34.07	118.965	14	2.5	8				Stierman and Ellsworth, 1976 (#15)
196	1973	2	21	34.063	118.976	15	2.6	7				Stierman and Ellsworth, 1976 (#16)
197	1973	2	21	34.061	118.988	13.8	2.6	9				Stierman and Ellsworth, 1976 (#17)
198	1973	2	21	34.053	119.012	16.6	2.3	7				Stierman and Ellsworth, 1976 (#18)

EQ Ref. No.	Year	Date Mo	Da	Hypocenter/Epicenter Location Lat (°N)	Long (°W)	Depth (km)	Mag	Reported Arrivals	Focal Mechanism Soln Dip Azim	Dip Angle	Slip Azim	Source
199	1973	2	21	34.1	119.034	17.5	2.7	9	360	54	214	Stierman and Ellsworth, 1976 (#19)
200	1973	2	21	34.089	118.997	12.8	2.4	8				Stierman and Ellsworth, 1976 (#20)
201	1973	2	21	34.083	118.994	16.6	3.4	9	34	54	272	Stierman and Ellsworth, 1976 (#21)
202	1973	2	22	34.094	118.972	14.4	3.4	9	60	45	222	Stierman and Ellsworth, 1976 (#22)
203	1973	2	22	34.087	118.992	15.6	2.5	8				Stierman and Ellsworth, 1976 (#23)
204	1973	2	22	34.09	118.996	13	2.4	9				Stierman and Ellsworth, 1976 (#24)
205	1973	2	22	34.055	119.056	13.1	2.4	9				Stierman and Ellsworth, 1976 (#25)
206	1973	2	22	34.067	118.984	13.7	3	9	18	54	148	Stierman and Ellsworth, 1976 (#26)
207	1973	2	22	34.067	118.966	14.2	2.5	9	18	50	196	Stierman and Ellsworth, 1976 (#27)
208	1973	2	22	34.064	119.013	14.5	2.2	9				Stierman and Ellsworth, 1976 (#28)
209	1973	2	22	34.056	118.993	14.2	2.5	9				Stierman and Ellsworth, 1976 (#29)
210	1973	2	22	34.072	118.985	12.7	2.5	9				Stierman and Ellsworth, 1976 (#30)
211	1973	2	22	34.055	119.005	15.6	2.2	7	62	50	51	Stierman and Ellsworth, 1976 (#31)
212	1973	2	22	34.072	118.993	14.2	2.4	9				Stierman and Ellsworth, 1976 (#32)
213	1973	2	22	34.089	119.049	15.9	4	12	356	36	204	Stierman and Ellsworth, 1976 (#33)
214	1973	2	22	34.077	118.992	13.8	2.3	11	335	80	242	Stierman and Ellsworth, 1976 (#34)
215	1973	2	22	34.067	118.967	14.5	2.3	11				Stierman and Ellsworth, 1976 (#35)
216	1973	2	22	34.063	118.991	13	2	8	10	60	190	Stierman and Ellsworth, 1976 (#36)
217	1973	2	22	34.043	119.006	13.5	2.5	11				Stierman and Ellsworth, 1976 (#37)
218	1973	2	22	33.983	118.957	3.2	2.1	6				Lee et al., 1979 (#234)
219	1973	2	22	34.067	118.993	13.7	2.9	10	335	30	136	Stierman and Ellsworth, 1976 (#38)
220	1973	2	22	34.071	118.984	13.8	1.7	10				Stierman and Ellsworth, 1976 (#39)
221	1973	2	22	34.069	118.981	14	1.9	8				Stierman and Ellsworth, 1976 (#40)
222	1973	2	22	34.058	118.986	13.9	2	10				Stierman and Ellsworth, 1976 (#41)
223	1973	2	23	34.069	118.987	13	1.3	6				Stierman and Ellsworth, 1976 (#42)
224	1973	2	23	34.073	118.98	11.9	1.1	6				Stierman and Ellsworth, 1976 (#43)
225	1973	2	23	34.092	118.983	12.3	1	8				Stierman and Ellsworth, 1976 (#44)
226	1973	2	23	34.061	118.982	13.7	3	19	0	84	264	Stierman and Ellsworth, 1976 (#45)
227	1973	2	23	34.061	118.983	12.3	0.5	9				Stierman and Ellsworth, 1976 (#46)
228	1973	2	23	34.057	118.988	13.4	1.2	7				Stierman and Ellsworth, 1976 (#47)
229	1973	2	23	34.07	118.988	14.4	0.9	10				Stierman and Ellsworth, 1976 (#48)
230	1973	2	23	34.087	119.011	10.1	1.3	7				Stierman and Ellsworth, 1976 (#49)
231	1973	2	23	34.073	118.974	12	1.1	6				Stierman and Ellsworth, 1976 (#50)
232	1973	2	23	34.047	119.017	13.4	1.4	7				Stierman and Ellsworth, 1976 (#51)
233	1973	2	23	34.051	118.983	11.9	1.4	10				Stierman and Ellsworth, 1976 (#52)
234	1973	2	23	34.058	119	14.7	1.6	9				Stierman and Ellsworth, 1976 (#53)
235	1973	2	23	34.08	118.973	13.2	1.5	10				Stierman and Ellsworth, 1976 (#54)
236	1973	2	23	34.081	119.028	15.1	1.5	9				Stierman and Ellsworth, 1976 (#55)
237	1973	2	24	34.075	119.062	10	2.1	15	353	90	262	Stierman and Ellsworth, 1976 (#56)
238	1973	2	24	34.055	118.981	14.1	1.6	11				Stierman and Ellsworth, 1976 (#57)
239	1973	2	24	34.084	119.013	14	1.7	14				Stierman and Ellsworth, 1976 (#58)
240	1973	2	24	34.063	118.981	14.7	0.7	6				Stierman and Ellsworth, 1976 (#59)
241	1973	2	24	34.057	118.989	14.8	1.5	13				Stierman and Ellsworth, 1976 (#60)
242	1973	2	24	34.08	118.982	16.4	2.1	22	1	50	228	Stierman and Ellsworth, 1976 (#61)
243	1973	2	24	34.066	118.998	16.5	1.7	16				Stierman and Ellsworth, 1976 (#62)
244	1973	2	24	34.093	118.975	10.8	0.9	7				Stierman and Ellsworth, 1976 (#63)
245	1973	2	24	34.085	118.98	13.3	0.9	10				Stierman and Ellsworth, 1976 (#64)
246	1973	2	24	34.073	119.051	16.6	1.8	14	0	60	256	Stierman and Ellsworth, 1976 (#65)
247	1973	2	24	34.078	118.957	14.5	1.9	20	6	50	230	Stierman and Ellsworth, 1976 (#66)
248	1973	2	24	34.068	118.973	12.8	2.2	21	340	52	224	Stierman and Ellsworth, 1976 (#67)
249	1973	2	24	34.082	118.962	13.2	1.6	10				Stierman and Ellsworth, 1976 (#68)
250	1973	2	24	34.095	119.018	14.2	1.5	14				Stierman and Ellsworth, 1976 (#69)
251	1973	2	24	34.08	118.977	11.5	1.7	13	22	52	216	Stierman and Ellsworth, 1976 (#70)
252	1973	2	24	34.054	118.986	14.3	1.6	9	133	42	249	Stierman and Ellsworth, 1976 (#71)
253	1973	2	25	34.072	119.002	15.3	1.1	13				Stierman and Ellsworth, 1976 (#72)
254	1973	2	25	34.091	118.98	11.8	0.9	9				Stierman and Ellsworth, 1976 (#73)
255	1973	2	25	34.074	118.963	14.1	0.9	20	332	70	230	Stierman and Ellsworth, 1976 (#74)
256	1973	2	25	34.084	118.979	13.4	0.8	21	356	70	240	Stierman and Ellsworth, 1976 (#75)
257	1973	2	25	34.052	118.997	14.3	1.2	14	348	82	252	Stierman and Ellsworth, 1976 (#76)
258	1973	2	25	34.076	118.986	12.6	1.5	13	13	50	193	Stierman and Ellsworth, 1976 (#77)
259a	1973	2	26	34.082	118.999	15.4	2.7	21	72	0	252	Stierman and Ellsworth, 1976 (#78)
259b	1973	2	26	34.082	118.999	15.4	2.7	21	65	0	245	Webb and Kanamori, 1985 (#62)
260	1973	2	26	34.062	118.99	15.2	1.2	9				Stierman and Ellsworth, 1976 (#79)
261	1973	2	26	34.058	118.983	14.4	1.7	19	58	33	218	Stierman and Ellsworth, 1976 (#80)
262	1973	2	27	34.089	118.995	14.7	1.5	19				Stierman and Ellsworth, 1976 (#81)
263	1973	2	27	34.047	118.996	17.2	2.3	22	177	85	85	Stierman and Ellsworth, 1976 (#82)
264	1973	2	27	34.09	118.975	14.1	2.5	25	330	38	201	Stierman and Ellsworth, 1976 (#83)
265	1973	2	27	34.066	118.969	14.6	1.9	17				Stierman and Ellsworth, 1976 (#84)
266	1973	2	27	34.042	119.002	13	1.9	17	332	90	222	Stierman and Ellsworth, 1976 (#85)

EQ Ref. No.	Year	Date Mo	Da	Hypocenter/Epicenter Location Lat (°N)	Long (°W)	Depth (km)	Mag	Reported Arrivals	Focal Mechanism Soln Dip Azim	Dip Angle	Slip Azim	Source
267	1973	2	28	34.089	119.003	13.8	0.8	7				Stierman and Ellsworth, 1976 (#86)
268	1973	2	28	34.051	118.991	15.8	1.6	14	176	65	262	Stierman and Ellsworth, 1976 (#87)
269	1973	2	28	34.067	118.98	15.9	0.7	11				Stierman and Ellsworth, 1976 (#88)
270	1973	2	28	34.048	118.995	17	2.7	26	192	55	268	Stierman and Ellsworth, 1976 (#89)
271	1973	3	1	34.054	118.994	16.4	1.1	13	119	80	218	Stierman and Ellsworth, 1976 (#90)
272	1973	3	1	34.056	118.97	14.3	0.9	12				Stierman and Ellsworth, 1976 (#91)
273a	1973	3	1	34.074	118.994	14.7	2.5	22	56	16	236	Stierman and Ellsworth, 1976 (#92)
273b	1973	3	1	34.074	118.994	14.7	2.5	22	60	5	240	Webb and Kanamori, 1985 (#63)
274	1973	3	1	34.074	118.967	13.4	1.2	12				Stierman and Ellsworth, 1976 (#93)
275	1973	3	1	34.075	118.968	13.4	0.8	12				Stierman and Ellsworth, 1976 (#94)
276	1973	3	1	34.074	118.975	12.9	0.5	11				Stierman and Ellsworth, 1976 (#95)
277	1973	3	2	34.093	119.026	15.2	1.9	20	332	62	230	Stierman and Ellsworth, 1976 (#96)
278	1973	3	2	34.071	119.048	15.1	1.1	13				Stierman and Ellsworth, 1976 (#97)
279	1973	3	2	34.075	118.976	15.7	1.3	12	322	70	232	Stierman and Ellsworth, 1976 (#98)
280	1973	3	2	34.095	119.003	14.9	1.2	13				Stierman and Ellsworth, 1976 (#99)
281	1973	3	3	34.017	119.085	9.5	1.3	22				Stierman and Ellsworth, 1976 (#100)
282	1973	3	3	34.076	119.028	14.2	0.8	16				Stierman and Ellsworth, 1976 (#101)
283	1973	3	4	34.063	118.982	13.3	0.8	14				Stierman and Ellsworth, 1976 (#102)
284	1973	3	5	34.074	118.993	12.2	1.3	20	329	34	171	Stierman and Ellsworth, 1976 (#103)
285	1973	3	5	34.041	118.99	16.7	3.5	24	102	60	208	Stierman and Ellsworth, 1976 (#104)
286	1973	3	5	34.066	118.982	13	1	8				Stierman and Ellsworth, 1976 (#105)
287	1973	3	6	34.065	118.977	12.5	0.9	9				Stierman and Ellsworth, 1976 (#106)
288	1973	3	6	34.061	118.979	12.9	0.2	6				Stierman and Ellsworth, 1976 (#107)
289	1973	3	6	33.93	118.522	16	2.3	11				Lee et al., 1979 (#275)
290	1973	3	6	34.073	118.976	11.6	0.8	12				Stierman and Ellsworth, 1976 (#108)
291	1973	3	7	34.043	119.001	17.8	2.5	19	100	70	202	Stierman and Ellsworth, 1976 (#109)
292	1973	3	7	34.058	118.975	12.3	1.1	16				Stierman and Ellsworth, 1976 (#110)
293	1973	3	7	34.079	119.023	15.2	1	16				Stierman and Ellsworth, 1976 (#111)
294	1973	3	7	34.095	119.041	13.8	1.9	17	114	54	82	Stierman and Ellsworth, 1976 (#112)
295	1973	3	7	34.063	118.979	12.5	1	10				Stierman and Ellsworth, 1976 (#113)
296	1973	3	7	34.068	119.007	13.1	0.8	17				Stierman and Ellsworth, 1976 (#114)
297	1973	3	7	34.068	118.979	12.4	0.8	12				Stierman and Ellsworth, 1976 (#115)
298	1973	3	10	34.078	118.964	13.3	2	22	172	72	260	Stierman and Ellsworth, 1976 (#116)
299	1973	3	16	34.074	118.997	13	3.5	18	88	34	234	Stierman and Ellsworth, 1976 (#117)
300	1973	3	17	34.071	118.992	13.7	3.7	18	342	74	244	Stierman and Ellsworth, 1976 (#118)
301	1973	3	21	34.089	119.001	15.7	1.3	16				Stierman and Ellsworth, 1976 (#119)
302	1973	3	22	34.076	119.043	17.2	1.6	11				Stierman and Ellsworth, 1976 (#120)
303	1973	3	22	34.086	119.018	14.8	1	12				Stierman and Ellsworth, 1976 (#121)
304	1973	3	23	34.074	118.995	13.7	1.9	9				Stierman and Ellsworth, 1976 (#122)
305	1973	3	25	34.065	118.971	15.3	1.1	15				Stierman and Ellsworth, 1976 (#123)
306	1973	3	26	34.062	118.973	12.5	1.7	10				Stierman and Ellsworth, 1976 (#124)
307	1973	3	26	34.058	118.978	13.4	2	9				Stierman and Ellsworth, 1976 (#125)
308	1973	3	26	34.073	118.983	13.2	3	17	314	44	196	Stierman and Ellsworth, 1976 (#126)
309	1973	3	26	34.074	118.99	11.5	1.7	20	14	30	194	Stierman and Ellsworth, 1976 (#127)
310	1973	3	27	34.071	118.986	12.2	1.9	7				Stierman and Ellsworth, 1976 (#128)
311	1973	3	28	34.09	118.988	4.3	0.5	8				Stierman and Ellsworth, 1976 (#129)
312	1973	3	28	34.061	118.957	11.7	1	6				Stierman and Ellsworth, 1976 (#130)
313	1973	3	28	34.072	118.977	11.6	1.6	8				Stierman and Ellsworth, 1976 (#131)
314	1973	3	29	34.056	118.984	13.2	1.4	8				Stierman and Ellsworth, 1976 (#132)
315	1973	3	29	33.98	118.547	2.4	2.6	23				Lee et al., 1979 (#298)
316	1973	3	31	34.038	118.772	8	1.6	7				Lee et al., 1979 (#299)
317	1973	3	31	34.048	118.969	13.5	1.6	9	320	50	321	Stierman and Ellsworth, 1976 (#133)
318	1973	4	1	34.067	119.01	6.1	0.9	7				Stierman and Ellsworth, 1976 (#134)
319	1973	4	2	34.042	118.978	8.2	0.8	13				Stierman and Ellsworth, 1976 (#135)
320	1973	4	2	34.077	118.981	11.5	1.3	13				Stierman and Ellsworth, 1976 (#136)
321	1973	4	2	34.089	119.013	14.6	1.3	14				Stierman and Ellsworth, 1976 (#137)
322	1973	4	4	34.138	118.988	10.9	1.4	6				Lee et al., 1979 (#302)
323	1973	4	5	34.031	119.022	12.2	1.9	16	348	52	210	Stierman and Ellsworth, 1976 (#138)
324	1973	4	5	34.073	118.986	12	1.6	9				Stierman and Ellsworth, 1976 (#139)
325a	1973	4	7	34.101	118.978	13.1	1.7	14	335	30	231	Stierman and Ellsworth, 1976 (#140)
325b	1973	4	7	34.101	118.978	13.1	1.7	14	50	10	230	Webb and Kanamori, 1985 (#64)
326	1973	4	8	34.038	119.067	10.6	1.8	15				Lee et al., 1979 (#310)
327	1973	4	11	34.098	119.027	14.7	1.2	16				Stierman and Ellsworth, 1976 (#141)
328	1973	4	12	34.097	119.039	13.9	1.6	11				Stierman and Ellsworth, 1976 (#142)
329	1973	4	19	33.95	118.715	1.9	2.1	11				Lee et al., 1979 (#317)
330	1973	4	20	33.998	118.932	7.3	2.1	7				Lee et al., 1979 (#318)
331	1973	5	11	33.973	118.55	3.7	2.5	17				Lee et al., 1979 (#324)
332	1973	5	12	34.013	119.032	6.4	3.1	14				Lee et al., 1979 (#326)
333	1973	5	14	34.032	119.042	10.7	2.2	8				Lee et al., 1979 (#327)

EQ Ref. No.	Year	Date Mo	Da	Hypocenter/Epicenter Location Lat (°N)	Long (°W)	Depth (km)	Mag	Reported Arrivals	Focal Mechanism Soln Dip Azim	Dip Angle	Slip Azim	Source
334	1973	6	21	34.053	118.835	3.6	1.4	6				Lee et al., 1979 (#339)
335	1973	6	22	34.055	118.805	1.5	1.7	6				Lee et al., 1979 (#340)
336	1973	6	27	34.05	118.992	2	1.9	9				Lee et al., 1979 (#342)
337	1973	7	5	34.058	119.018	13.3	2.1	9				Lee et al., 1979 (#343)
338	1973	7	8	34.06	118.99	12.2	2	12				Lee et al., 1979 (#344)
339	1973	7	14	34.012	118.82	13.5	2	13				Lee et al., 1979 (#345)
340	1973	7	14	34.035	119.033	13.1	2	13				Lee et al., 1979 (#346)
341	1973	7	15	34.067	119.063	17.6	1.6	10				Lee et al., 1979 (#347)
342	1973	7	18	34.035	118.74	5.7	1.6	10				Lee et al., 1979 (#350)
343	1973	7	24	34.038	119.018	12.5	2.5	21				Lee et al., 1979 (#351)
344	1973	7	26	33.995	118.732	2.4	1.6	8				Lee et al., 1979 (#353)
345	1973	7	29	34.053	118.96	11.8	2.3	15				Lee et al., 1979 (#354)
346	1973	8	3	34.062	119.083	16.2	1.6	12				Lee et al., 1979 (#356)
347	1973	8	13	34.047	118.98	15.8	1.9	14				Lee et al., 1979 (#363)
348	1973	8	16	34.062	118.813	2.6	1.4	9				Lee et al., 1979 (#367)
349	1973	8	19	34.065	119.038	7.5	1.8	11				Lee et al., 1979 (#369)
350	1973	8	21	34.073	118.997	11.7	1.3	7				Lee et al., 1979 (#372)
351	1973	8	23	34.075	119.072	17.8	1.8	8				Lee et al., 1979 (#374)
352	1973	8	23	34.052	118.965	12.5	1.8	8				Lee et al., 1979 (#375)
353	1973	8	27	34.047	118.99	3.6	2	10				Lee et al., 1979 (#378)
354	1973	8	27	34.042	118.987	2.6	1.9	9				Lee et al., 1979 (#379)
355	1973	8	28	34.045	118.79	6	1.5	8				Lee et al., 1979 (#380)
356	1973	8	29	34.052	118.998	2.4	1.8	9				Lee et al., 1979 (#381)
357	1973	9	2	34.018	118.748	13.9	2.3	17	316	44	181	Lee et al., 1979 (#385)
358	1973	9	3	34.033	118.84	13.7	1.2	9				Lee et al., 1979 (#387)
359	1973	9	4	34.037	118.802	6.1	1.7	7				Lee et al., 1979 (#390)
360	1973	9	20	34.017	119.012	11.1	2	19				Lee et al., 1979 (#400)
361	1973	10	6	34.033	119.01	8	1.8	17				Lee et al., 1979 (#403)
362	1973	10	10	34.053	118.797	1.1	1.3	6				Lee et al., 1979 (#405)
363	1973	10	12	34.053	118.898	10.7	2.2	17				Lee et al., 1979 (#406)
364	1973	10	15	34.05	118.795	2.2	1.1	7				Lee et al., 1979 (#408)
365	1973	10	21	34.078	118.965	14.6	1.1	9				Lee et al., 1979 (#410)
366	1973	10	24	34.043	118.798	6	1.1	6				Lee et al., 1979 (#411)
367	1973	10	26	34.031	118.898	4.5	1.9	8				Lee et al., 1979 (#413)
368	1973	10	30	34.042	118.98	14.1	1.3	9				Lee et al., 1979 (#414)
369	1973	11	6	34.04	119.02	16.4	1.4	9				Lee et al., 1979 (#416)
370	1973	11	8	34.048	118.798	4.9	1	7				Lee et al., 1979 (#417)
371	1973	12	5	34.062	119.042	7.9	1.4	12				Lee et al., 1979 (#422)
372	1973	12	12	34.068	118.98	12.3	1.8	11				Lee et al., 1979 (#424)
373	1973	12	20	34.073	118.933	13.3	2.1	18	62	50	276	Lee et al., 1979 (#426)
374	1973	12	28	34.053	118.797	2.4	1.3	7				Lee et al., 1979 (#431)
375	1973	12	30	33.972	118.772	16.3	1.7	9				Lee et al., 1979 (#432)
376	1974	1	10	34.06	119.055	13.7	2.1	12				Lee et al., 1979 (#434)
377	1974	1	10	34.092	119.013	11.3	1.5	8				Lee et al., 1979 (#435)
378	1974	1	12	34.063	118.965	15.7	2.2	9				Lee et al., 1979 (#436)
379	1974	1	17	34.095	119.045	13.8	1.5	8				Lee et al., 1979 (#437)
380	1974	1	18	34.085	118.863	17.2	1.5	8				Lee et al., 1979 (#438)
381	1974	1	25	34.06	118.903	12.7	1.2	8				Lee et al., 1979 (#441)
382	1974	1	25	33.917	118.715	8	1.9	14				Lee et al., 1979 (#442)
383	1974	2	1	34.062	119.005	2.3	1.3	8				Lee et al., 1979 (#443)
384	1974	2	1	34.038	119.005	8	1.5	10				Lee et al., 1979 (#444)
385	1974	2	23	34.055	118.938	14.9	1.3	7				Lee et al., 1979 (#448)
386	1974	3	3	34.033	118.993	9.2	2.3	14				Lee et al., 1979 (#451)
387	1974	3	3	34.055	119.005	8.9	2.3	14				Lee et al., 1979 (#452)
388	1974	3	6	33.924	118.671	5	2.1					CDMG via NEIC, 1995
389	1974	3	7	33.925	118.71	8	1.9	11				Lee et al., 1979 (#455)
390	1974	3	17	34.058	118.997	1.9	1.5	8				Lee et al., 1979 (#458)
391	1974	3	18	34.047	118.912	12.7	2	15				Lee et al., 1979 (#459)
392	1974	3	30	34.085	118.847	13.1	1.8	11				Lee et al., 1979 (#461)
393a	1974	3	31	34.02	118.748	5.9	2.6	16				Lee et al., 1979 (#462)
393b	1974	3	31	34.018	118.744	5.1	1.6	17	358	60	16	Buika and Teng, 1979 (#24/210)
394	1974	4	1	34.068	118.992	14.5	2.2	17				Lee et al., 1979 (#463)
395	1974	4	2	34.052	118.965	13.7	1.5	8				Lee et al., 1979 (#464)
396	1974	4	3	34.055	118.897	11.3	2.5	14				Lee et al., 1979 (#466)
397	1974	4	5	34.047	118.938	11.4	2.5	14				Lee et al., 1979 (#467)
398	1974	4	11	34.07	119.01	15.7	1.4	6				Lee et al., 1979 (#468)
399	1974	4	14	34.095	119.04	19.2	1.6	10				Lee et al., 1979 (#469)
400	1974	4	24	34.095	118.862	1.7	1.2	8				Lee et al., 1979 (#471)
401	1974	4	25	34.03	119.083	9.9	1.9	16				Lee et al., 1979 (#473)

EQ Ref. No.	Year	Date Mo	Da	Hypocenter/Epicenter Location Lat (°N)	Long (°W)	Depth (km)	Mag	Reported Arrivals	Focal Mechanism Soln Dip Azim	Dip Angle	Slip Azim	Source
402	1974	5	10	34.063	118.905	13.8	1.1	8				Lee et al., 1979 (#475)
403	1974	5	22	34.052	118.977	14.1	1.5	11				Lee et al., 1979 (#477)
404	1974	5	22	34.038	119	9	1.4	8				Lee et al., 1979 (#478)
405	1974	6	21	34.092	119.018	15.8	2.3	17				Lee et al., 1979 (#480)
406	1974	7	6	34.047	119.03	16.4	1.8	12				Lee et al., 1979 (#481)
407	1974	7	12	34.007	118.815	9.8	1.9	16				Lee et al., 1979 (#483)
408	1974	7	23	34.063	118.98	14.2	1.5	9				Lee et al., 1979 (#484)
409	1974	7	25	33.937	118.862	7.2	2.3	12				Lee et al., 1979 (#485)
410	1974	8	25	33.937	118.672	10.8	2	11				Lee et al., 1979 (#491)
411	1974	10	8	34.038	118.983	2.1	3.4	14				Lee et al., 1979 (#509)
412	1974	10	8	34.057	119	1.7	1.4	6				Lee et al., 1979 (#510)
413	1974	10	8	34.057	118.997	1.9	1.4	7				Lee et al., 1979 (#511)
414	1974	10	8	34.06	118.998	1.9	1.7	7				Lee et al., 1979 (#512)
415	1974	10	8	34.062	119.002	1.6	1.2	6				Lee et al., 1979 (#513)
416	1974	10	8	34.057	118.997	2.1	1.7	7				Lee et al., 1979 (#514)
417	1974	10	8	34.06	119	1.9	1.6	7				Lee et al., 1979 (#515)
418	1974	10	8	34.057	118.998	1.8	1.5	7				Lee et al., 1979 (#516)
419	1974	10	8	34.057	118.992	2	1.7	7				Lee et al., 1979 (#517)
420	1974	10	8	34.058	118.993	2	1.7	7				Lee et al., 1979 (#518)
421	1974	10	8	34.058	118.99	2	1.5	5				Lee et al., 1979 (#519)
422	1974	10	8	34.055	118.997	2.5	1.5	7				Lee et al., 1979 (#520)
423	1974	10	9	34.053	118.998	2.1	1.1	6				Lee et al., 1979 (#521)
424	1974	10	9	34.058	118.998	1.7	1.1	7				Lee et al., 1979 (#522)
425	1974	10	9	34.055	118.993	2	1.1	6				Lee et al., 1979 (#523)
426	1974	10	9	34.058	118.997	2.2	1.7	8				Lee et al., 1979 (#524)
427	1974	10	10	34.06	118.995	1.9	1.3	7				Lee et al., 1979 (#525)
428	1974	10	12	34.055	118.988	3.3	2.9	17				Lee et al., 1979 (#526)
429	1974	10	12	34.075	118.988	4.4	1.6	9				Lee et al., 1979 (#527)
430	1974	10	12	34.058	118.997	1.9	1.8	8				Lee et al., 1979 (#528)
431	1974	10	12	34.048	119.005	1.2	1	7				Lee et al., 1979 (#529)
432	1974	10	18	34.058	119.003	1.7	1.2	7				Lee et al., 1979 (#531)
433	1974	10	22	34.057	119.007	2.3	1.1	7				Lee et al., 1979 (#532)
434	1974	11	6	34.055	118.998	3.9	1.1	7				Lee et al., 1979 (#533)
435	1974	11	11	34.065	118.993	14.9	1.6	10				Lee et al., 1979 (#534)
436	1974	11	14	34.06	118.998	1.9	1.3	7				Lee et al., 1979 (#535)
437	1974	11	14	34.058	118.998	1.9	1	7				Lee et al., 1979 (#536)
438	1974	11	14	34.06	118.998	1.9	1	7				Lee et al., 1979 (#537)
439	1974	11	15	34.055	119.003	2.1	1.2	7				Lee et al., 1979 (#538)
440	1974	11	27	34.088	118.965	16.8	1.4	8				Lee et al., 1979 (#540)
441	1974	12	4	34.067	119.002	14.7	1.2	6				Lee et al., 1979 (#542)
442	1974	12	7	34.09	119.007	8	1	6				Lee et al., 1979 (#543)
443	1974	12	19	34.063	118.742	4	1.3	8				Lee et al., 1979 (#545)
444	1974	12	20	34.092	118.867	12.5	2.1	12				Lee et al., 1979 (#547)
445	1974	12	25	34.038	119.008	8.7	1.8	7				Lee et al., 1979 (#548)
446	1975	1	7	34.113	119.025	17.3	1.2	9				Lee et al., 1979 (#552)
447	1975	1	11	33.99	118.862	13	2.5	14	5	45	185	Lee et al., 1979 (#553)
448	1975	1	23	33.917	118.633	12	3					PDE via NEIC, 1995
449	1975	1	24	34.023	119.018	10.9	2.1	13				Lee et al., 1979 (#556)
450	1975	2	4	34.065	118.793	8.3	1.4	9				Lee et al., 1979 (#562)
451	1975	2	8	34.067	118.787	7	1.8	12				Lee et al., 1979 (#563)
452	1975	2	23	34.063	118.985	13.3	2.7	21				Lee et al., 1979 (#566)
453	1975	3	1	34.02	118.72	6.6	2	13	38	56	162	Lee et al., 1979 (#570)
454	1975	4	11	34.052	118.997	9.6	3.1	22				Lee et al., 1979 (#578)
455	1975	4	12	34.053	118.992	11.9	2.1	13				Lee et al., 1979 (#579)
456	1975	4	14	34.033	119.025	16.6	1.7	12				Lee et al., 1979 (#580)
457	1975	4	24	34.048	118.992	1.9	2	8				Lee et al., 1979 (#582)
458	1975	4	25	34.048	118.988	16.5	1.4	9				Lee et al., 1979 (#583)
459	1975	4	27	34.09	119.007	14.3	1.4	8				Lee et al., 1979 (#584)
460	1975	5	26	34.078	118.98	16.8	1.5	8				Lee et al., 1979 (#588)
461	1975	5	28	34.035	118.993	12.5	2.1	14				Lee et al., 1979 (#590)
462	1975	6	9	34.038	119.032	13.3	1.5	10				Lee et al., 1979 (#594)
463	1975	6	10	34.015	118.752	8.7	2.1	11				Lee et al., 1979 (#595)
464	1975	6	21	34.027	119.018	4.6	1.9	10				Lee et al., 1979 (#596)
465	1975	7	6	34.062	118.885	9.9	2.3	8				Lee et al., 1979 (#600)
466	1975	7	12	34.077	118.975	10.9	1.4	9				Lee et al., 1979 (#602)
467	1975	7	13	34.073	118.968	11.3	1.6	10				Lee et al., 1979 (#603)
468	1975	9	2	34.047	118.973	6.9	1.4	9				Lee et al., 1979 (#611)
469	1975	9	25	34.935	118.925	13	1.5	9				Lee et al., 1979 (#613)
470	1975	9	26	34.047	119.018	8	1.3	8				Lee et al., 1979 (#614)

EQ Ref. No.	Year	Date Mo	Da	Hypocenter/Epicenter Location Lat (°N)	Long (°W)	Depth (km)	Mag	Reported Arrivals	Focal Mechanism Soln Dip Azim	Dip Angle	Slip Azim	Source
471	1975	10	5	34.042	118.952	13.4	2	13				Lee et al., 1979 (#617)
472	1975	12	25	34.018	119.075	9.9	2.1	11				Lee et al., 1979 (#627)
473	1976	2	12	33.999	118.829	8	2.6					DNAG via NEIC, 1995
474	1976	5	4	34.09	119.014	13.4	3.1	21	222	70	224	Buika and Teng, 1979 (#25/358)
475	1976	6	9	34.041	118.973	11	2.5					DNAG via NEIC, 1995
476	1976	6	20	33.998	118.818	8	3.8	26	341	50	224	Buika and Teng, 1979 (#23/365)
477	1976	11	22	33.956	118.621	2	3.8					DNAG via NEIC, 1995
478	1976	11	22	33.937	118.626	8	4.2	37	350	90	260	Buika and Teng, 1979 (#12/410)
479	1976	11	22	33.977	118.581	8	2.9					DNAG via NEIC, 1995
480	1976	12	11	33.953	118.664	10	2.8					DNAG via NEIC, 1995
481	1976	12	13	34.042	119.031	8	2.5					DNAG via NEIC, 1995
482	1977	7	29	33.986	118.9	7	2.7					DNAG via NEIC, 1995
483	1977	9	10	34.049	118.989	9	2.7					DNAG via NEIC, 1995
484	1977	9	10	34.044	118.99	5	2.7					DNAG via NEIC, 1995
485	1977	10	14	34.051	118.811	10	2.8					DNAG via NEIC, 1995
486	1977	12	7	34.047	118.913	11	2.9					DNAG via NEIC, 1995
487	1978	3	14	34.001	118.674	13.6	3.1	28	3	35	219	Hauksson, 1990
488	1978	4	22	34.06	118.978	13	3.4					DNAG via NEIC, 1995
489	1978	5	1	33.947	118.737	12.9	2.5	37	320	41	189	Hauksson, 1990
490	1978	7	21	34.055	118.901	15	3					DNAG via NEIC, 1995
491	1978	11	19	34.013	118.628	11.8	2.8	76	64	24	190	Hauksson, 1990
492a	1979	1	1	33.951	118.673	12.1	5	80	20	52	175	Hauksson, 1990
492b	1979	1	1	33.948	118.688	9.6	5		10	60	200	Hauksson and Saldivar, 1986 (#1)
492c	1979	1	1	33.944	118.681	11.1	5		10	60	200	Hill et al., 1990 (#60)
492d	1979	1	1	33.944	118.681		5.2					Hutton and Jones, 1993
493	1979	1	1	33.97	118.72	8.5	3.2		10	45	200	Hauksson and Saldivar, 1986 (#2)
494	1979	1	1	33.96	118.692	6.3	3.1		15	40	179	Hauksson and Saldivar, 1986 (#3)
495a	1979	1	1	33.937	118.698	9.4	3.4		350	65	220	Hauksson and Saldivar, 1986 (#4)
495b	1979	1	1	33.933	118.714	13	3.4		63	22	289	Webb and Kanamori, 1985 (#24)
496	1979	1	1	33.95	118.665	7.3	3		355	52	196	Hauksson and Saldivar, 1986 (#5)
497	1979	1	1	33.958	118.673	3.5	3		10	62	240	Hauksson and Saldivar, 1986 (#6)
498	1979	1	1	33.95	118.673	7.7	3.9		360	50	225	Hauksson and Saldivar, 1986 (#7)
499	1979	1	1	33.952	118.682	7	3		20	72	224	Hauksson and Saldivar, 1986 (#8)
500	1979	1	1	33.996	118.638	5	3					DNAG via NEIC, 1995
501	1979	1	1	33.942	118.692	9	2.5					Hauksson and Saldivar, 1986
502	1979	1	1	33.943	118.673	7.2	2.6					Hauksson and Saldivar, 1986
503	1979	1	1	33.937	118.677	10.1	3.7		10	60	225	Hauksson and Saldivar, 1986 (#9)
504	1979	1	2	33.948	118.688	8.8	3		20	56	236	Hauksson and Saldivar, 1986 (#10)
505	1979	1	2	33.96	118.693	8.9	2.9					Hauksson and Saldivar, 1986
506	1979	1	2	33.95	118.693	9.3	2.6					Hauksson and Saldivar, 1986
507	1979	1	2	33.94	118.695	9.3	2.7					Hauksson and Saldivar, 1986
508	1979	1	2	33.96	118.692	9.5	2.7					Hauksson and Saldivar, 1986
509	1979	1	2	33.953	118.697	9.9	3		25	48	230	Hauksson and Saldivar, 1986 (#11)
510	1979	1	2	33.943	118.708	8.2	3.7		10	51	206	Hauksson and Saldivar, 1986 (#12)
511	1979	1	2	33.948	118.705	5.9	2.7					Hauksson and Saldivar, 1986
512	1979	1	2	33.94	118.687	8.6	2.5					Hauksson and Saldivar, 1986
513	1979	1	2	33.935	118.665	8.2	2.7					Hauksson and Saldivar, 1986
514	1979	1	2	33.953	118.682	9.8	2.9					Hauksson and Saldivar, 1986
515	1979	1	2	33.933	118.685	8.3	3.4		10	50	190	Hauksson and Saldivar, 1986 (#13)
516	1979	1	2	33.935	118.677	9	2.5					Hauksson and Saldivar, 1986
517	1979	1	2	33.955	118.678	8.2	2.6					Hauksson and Saldivar, 1986
518	1979	1	3	33.94	118.662	7.3	2.8					Hauksson and Saldivar, 1986
519	1979	1	3	33.938	118.702	9.3	2.7					Hauksson and Saldivar, 1986
520	1979	1	3	33.928	118.695	7.8	2.5					Hauksson and Saldivar, 1986
521	1979	1	3	33.943	118.682	7.7	2.6					Hauksson and Saldivar, 1986
522	1979	1	3	33.998	118.705	9.2	2.9					Hauksson and Saldivar, 1986
523	1979	1	3	33.967	118.685	7.9	3		360	51	196	Hauksson and Saldivar, 1986 (#14)
524	1979	1	4	33.942	118.672	8.7	3		355	62	225	Hauksson and Saldivar, 1986 (#15)
525	1979	1	5	33.935	118.662	8.4	2.6					Hauksson and Saldivar, 1986
526	1979	1	6	33.94	118.695	9.4	2.5					Hauksson and Saldivar, 1986
527	1979	1	6	33.963	118.67	9.1	2.6					Hauksson and Saldivar, 1986
528	1979	1	8	33.95	118.682	9.4	2.7					Hauksson and Saldivar, 1986
529	1979	1	8	33.928	118.673	8.1	2.8					Hauksson and Saldivar, 1986
530	1979	1	9	33.935	118.688	7.2	2.6					Hauksson and Saldivar, 1986
531	1979	1	13	33.953	118.667	7.2	2.8					Hauksson and Saldivar, 1986
532	1979	1	15	33.952	118.7	9.3	3.7		15	62	236	Hauksson and Saldivar, 1986 (#16)
533	1979	1	16	33.96	118.682	9	2.9					Hauksson and Saldivar, 1986
534	1979	1	29	33.943	118.663	10.8	3.1		10	62	211	Hauksson and Saldivar, 1986 (#17)
535	1979	2	18	33.997	118.925	7	2.6					DNAG via NEIC, 1995

EQ Ref. No.	Year	Date Mo	Da	Hypocenter/Epicenter Location Lat (°N)	Long (°W)	Depth (km)	Mag	Reported Arrivals	Focal Mechanism Soln Dip Azim	Dip Angle	Slip Azim	Source
536	1979	2	20	34.046	119	16	2.8					DNAG via NEIC, 1995
537	1979	2	28	33.958	118.7	6.5	2.5					Hauksson and Saldivar, 1986
538	1979	3	5	33.948	118.712	10.1	3.7		15	60	189	Hauksson and Saldivar, 1986 (#18)
539	1979	3	13	33.926	118.975	5	2.8					DNAG via NEIC, 1995
540	1979	6	29	34.006	118.988	5	2.7					DNAG via NEIC, 1995
541	1979	8	29	33.967	118.698	8.8	2.7					Hauksson and Saldivar, 1986
542	1979	9	5	34.029	118.935	14	3.4					DNAG via NEIC, 1995
543	1979	9	5	34.017	118.932	14	2.5					DNAG via NEIC, 1995
544	1979	9	6	33.958	118.698	6.3	2.5					Hauksson and Saldivar, 1986
545	1979	10	17	33.932	118.667	9.4	4.2		5	57	205	Hauksson and Saldivar, 1986 (#19)
546	1979	10	18	33.943	118.667	5.8	2.6					Hauksson and Saldivar, 1986
547a	1979	10	18	33.938	118.662	8.4	3		10	70	184	Hauksson and Saldivar, 1986 (#20)
547b	1979	10	18	33.932	118.676	12.8	3		177	15.2	7	Webb and Kanamori, 1985 (#37)
548	1979	10	26	33.935	118.657	3.6	2.5					Hauksson and Saldivar, 1986
549	1979	11	28	33.952	118.662	7.3	2.7					Hauksson and Saldivar, 1986
550	1979	12	2	33.932	118.668	7.2	2.7					Hauksson and Saldivar, 1986
551	1979	12	16	33.953	118.66	8.7	3.2		360	62	230	Hauksson and Saldivar, 1986 (#21)
552	1979	12	18	33.945	118.657	11.8	2.8	89	20	31	220	Hauksson, 1990
553	1980	2	20	34.038	118.971	13	3.2					DNAG via NEIC, 1995
554	1980	3	16	33.995	118.885	18	2.5					DNAG via NEIC, 1995
555	1980	3	25	33.945	118.682	13	2.9					DNAG via NEIC, 1995
556	1980	4	1	34.009	118.662	14	2.8	31	34	41	166	Hauksson, 1990
557	1980	4	12	34.052	118.717	11	2.9	16	37	39	185	Hauksson, 1990
558	1980	8	30	34.052	118.999	12	2.6					DNAG via NEIC, 1995
559	1980	11	18	34.059	118.809	11	2.6					DNAG via NEIC, 1995
560	1980	12	1	34.068	118.966	15	2.6					DNAG via NEIC, 1995
561	1981	1	8	33.939	118.677	12	3.3					DNAG via NEIC, 1995
562	1981	2	24	33.95	118.667	6	2.4					PDE via NEIC, 1995
563	1981	2	27	34.156	118.594	14.3	3.5	84	255	75	345	Hauksson, 1990
564	1981	6	18	33.931	118.668	5	2.6					DNAG via NEIC, 1995
565	1981	8	12	34.126	118.608	3.3	2.7	67	129	67	85	Hauksson, 1990
566	1981	8	14	33.963	118.572	8.3	3.4	94	225	75	327	Hauksson, 1990
567	1982	4	13	34.054	118.964	16	4.3					DNAG via NEIC, 1995
568	1982	5	3	33.952	118.763	14	3.2					DNAG via NEIC, 1995
569	1982	7	29	34.084	119.012	12	3					DNAG via NEIC, 1995
570	1982	7	29	33.947	118.72	11	3.4					DNAG via NEIC, 1995
571	1982	12	30	33.955	118.823	0	4					DNAG via NEIC, 1995
572	1983	1	10	33.979	118.731	8	3.1					DNAG via NEIC, 1995
573	1983	1	28	33.941	118.719	12	3.8					DNAG via NEIC, 1995
574	1983	2	24	34.094	118.885	13	3.1					DNAG via NEIC, 1995
575	1983	3	6	34.064	118.881	13	2.5					DNAG via NEIC, 1995
576	1983	6	14	34.083	118.85	3	2.2					PDE via NEIC, 1995
577	1983	11	23	34.031	118.569	8.1	2.5	55	71	50	169	Hauksson, 1990
578	1984	1	23	33.943	118.825	12	2.7					DNAG via NEIC, 1995
579	1984	3	24	34.124	118.546	14.9	2.6	75	300	57	170	Hauksson, 1990
580	1984	6	10	33.987	118.763	10	2.6					DNAG via NEIC, 1995
581	1984	10	3	33.983	118.653	13.2	3.3	123	337	56	224	Hauksson, 1990
582	1984	10	26	34.016	118.988	13	4.6					USHIS via NEIC, 1995
583	1984	11	3	33.961	118.789	9	2.5					DNAG via NEIC, 1995
584	1985	3	4	33.993	118.575	9.8	3.2	107	59	48	180	Hauksson, 1990
585	1985	3	5	34.078	118.966	15	2.9					DNAG via NEIC, 1995
586	1985	3	18	33.989	118.576	8.9	2.7	135	65	60	145	Hauksson, 1990
587	1985	4	8	34.05	118.922	13	3.4					DNAG via NEIC, 1995
588	1985	4	8	34.055	118.932	9	2.8					DNAG via NEIC, 1995
589	1985	4	8	34.049	118.922	13	3					DNAG via NEIC, 1995
590	1985	4	20	34.046	118.925	11	2.6					DNAG via NEIC, 1995
591	1985	9	26	33.944	118.591	10.3	2.5	108	42	48	196	Hauksson, 1990
592	1986	4	5	33.991	118.721	12.4	2.7	121	354	51	230	Hauksson, 1990
593	1986	5	20	33.94	118.659	12.4	2.8	110	30	45	210	Hauksson, 1990
594	1986	7	11	33.993	118.699	11.6	2.6	72	14	43	165	Hauksson, 1990
595	1986	9	5	33.988	118.549	4.6	2.5	98	4	57	135	Hauksson, 1990
596	1987	7	2	33.918	118.64	12.8	2.8	95	30	70	120	Hauksson, 1990
597	1987	10	17	33.989	118.687	9	2.7	104	355	43	205	Hauksson, 1990
598	1988	3	26	33.99	118.701	13.1	3.7	127	27	55	219	Hauksson, 1990
599	1988	9	9	33.974	118.762	12.5	2.5	55	358	20	255	Hauksson, 1990
600	1989	1	19	33.917	118.623	13.8	5	139	19	45	186	Hauksson, 1990
601	1989	1	19	33.92	118.62	12	3.1					PDE via NEIC, 1995
602	1989	1	19	33.917	118.622	10	2					PDE via NEIC, 1995
603	1989	1	19	33.929	118.657	10	2					PDE via NEIC, 1995

EQ Ref. No.	Year	Date Mo	Da	Hypocenter/Epicenter Location Lat (°N)	Long (°W)	Depth (km)	Mag	Reported Arrivals	Focal Mechanism Soln Dip Azim	Dip Angle	Slip Azim	Source
604	1989	1	19	33.92	118.62	12	3.2					PDE via NEIC, 1995
605	1989	1	19	33.92	118.61	11	3.3					PDE via NEIC, 1995
606	1989	1	19	33.923	118.622	10	2					PDE via NEIC, 1995
607	1989	1	19	33.92	118.62	11	3.1					PDE via NEIC, 1995
608	1989	1	19	33.92	118.64	12	3.8					PDE via NEIC, 1995
609	1989	1	19	33.92	118.64	12	3.5					PDE via NEIC, 1995
610	1989	1	27	33.947	118.588	5	3.1					PDE via NEIC, 1995
611	1989	2	2	33.94	118.86	8	3.8					PDE via NEIC, 1995
612	1989	2	2	33.94	118.82	5	3					PDE via NEIC, 1995
613	1989	2	25	33.93	118.63	11	3.7					PDE via NEIC, 1995
614	1989	3	8	34.107	118.513	5	3.1					PDE via NEIC, 1995
615	1989	4	11	33.93	118.628	6	3.1					PDE via NEIC, 1995
616	1989	4	26	33.93	118.58	11	3.4					PDE via NEIC, 1995
617	1990	6	18	34.046	118.958	10	3					PDE via NEIC, 1995
618	1991	4	12	33.976	118.794	10	2.7					PDE via NEIC, 1995
619	1992	1	22	33.995	118.725	10	2.5					PDE via NEIC, 1995
620	1992	2	28	33.986	118.676	13	2.4					PDE via NEIC, 1995
621	1992	9	5	34.085	119.025	16	2.8					PDE via NEIC, 1995
622	1993	7	26	33.982	118.737	13	3.5					PDE via NEIC, 1995
623	1994	1	9	33.988	118.504	2	3.7					PDE via NEIC, 1995
624	1994	1	12	33.988	118.501	2	2.2					PDE via NEIC, 1995
625	1994	1	12	33.984	118.504	11	3.5					PDE via NEIC, 1995
626	1994	1	12	33.985	118.508	11	3.2					PDE via NEIC, 1995
627	1994	1	18	34.128	118.559	10	3.1					PDE via NEIC, 1995
628	1994	1	18	34.127	118.723	10	2.9					PDE via NEIC, 1995
629	1994	1	20	34.104	118.678	10	2.6					PDE via NEIC, 1995
630	1994	2	3	34.141	118.632	10	2.9					PDE via NEIC, 1995
631	1994	2	3	34.023	118.929	8	2.6					PDE via NEIC, 1995
632	1994	2	5	34.116	118.5	16	3					PDE via NEIC, 1995
633	1994	2	16	34.097	118.51	5	3.2					PDE via NEIC, 1995
634	1995	2	19	34.049	118.915	15	4.3					PDE-W via NEIC, 1995
635	1995	2	19	34.046	118.922	15	3.7					PDE-W via NEIC, 1995
636	1995	7	22	34.053	118.927	15	2.7					PDE-W via NEIC, 1995
637	1995	12	9	34.035	118.937	13.8	3.5		24	38	150	Kate Hutton, pers. com. 1995
638	1995	12	9	34.038	118.938	15.3	3		24	35	135	Kate Hutton, pers. com. 1995

REFERENCES CITED

Aki, K., and Richards, P. G., 1980, Quantitative seismology—theory and methods. Vol. 1: San Francisco, California, W. C. Freeman, 557 p.

Allen, C. R., 1975, Geologic criteria for evaluating seismicity: Geological Society of America Bulletin, v. 86, p. 1041–1057.

Allen, C. R., 1976, Responsibilities in earthquake prediction: Bulletin of the Seismological Society of America, v. 66, p. 2069–2074.

Anderson, D. L., 1971, The San Andreas fault: Scientific American, v. 225, November, p. 52–66.

Atwater, T., 1970, Implications of plate tectonics for the Cenozoic tectonic evolution of western North America: Geological Society of America Bulletin, v. 81, p. 3513–3536.

Bent, A. L., and Helmberger, D. V., 1991, Seismic characteristics of earthquakes along the offshore extension of the western Transverse Ranges, California: Bulletin of the Seismological Society of America, v. 81, p. 399–422.

Berberian, M., 1982, Aftershock tectonics of the 1978 Tabas-e-Golshan (Iran) earthquake sequence: A documented active 'thin- and thick-skinned tectonic' case: Geophysical Journal, Royal Astronomical Society, v. 68, p. 499–530.

Bird, P., and Rosenstock, R. W., 1984, Kinematics of present crust and mantle flow in southern California: Geological Society of America Bulletin, v. 95, p. 946–957.

Birkeland, P. W., 1972, Late Quaternary eustatic sea-level changes along the Malibu coast, Los Angeles County, California: Journal of Geology, v. 80, p. 432–448.

Bohannon, R. G., and Parsons, T., 1995, Tectonic implications of post-30 Ma Pacific and North American relative plate motions: Geological Society of America Bulletin, v. 107, p. 937–959.

Bonilla, M. B., 1970, Surface faulting and related effects, in Weigel, R. L., ed., Earthquake engineering: Englewood Cliffs, New Jersey, Prentice-Hall, p. 47–74.

Bonilla, M. B., 1982, Evaluation of potential surface faulting and other tectonic deformation: U.S. Geological Survey Open-File Report 82-732, 58 p.

Bonilla, M. G., Mark, R. K., and Lienkaemper, J. J., 1984, Statistical relations among earthquake magnitude, surface rupture length, and surface fault displacement: Bulletin of the Seismological Society of America, v. 74, p. 2379–2411.

Boyer, S. E., and Elliott, D., 1982, Thrust systems: American Association of Petroleum Geologists Bulletin, v. 66, p. 1196–1230.

Bronowski, J., 1965, Science and human values (revised edition): New York, Harper & Row Publishers, 119 p.

Bronowski, J., 1978, The common sense of science: Cambridge, Harvard University Press, 154 p.

Bryant, A. S., and Jones, L. M., 1992, Anomalously deep crustal earthquakes in the Ventura basin, southern California: Journal of Geophysical Research, v. 97, p. 437–447.

Buika, J. A., and Teng, T. L., 1979, A seismicity study for portions of the Los Angeles basin, Santa Monica basin, and Santa Monica Mountains, California: University of Southern California, Geophysical Laboratory, Technical Report 79-9, 191 p.

Bullen, K. E., and Bolt, B. A., 1985, An introduction to the theory of seismology (fourth edition): Cambridge, Cambridge University Press, 499 p.

Campbell, R. H., 1990, Geology and tectonic evolution of the western Transverse Ranges: unpublished report for California Coastal Commission workshop on seismic activity of the Malibu Coast Fault Zone, May 9, 1990, 6 p.

Campbell, R. H., and Yerkes, R. F., 1976, Cenozoic evolution of the Los Angeles basin area—relation to plate tectonics, *in* Howell, D. G., ed., Aspects of the geologic history of the California continental borderland: American Association of Petroleum Geologists, Pacific Section, Miscellaneous Publication 24, p. 541–558.

Campbell, R. H., Yerkes, R. F., and Wentworth, C. M., 1966, Detachment faults in the central Santa Monica Mountains, California, *in* Geological Survey Research, 1966: U.S. Geological Survey Professional Paper 550-C, p. C1–C11.

Campbell, R. H., Blackerby, B. A., Yerkes, R. F., Schoellhamer, J. E., Birkeland, P. W., and Wentworth, C. M., 1970, Preliminary geologic map of the Point Dume Quadrangle, Los Angeles County, California: U.S. Geological Survey Open-File Map, scale 1:12,000 and 1:24,000.

Castle, R. O., Church, J. P. Elliott, M. R., and Savage, J. C., 1977, Preseismic and coseismic elevation changes in the epicentral region of the Point Mugu earthquake of February 21, 1973: Bulletin of the Seismological Society of America, v. 67, p. 219–231.

Clark, M. M., and 12 others, 1984, Preliminary slip-rate table and map of late-Quaternary faults of California: U.S. Geological Survey Open-File Report 84-106, 12 p., 5 plates, map scale 1:1,000,000.

Cleveland, G. B., and Troxel, B. W., 1965, Geology related to the safety of the Corral Canyon nuclear reactor site, Malibu, Los Angeles County, California: unpublished report, California Department of Conservation, Division of Mines and Geology, February 1965, 36 p.

Colburn, I. P., 1973, Stratigraphic relations of the southern California Cretaceous strata, *in* Colburn, I. P., and Fritsche, A. E., eds., Cretaceous stratigraphy of the Santa Monica Mountains and Simi Hills: Society of Economic Paleontologists and Mineralogists, Pacific Section, Fall Field Trip Guidebook, p. 45–73.

Crook, R., Jr., and Proctor, R. J., 1992, The Santa Monica and Hollywood faults and the southern boundary of the Transverse Ranges Province, *in* Pipkin, B., and Proctor, R., eds., Engineering geology practice in southern California: Association of Engineering Geologists, Southern California Section, Special Publication 4, p. 233–246.

Crook, R., Jr., Proctor, R. J., and Lindvall, C. E., 1983, Seismicity of the Santa Monica and Hollywood faults determined by trenching: Menlo Park, California, Technical report to the U.S. Geological Survey under contract 14-08-0001-20523, 26 p.

Crouch, J. K., Bachman, S. B., and Shay, J. T., 1984, Post-Miocene compressional tectonics along the central California margin, *in* Crouch, J. K., and Bachman, S. B., eds., Tectonics and sedimentation along the California margin: Bakersfield, California, Society of Economic Paleontologists and Mineralogists, Pacific Section, v. 38, p. 37–54.

Dahlen, F. A., 1984, Noncohesive critical Coulomb wedges—An exact solution: Journal of Geophysical Research, v. 89, p. 10125–10133.

Dahlen, F. A., Suppe, J., and Davis, D., 1984, Mechanics of fold-and-thrust belts and accretionary wedges—Cohesive Coulomb theory: Journal of Geophysical Research, v. 89, p. 10087–10101.

Davis, W. M., 1933, Glacial epochs of the Santa Monica Mountains, California: Geological Society of America Bulletin, v. 44, p. 1041–1133.

Davis, D., Dahlen, F. A., and Suppe, J., 1983, Mechanics of fold-and-thrust belts and accretionary wedges: Journal of Geophysical Research, v. 88, p. 1153–1172.

Davis, T. L., Namson, J., and Yerkes, R. F., 1989, A cross section of the Los Angeles area: Seismically active fold and thrust belt, the 1987 Whittier Narrows earthquake, and earthquake hazard: Journal of Geophysical Research, v. 94, p. 9644–9664.

DeMets, C., Gordon, R. G., Argus, D. F., and Stein, S., 1994, Effect of recent revisions to the geomagnetic reversal time scale on estimates of current plate motions: Geophysical Research Letters, v. 21, p. 2191–2194.

Dibblee, T. W., Jr., 1991a, Geologic map of the Hollywood and Burbank (South ½) Quadrangles, Los Angeles County, California: Dibblee Geological Foundation Map DF-30, scale 1:24,000.

Dibblee, T. W., Jr., 1991b, Geologic map of the Beverly Hills and Van Nuys (South ½) Quadrangles, Los Angeles County, California: Dibblee Geological Foundation Map DF-31, scale 1:24,000.

Dibblee, T. W., Jr., 1992, Geologic map of the Topanga and Canoga Park (south ½) Quadrangles, Los Angeles County, California: Dibblee Geological Foundation Map DF-35, scale 1:24,000.

Dibblee, T. W., Jr., 1993, Geologic map of the Malibu Beach Quadrangle, Los Angeles County, California: Dibblee Geological Foundation Map DF-47, scale 1:24,000.

Dibblee, T. W., Jr., and Ehrenspeck, H. E., 1990, Geologic map of the Point Mugu and Triunfo Pass Quadrangles, Ventura and Los Angeles Counties, California: Dibblee Geological Foundation Map DF-29, scale 1:24,000.

Dibble, T. W., Jr., and Ehrenspeck, H. E., 1993, Geologic map of the Point Dume Quadrangle, Los Angeles and Ventura Counties, California: Dibblee Geological Foundation Map DF-48, scale 1:24,000.

Dill, R., 1993, Castellammare offshore seismic survey, Santa Monica, California: unpublished report for Slosson and Associates, Van Nuys, California, 48 p.

Division of Mines and Geology, 1975a, Recommended guidelines for determining the maximum credible and the maximum probable earthquakes: California Department of Conservation, Division of Mines and Geology, Note 43, 1 p.

Division of Mines and Geology, 1975b, Checklists for the review of geologic/seismic reports: California Department of Conservation, Division of Mines and Geology, Note 48, 2 p.

Division of Mines and Geology, 1982, Guidelines for geologic/seismic considerations in environmental impact reports: California Department of Conservation, Division of Mines and Geology, Note 46, 2 p.

Division of Mines and Geology, 1986a, Guidelines to geologic/seismic reports: California Department of Conservation, Division of Mines and Geology, Note 42, 2 p.

Division of Mines and Geology, 1986b, Guidelines for preparing engineering geologic reports: California Department of Conservation, Division of Mines and Geology, Note 44, 2 p.

Division of Mines and Geology, 1986c, Guidelines for evaluating the hazard of surface fault rupture: California Department of Conservation, Division of Mines and Geology, Note 49, 2 p.

Division of Mines and Geology, 1995a, Earthquake Fault Zone map, Point Dume Quadrangle: California Department of Conservation, Division of Mines and Geology, scale 1:24,000.

Division of Mines and Geology, 1995b, Earthquake Fault Zone map, Malibu Quadrangle: California Department of Conservation, Division of Mines and Geology, scale 1:24,000.

Dolan, J. F., Sieh, K., Rockwell, T. K., Yeats, R. S., Shaw, J., Suppe, J., Huftile, G. J., and Gath, E. M., 1995, Prospects for larger or more frequent earthquakes in the Los Angeles metropolitan region: Science, v. 267, p. 199–205.

Donnelan, A., Hager, B. H., and King, R. W., 1993a, Discrepancy between geologic and geodetic deformation rates in the Ventura basin: Nature, v. 336, p. 333–336.

Donnellan, A., Hager, B. H., King, R. W., and Herring, T. A., 1993b, Geodetic measurement of deformation in the Ventura basin region, southern California: Journal of Geophysical Research, v. 98, p. 21727–21739.

Drumm, P. L., 1992, Holocene displacement of the central splay of the Malibu Coast Fault Zone, Latigo Canyon, Malibu, *in* Pipkin, B., and Proctor, R., eds., Engineering geology practice in southern California: Association of Engineering Geologists, Southern California Section, Special Publication 4, p. 247–254.

Ellsworth, W. L., 1990, Earthquake history, 1769–1989, *in* Wallace, R. E., ed., The San Andreas fault system, California: U.S. Geological Survey, Professional Paper 1515, p. 153–187.

Ellsworth, W. L., and 10 others, 1973, Point Mugu, California, earthquake of 21 February, 1973, and its aftershocks: Science, v. 182, p. 1127–1129.

Engdahl, E. R., and Rinehart, W. A., 1988, Seismicity map of North America:

Boulder, Colorado, The Geological Society of America, Centennial Special Map CSM-4, scale 1:5,000,000.

Engdahl, E. R., and Rinehart, W. A., 1991, Seismicity map of North America, *in* Slemmons, D. B., Engdahl, E. R., and Blackwell, D., eds., Neotectonics of North America: Boulder, Colorado, The Geological Society of America Decade Map Volume 1, p. 21–27.

Evernden, J. F., Kohler, W. M., and Clow, G. D., 1981, Seismic intensities of earthquakes of conterminous United States—their prediction and interpretation: U.S. Geological Survey Professional Paper 1223, 56 p.

Feigl, K. L., and 14 others, 1993, Space geodetic measurement of crustal deformation in central and southern California, 1984–1992: Journal of Geophysical Research, v. 98, p. 21677–21712.

Gilluly, J., 1949, Distribution of mountain building in geologic time: Geological Society of America Bulletin, v. 60, p. 561–590.

Gilluly, J., 1962, The tectonic evolution of the western United States: Geological Society of London Quarterly Journal, v. 119, p. 133–174.

Gilluly, J., 1979, Cenozoic tectonics and regional geophysics of the western Cordillera (Review), *in* Smith, R. E., and Eaton, G. P., eds., Geological Society of America Memoir 152, 1978: Eos (Transactions, American Geophysical Union) v. 60–22, p. 475.

Greene, H. G., and Kennedy, M. P., eds., 1986, Geology of the mid-southern California continental margin: California Department of Conservation, Division of Mines and Geology, California Continental Margin Geologic Map Series, Area 2, 4 sheets, scale 1:250,000.

Greene, H. G., Clarke, S. H., Field, M. E., Linker, F. I., and Wagner, H. C., 1975, Preliminary report on the environmental geology of selected areas of the southern California borderland: U.S. Geological Survey Open-File Report 75-596, 70 p., 16 pl.

Greensfelder, R. W., 1972, Maximum credible bedrock acceleration from earthquakes in California: California Department of Conservation, Division of Mines and Geology Map Sheet 23, scale 1:2,000,000. (Revised August 1974; modified by California Department of Transportation Office of Structures, October 1974.)

Greensfelder, R. W., 1973, A map of maximum expected bedrock acceleration from earthquakes in California: California Department of Conservation, Division of Mines and Geology, Report accompanying Map Sheet 23, 19 p.

Griggs, D., 1939, A theory of mountain-building: American Journal of Science, v. 237, p. 611–650.

Griscom, A., and Jachens, R. C., 1990, Crustal and lithospheric structure from gravity and magnetic studies, *in* Wallace, R. E., ed., The San Andreas fault system, California: U.S. Geological Survey, Professional Paper 1515, p. 239–259.

Gutenberg, B., Richter, C. F., and Wood, H. O., 1932, The earthquake in Santa Monica Bay, California, on August 30, 1930: Bulletin of the Seismological Society of America, v. 22, no. 2, p. 138–154.

Hadley, D. M., and Kanamori, H., 1977, Seismic structure of the Transverse Ranges, California: Geological Society of America Bulletin, v. 88, no. 10, p. 1469–1478.

Hadley, D. M., and Kanamori, H., 1978, Recent seismicity in the San Fernando region and tectonics in the west-central Transverse Ranges, California: Bulletin of the Seismological Society of America, v. 68, p. 1449–1457.

Hanks, T. C., and Kanamori, H., 1979, A moment magnitude scale: Journal of Geophysical Research, v. 84, p. 2348–2350.

Harman, G., 1977, The nature of morality, an introduction to ethics: New York, Oxford University Press, 165 p.

Hart, E. W., 1994, Fault-rupture hazard zones in California: California Department of Conservation, Division of Mines and Geology, Special Publication 42, Revised 1994, 34 p.

Hatheway, A. W., and Leighton, F. B., 1979, Trenching as an exploratory tool, *in* Hatheway, A. W., and McClure, C. R., Jr., eds., Geology in the siting of nuclear power plants: Geological Society of America Reviews in Engineering Geology, v. IV, p. 169–195.

Hauksson, E., 1990, Earthquakes, faulting and stress in the Los Angeles basin: Journal of Geophysical Research, v. 95, p. 15365–15391.

Hauksson, E., 1992, Seismicity, faults, and earthquake potential in Los Angeles, southern California, *in* Pipkin, B., and Proctor, R., eds., Engineering geology practice in southern California: Association of Engineering Geologists, Southern California Section, Special Publication 4, p. 167–179.

Hauksson, E., and Saldivar, G. V., 1986, The 1930 Santa Monica and the 1979 Malibu, California, earthquakes: Bulletin of the Seismological Society of America, v. 76, p. 1542–1559.

Hauksson, E., and Saldivar, G. V., 1989, Seismicity and active compressional tectonics in Santa Monica Bay, southern California: Journal of Geophysical Research, v. 94, p. 9591–9606.

Hearn, T. M., 1984, *Pn* travel times in southern California: Journal of Geophysical Research, v. 89, p. 1843–1855.

Hearn, T. M., and Clayton, R. W., 1986a, Lateral velocity variations in southern California: I. Results for the upper crust from *Pg* waves: Bulletin of the Seismological Society of America, v. 76, p. 495–509.

Hearn, T. M., and Clayton, R. W., 1986b, Lateral velocity variations in southern California: II. Results for the lower crust from *Pn* waves: Bulletin of the Seismological Society of America, v. 76, p. 511–520.

Hileman, J. A., Allen, C. R., and Nordquist, J. M., 1973, Seismicity of the southern California region: California Institute of Technology, Division of Geological and Planetary Sciences, Contribution No. 2385, 83 p., 404 p. appendix.

Hill, D. P., Eaton, J. P., and Jones, L. M., 1990, Seismicity, 1980-86, *in* Wallace, R. E., ed., The San Andreas fault system, California: U.S. Geological Survey, Professional Paper 1515, p. 115–151.

Hill, M. L., 1981, San Andreas fault: History of concepts: Geological Society of America Bulletin, v. 92, p. 112–131.

Hill, M. L., and Dibblee, T. W., Jr., 1953, San Andreas, Garlock and Big Pine faults, California—A study of the character, history, and tectonic significance of their displacement: Geological Society of America Bulletin, v. 64, p. 443–458.

Hill, R. L., 1979, Potrero Canyon fault and University High School escarpment, *in* Field guide to selected engineering geologic features, Santa Monica Mountains, Association of Engineering Geologists, Southern California Section, Guidebook to May 19, 1979, field trip: Los Angeles, California, Association of Engineering Geologists, p. 83–103.

Hill, R. L., Sprotte, E. C., Bennett, J. H., Real, C. R., and Slade, R. C., 1979, Location and activity of the Santa Monica fault, Beverly Hills–Hollywood area, California, *in* Earthquake hazards associated with faults in the greater Los Angeles metropolitan area, Los Angeles County, California, including faults in the Santa Monica–Raymond, Verdugo–Eagle Rock, and Benedict Canyon fault zones: California Department of Conservation, Division of Mines and Geology Open-File Report 79-16 LA, p. B1–B43.

Hornafius, J. S., Luyendyk, B. P., Terres, R. R., and Kamerling, M. J., 1986, Timing and extent of Neogene tectonic rotation in the western Transverse Ranges, California: Geological Society of America Bulletin, v. 97, no. 12, p. 1476–1487.

Humphreys, E. D., and Clayton, R. W., 1988, Adaptation of tomographic reconstruction to seismic travel time problems: Journal of Geophysical Research, v. 93, p. 1073–1085.

Humphreys, E. D., and Clayton, R. W., 1990, Tomographic image of the southern California mantle: Journal of Geophysical Research, v. 95, p. 19725–19746.

Humphreys, E. D., and Hager, B. H., 1990, A kinematic model for the late Cenozoic development of southern California crust and upper mantle: Journal of Geophysical Research, v. 95, p. 19747–19762.

Humphreys, E. D., Clayton, R. W., and Hager, B. H., 1984, A tomographic image of mantle structure beneath southern California: Geophysical Research Letters, v. 11, no. 7, p. 625–627.

Hutton, L. K., and Jones, L. M., 1993, Local magnitudes and apparent variations in seismicity rates in southern California: Bulletin of the Seismological Society of America, v. 83, p. 313–329.

Hutton, L. K., Jones, L. M., Hauksson, E., and Given, D. D., 1991, Seismotectonics of southern California, *in* Slemmons, D. B., Engdahl, E. R., Zoback, M. D., and Blackwell, D. D., eds., Neotectonics of North America: Boulder, Colorado, Geological Society of America, Decade Map Volume 1, p. 133–152.

Jachens, R. C., and Griscom, A., 1985, An isostatic residual gravity map of California; A residual map for interpretation of anomalies from intracrustal sources, *in* Hinze, W. J., ed., The utility of regional gravity and magnetic anomaly maps: Tulsa, Oklahoma, Society of Exploration Geophysicists, p. 347–360.

Jachens, R. C., Simpson, R. W., Blakely, R. J., and Saltus, R. W., 1989, Isostatic residual gravity and crustal geology of the United States, *in* Pakiser, L. C., and Mooney, W. D., eds., Geophysical framework of the continental United States: Boulder, Colorado, Geological Society of America Memoir 172, p. 405–424.

Jackson, J., and Molnar, P., 1990, Active faulting and block rotations in the western Transverse Ranges, California: Journal of Geophysical Research, v. 95, p. 22073–22087. Erratum: 1991, Journal of Geophysical Research, v. 96, p. 2203.

Jahns, R. H., ed., 1954, Geology of southern California: California Department of Conservation, Division of Mines and Geology Bulletin 170.

Jennings, C. W., compiler, 1994, Fault activity map of California and adjacent areas with locations and ages of recent volcanic eruptions: California Department of Conservation, Division of Mines and Geology, California Geologic Data Map Series Map No. 6, scale 1:750,000, 92 p. explanatory text.

Jennings, C. W., and Strand, R. G., 1969, Geologic map of California, Los Angeles sheet: California Department of Conservation, Division of Mines and Geology, scale 1:250,000.

Johnson, H. R., 1932, Folio of plates to accompany geologic report on Quelinda Estate: unpublished consulting report for Quinton, Code, Hill, Leeds and Barnard, Engineers Consolidated, 25 pl.

Junger, A., 1976, Tectonics of the southern California borderland, *in* Howell, D. G., ed., Aspects of the geologic history of the California continental borderland: American Association of Petroleum Geologists, Pacific Section, Miscellaneous Publication 24, p. 486–498.

Junger, A., 1979, Maps and seismic profiles showing geologic structure of the northern Channel Islands platform, California Continental Borderland: U.S. Geological Survey Miscellaneous Field Studies Map MF-991, scale 1:250,000.

Junger, A., and Wagner, H. C., 1977, Geology of the Santa Monica and San Pedro basins, California continental borderland: U.S. Geological Survey Map, MF-820, scale 1:250,000.

Kanamori, H., 1977, The energy release in great earthquakes: Journal of Geophysical Research, v. 82, p. 2981–2987.

Kant, I., 1785, Foundations of the metaphysics of morals (Beck, L. W., translator, 1981): Indianapolis, Indiana, Bobbs-Merrill Educational Publishing, 92 p.

Kant, I., 1788, Critique of practical reason (Beck, L. W., editor and translator, 1993, third edition): New York, Macmillan Publishing Co., 171 p.

Keller, B., and Prothero, W., 1987, Western Transverse Ranges crustal structure: Journal of Geophysical Research, v. 92, p. 7890–7906.

Keller, E. A., and Pinter, N., 1996, Active tectonics—earthquakes, uplift, and landscape: Upper Saddle River, New Jersey, Prentice Hall, 338 p.

Kew, W. S. W., 1927, Geologic sketch of Santa Rosa Island, Santa Barbara County, California: Geological Society of America Bulletin, v. 38, p. 645–653.

Kockelman, W. J., 1985, Using earth-science information for earthquake hazard reduction, *in* Ziony, J. I., ed., Evaluating earthquake hazards in the Los Angeles region—An Earth-science perspective: U.S. Geological Survey, Professional Paper 1360, p. 443–468.

Lajoie, K. R., Kern, J. P., Wehmiller, J. F., Kennedy, G. L., Mathieson, S. A., Sarna-Wojcicki, A. M., Yerkes, R. F., and McCrory, P. F., 1979, Quaternary marine shorelines and crustal deformation, San Diego to Santa Barbara, California, *in* Abbott, P. L., ed., Geological excursions in the southern California area. Guidebook for field trips, Geological Society of America Annual Meeting, Nov. 1979: San Diego, California, Department of Geological Sciences, San Diego State University, p. 3–15.

Lamar, D. L., 1961, Structural evolution of the northern margin of the Los Angeles basin [Ph.D. thesis]: Los Angeles, California, University of California at Los Angeles, 106 p.

Lamb, S. H., 1987, A model for tectonic rotations about a vertical axis: Earth and Planetary Science Letters, v. 84, p. 75–86.

Larson, R. A., and Slosson, J. E., 1992, The role of seismic hazard evaluation in engineering geology reports, *in* Pipkin, B., and Proctor, R., eds., Engineering geology practice in southern California: Association of Engineering Geologists, Southern California Section, Special Publication 4, p. 191–194.

Lee, W. H. K., Yerkes, R. F., and Simirenko, M., 1979, Recent earthquake activity and focal mechanisms in the western Transverse Ranges, California: U.S. Geological Survey Circular 799-A, 26 p.

Link, M. H., Squires, R. L., and Colburn, I. P., 1984, Slope and deep-sea fan facies and paleogeography of Upper Cretaceous Chatsworth Formation, Simi Hills, California: American Association of Petroleum Geologists Bulletin, v. 68, p. 850–873.

Lyon-Caen, H., and Molnar, P., 1983, Constraints on the structure of the Himalaya from an analysis of gravity and flexural model of the lithosphere: Journal of Geophysical Research, v. 88, p. 8171–8192.

Mackay, A. L., 1991, A dictionary of scientific quotations: Philadelphia, Institute of Physics Publishing, 297 p.

Martin, M. W., and Schinzinger, R., 1989, Ethics in engineering (second edition): New York, McGraw-Hill Book Company, 404 p.

McGill, J. T., 1981, Recent movement on the Potrero Canyon fault, Pacific Palisades area, Los Angeles, *in* Geological Survey research 1980: U.S. Geological Survey Professional Paper 1175, p. 258–259.

McGill, J. T., 1982, Preliminary geologic map of the Pacific Palisades area, City of Los Angeles, California: U.S. Geological Survey, Open-File Report 82-194, scale 1:4,800, 15 p. text.

McGill, J. T., 1989, Geologic maps of the Pacific Palisades area, Los Angeles, California: U.S. Geological Survey Map I-1828, 2 sheets, scale 1:4,800.

McGill, J. T., Lamar, D. L., Hill, R. L., and Michael, E. D., 1987, Potrero Canyon fault, landslides and oil drilling site, Pacific Palisades, Los Angeles, California: Geological Society of America, Centennial Field Guide Volume 1, p. 213–216.

Molnar, P., Burchfiel, B. C., Liang K'uangyi, and Zhao Ziyun, 1987, Geomorphic evidence for active faulting in the Altyn Tagh and northern Tibet and qualitative estimates of its contribution to the convergence of India and Eurasia: Geology, v. 15, p. 249–253.

Mooney, W. D., and Braile, L. W., 1989, The seismic structure of the continental crust and upper mantle of North America, *in* Bally, A. W., and Palmer, A. R., eds., The Geology of North America—An overview: Boulder, Colorado, Geological Society of America, The Geology of North America, v. A, p. 39–52.

Mooney, W. D., and Weaver, C. S., 1989, Regional crustal structure and tectonics of the Pacific Coastal States; California, Oregon, and Washington, *in* Pakiser, L. C., and Mooney, W. D., eds., Geophysical framework of the continental United States: Boulder, Colorado, Geological Society of America Memoir 172, p. 129–161.

Morton, D. M., and Matti, J. C., 1987, The Cucamonga Fault Zone: Geologic setting and Quaternary history, *in* Morton, D. M., and Yerkes, R. F., eds., Recent reverse faulting in the Transverse Ranges, California: U.S. Geological Survey Professional Paper 1339, p. 179–203, plate 12.1, scale 1:24,000.

Mualchin, L., and Jones, A. L., 1992, Peak acceleration from maximum credible earthquakes in California (rock and stiff-soil sites): California Department of Conservation, Division of Mines and Geology, Open-File Report 92-1, 53 p. text, map scale 1:1,000,000, 2 sheets.

Murbach, D., 1994, Characteristics of the 1992 fault rupture adjacent to distressed structures, Landers, California: Oakland, California, Earthquake Engineering Research Institute, 73 p., 6 plates.

Namson, J. S., and Davis, T. L., 1988, Structural transect of the western Transverse Ranges, California—Implications for lithospheric kinematics and seismic risk evaluation: Geology, v. 16, no. 8, p. 675–679.

Patterson, R. H., 1979, Tectonic geomorphology and neotectonics of the Santa Cruz Island fault, Santa Barbara County, California [M.S. thesis]: Santa Barbara, California, University of California at Santa Barbara, 141 p.

Pinter, N., and Sorlien, C., 1991, Evidence for latest Pleistocene to Holocene movement on the Santa Cruz Island fault, California: Geology, v. 19, p. 909–912.

Quinton, A., 1988, Utilitarian ethics: La Salle, Illinois, Open Court, 116 p.

Raikes, S. A., 1980, Regional variations in upper mantle structure beneath southern California: Royal Astronomical Society Geophysical Journal, v. 63, p. 187–216.

Raikes, S. A., and Hadley, D. M., 1979, The azimuthal variation of telesceismic P-residuals in southern California: Implications for upper mantle structure: Tectonophysics, v. 56, p. 89–96.

Rawls, J., 1971, A theory of justice: Cambridge, Harvard University Press, 607 p.

Real, C. R., 1987, Seismicity and tectonics of the Santa Monica—Hollywood—Raymond Hill fault zone and northern Los Angeles basin, *in* Morton, D. M., and Yerkes, R. F., eds., Recent reverse faulting in the Transverse Ranges, California: U.S. Geological Survey Professional Paper 1339, p. 113–124.

Real, C. R., Toppozada, T. R., and Parke, D. L., 1978, Earthquake epicenter map of California, 1900 through 1974: California Department of Conservation, Division of Mines and Geology Map Sheet 39, scale 1:1,000,000.

Roberts, C. W., Jachens, R. C., and Oliver, H. W., 1990, Isostatic residual gravity map of California and offshore southern California: California Department of Conservation, Division of Mines and Geology, California Geologic Data Map Series, Map 7, scale 1:750,000.

Rockwell, T. K., 1983, Soil chronology, geology and neotectonics of the north-central Ventura basin, California [Ph.D. thesis]: Santa Barbara, California, University of California at Santa Barbara, 424 p.

Rzonca, G. F., Spellman, H. A., Fall, E. W., and Schlemon, R. J., 1991, Holocene displacement of the Malibu Coast Fault Zone, Winter Mesa, Malibu, California—Engineering geologic implications: Association of Engineering Geologists Bulletin, v. 28, p. 147–158.

Sage, O. G., Jr., 1973, Paleocene geography of the Los Angeles region, *in* Kovach, R. L., and Nur, A., eds., Proceedings, Conference on tectonic problems of the San Andreas fault system: Palo Alto, California, Stanford University Publications, Geological Sciences, v. XIII, p. 348–357.

Scullin, C. M., 1983, Excavation and grading code administration, inspection, and enforcement: Englewood Cliffs, New Jersey, Prentice-Hall, 405 p.

Shackleton, N. J., and Opdyke, N. D., 1973, Oxygen isotope and palaeomagnetic stratigraphy of equatorial Pacific core V23-238—Oxygen isotope temperatures and ice volumes on a 10^5 year and 10^6 year time scale: Quaternary Research, v. 3, p. 39–55.

Sheffels, B., and McNutt, M., 1986, Role of subsurface loads and regional compensation in the isostatic balance of the Transverse Ranges, California: Evidence for intracontinental subduction: Journal of Geophysical Research, v. 91, p. 6419–6431.

Sibson, R. H., 1983, Continental fault structure and the shallow earthquake source: Journal of the Geological Society of London, v. 140, p. 741–767.

Simpson, R. W., Jachens, R. C., Blakely, R. J., and Saltus, R. W., 1986, A new isostatic residual gravity map of the conterminous United States with a discussion on the significance of isostatic residual anomalies: Journal of Geophysical Research, v. 91, p. 8348–8372.

Slemmons, D. B., 1977, State-of-the-art for assessing earthquake hazards in the United States: Report 6, faults and earthquake magnitude: U.S. Army Engineer Waterways Experiment Station Miscellaneous Paper S-73-1, 129 p., 37 p. appendix.

Slemmons, D. B., and dePolo, C. M., 1992, Evaluation of active faulting and associated hazards, *in* Studies in geophysics—Active tectonics: Washington, D.C., National Academy Press, p. 45–62.

Slosson, J. E., 1984, Genesis and evolution of guidelines for geologic reports: Bulletin of the Association of Engineering Geologists, v. XXI, p. 295–316.

Stierman, D. J., and Ellsworth, W. L., 1976, Aftershocks of the February 21, 1973, Point Mugu, California, earthquake: Bulletin of the Seismological Society of America, v. 66, p. 1931–1952.

Stover, C. W., and Coffman, J. L., 1993, Seismicity of the United States, 1568–1989: U.S. Geological Survey Professional Paper 1527, 418 p.

Szabo, B. J., and Rosholt, J. N., 1969, Uranium series dating of Pleistocene molluscan shells from southern California—an open system model: Journal

of Geophysical Research, v. 74, p. 3253–3260.

Taylor, C. L., and Cluff, L. S., 1973, Fault activity and its significance assessed by exploratory excavation, *in* Kovach, R. L., and Nur, A., eds., Proceedings, Conference on tectonic problems of the San Andreas fault system: Palo Alto, California, Stanford University Publication, Geological Sciences, v. XIII, p. 239–247.

Toppozada, T. R., Real, C. R., and Parke, D. L., 1981, Preparation of isoseismal maps and summaries of reported effects for pre-1900 California earthquakes: California Department of Conservation, Division of Mines and Geology Open-File Report 81-11 SAC, 182 p.

Toppozada, T. R., Real, C. R., Bezore, S. P., and Parke, D. L., 1984, Preparation of isoseismal maps and summaries of reported effects for pre-1900 California earthquakes: California Department of Conservation, Division of Mines and Geology, Contract Number 14-08-0001-18243.

Treiman, J. A., 1994, Malibu Coast fault, Los Angeles County, California: California Department of Conservation, Division of Mines and Geology, Fault Evaluation Report FER-229, 33 p.

Vedder, J. G., Beyer, L. A., Junger, A., Moore, G. W., Roberts, A. E., Taylor, J. C., and Wagner, H. C., 1974, Preliminary report on the geology of the continental borderland of southern California: U.S. Geological Survey Map MF-624, 34 p., scale 1:500,000.

Vedder, J. G., Greene, H. G., Clarke, S. H., and Kennedy, M. P., 1986, Geologic map of the mid-southern California continental margin, *in* Greene, H. G., and Kennedy, M. P., eds., Geology of the mid-southern California continental margin: California Department of Conservation, Division of Mines and Geology, Map 2A, scale 1:250,000.

Vedder, J. G., Crouch, J. K., and Junger, A., 1987, Geologic map of the outer-southern California continental margin, *in* Greene, H. G., and Kennedy, M. P., eds., Geology of the mid-southern California continental margin: California Department of Conservation, Division of Mines and Geology, Map 3A, scale 1:250,000.

Walck, M. C., and Minster, J. B., 1982, Relative array analysis of upper mantle velocity variations in southern California: Journal of Geophysical Research, v. 87, p. 1757–1772.

Wallace, R. E., 1977, Profiles and ages of young fault scarps, north-central Nevada: Geological Society of America Bulletin, v. 88, p. 1267–1281.

Wallace, R. E., ed., 1990, San Andreas fault system in California: U.S. Geological Survey, Professional Paper 1515, 283 p.

Webb, T. H., and Kanamori, H., 1985, Earthquake focal mechanisms in the eastern Transverse Ranges and San Emigdio Mountains, southern California and evidence for a regional decollement: Bulletin of the Seismological Society of America, v. 75, p. 737–757.

Weber, F. H., Jr., 1980, Geological features related to character and recency of movement along faults, north-central [Los Angeles area] Los Angeles County, California, *in* Weber, F. H., Jr., Bennett, J. H., Chapman, R. H., Chase, G. W., and Saul, R. B., eds., Earthquake hazards associated with the Verdugo–Eagle Rock and Benedict Canyon fault zones, Los Angeles County, California: California Department of Conservation, Division of Mines and Geology Open-File Report 80-10 LA, p. B1–B116.

Weldon, R. J., and Humphreys, E. D., 1986, A kinematic model of southern California: Tectonics, v. 5, no. 1, p. 33–48.

Wells, D. L., and Coppersmith, K. J., 1994, New empirical relationships among magnitude, rupture length, rupture width, rupture area, and surface displacement: Bulletin of the Seismological Society of America, v. 84, no. 4, p. 974–1002.

Wesnousky, S. G., 1986, Earthquakes, Quaternary faults and seismic hazard in California: Journal of Geophysical Research, v. 91, p. 12587–12632.

Wesson, R. L., Page, R. A., Boore, D. M., and Yerkes, R. F., 1974, Expectable earthquakes and their ground motions in the Van Norman reservoirs area, *in* The Van Norman reservoirs area, northern San Fernando Valley, California: U.S. Geological Survey Circular 691-B, p. B1–B9.

Woodford, A. O., 1956, What is geologic truth?—Response on receiving the Neil Miner Teaching Award: Journal of Geological Education, v. 4, no. 1, p. 5–8.

Wright, T. L., 1991, Structural geology and tectonic evolution of the Los Angeles basin, California, *in* Biddle, K. T., ed., Active margin basins: American Association of Petroleum Geologists Memoir 52, p. 35–134.

Yeats, R. S., 1968, Rifting and rafting in the southern California borderland, *in* Dickinson, W. R., and Grantz, A., eds., Proceedings, Conference on tectonic problems of the San Andreas fault system: Palo Alto, California, Stanford University Publications, Geological Sciences, v. XI, p. 307–322.

Yeats, R. S., 1981, Quaternary flake tectonics of the California Transverse Ranges: Geology, v. 9, no. 1, p. 16–20.

Yeats, R. S., 1983, Large-scale Quaternary detachments in Ventura basin, southern California: Journal of Geophysical Research, v. 88, no. 1, p. 569–583.

Yeats, R. S., Clark, M. N., Keller, E. A., and Rockwell, T. K., 1981, Active fault hazard in southern California—Ground rupture versus seismic shaking: Geological Society of America Bulletin, v. 92, p. 189–196.

Yerkes, R. F., and Campbell, R. H., 1980, Geologic map of east-central Santa Monica Mountains, Los Angeles County, California: U.S. Geological Survey Miscellaneous Investigations Series, Map I-1146, scale 1:24,000.

Yerkes, R. F., and Lee, W. H. K., 1979a, Late Quaternary deformation in the western Transverse Ranges of California: U.S. Geological Survey Circular 799-B, p. 27–37.

Yerkes, R. F., and Lee, W. H. K., 1979b, Faults, fault activity, epicenters, focal depths, and focal mechanisms, 1970–75 earthquakes, western Transverse Ranges, California: U.S. Geological Survey Miscellaneous Field Studies Map MF-1032, 2 sheets, scale 1:250,000.

Yerkes, R. F., and Lee, W. H. K., 1987, Late Quaternary deformation in the western Transverse Ranges, *in* Morton, D. M., and Yerkes, R. F. eds., Recent reverse faulting in the Transverse Ranges, California: U.S. Geological Survey Professional Paper 1339, p. 71–82.

Yerkes, R. F., and Wentworth, C. M., 1965, Structure, Quaternary history, and general geology of the Corral Canyon area, Los Angeles County, California: U.S. Geological Survey Open-File Report 864, 214 p.

Yerkes, R. F., Campbell, R. H., Blackerby, B. A., Wentworth, C. M., Birleland, P. W., and Schoellhamer, J. E., 1971, Preliminary geologic map of the Malibu Beach Quadrangle, Los Angeles County, California: U.S. Geological Survey Open-File Map, scale 1:12,000.

Yerkes, R. F., Sarna-Wojcicki, A. M., and Lajoie, K. R., 1987, Geology and Quaternary deformation of the Ventura area, *in* Morton, D. M., and Yerkes, R. F., eds., Recent reverse faulting in the Transverse Ranges, California: U.S. Geological Survey Professional Paper 1339, p. 169–178.

Zeitler, P. K., 1985, Cooling history of the NW Himalaya, Pakistan: Tectonics, v. 4, p. 127–151.

Ziony, J. K., and Jones, L. M., 1989, Map showing late Quaternary faults and 1978–84 seismicity of the Los Angeles region, California: U.S. Geological Survey Miscellaneous Field Studies Map MF–1964, scale 1:250,000.

Ziony, J. K., and Yerkes, R. F., 1985, Evaluating earthquake and surface faulting potential, *in* Ziony, J. I., ed., Evaluating earthquake hazards in the Los Angeles region—An Earth-science perspective: U.S. Geological Survey, Professional Paper 1360, p. 43–91.

Zoback, M. L., Zoback, M. D., Adams, J., Bell, S., Suter, M., Suarez, G., Jacob, K., Estabrook, C., and Magee, M., 1990, Stress map of North America, southwest sheet: Boulder, Colorado, Geological Society of America, scale 1:5,000,000.

MANUSCRIPT ACCEPTED BY THE SOCIETY JUNE 5, 1997

Geological Society of America
Reviews in Engineering Geology, Volume XII
1998

Glacial geology, law, and the Love Canal trial

Jodi A. Feld and Robert Emmet Hernan
New York State Department of Law, 120 Broadway, New York, New York 10271
David M. Mickelson
Department of Geology and Geophysics, University of Wisconsin, 1215 West Dayton Street, Madison, Wisconsin 53706

ABSTRACT

When scientists and lawyers meet in the litigation arena their backgrounds and perspectives set them apart. Each has different expectations of the process and criteria by which the court searches for truth. In the Love Canal trial, the worlds of the scientist and lawyer came together as data and expert opinions from soil scientists, hydrologists, engineers, and geologists were integrated to develop an understanding of the migration of contaminants away from the site. Issues related to the age and genesis of the fractured clay that forms the walls of the Love Canal landfill were important to the State of New York in proving that the chemical company, which disposed of the chemicals in the canal, was liable for the migration of dense nonaqueous phase liquids (DNAPLs) through the fractures to the surrounding properties. In particular, it was important to know whether the fractures were formed only as the result of recent excavations for sewers and homes in the 1960s and 1970s, or whether the fractures were present at the site when the chemical company was disposing of chemical wastes in the canal in the 1940s and 1950s. It was concluded that these fractures have been present for at least hundreds of years, and probably were formed during the mid-Holocene. The level of confidence in these conclusions differed between the scientist and lawyer, and those differences had to be reconciled through trial preparation.

INTRODUCTION

Lawyers and scientists often live in different worlds: they speak different languages, they dress differently, and they have differing versions of what constitutes "truth." When a lawyer hires a scientist to serve as an expert witness in a lawsuit, what does the lawyer expect from that witness? Certainty. What does a lawyer fear of such a witness? Equivocation. On the other hand, the scientist fears being pressured by the lawyer to exaggerate or to place too much confidence in a conclusion. This is because stating the "truth" without qualification is contrary to the discipline of science and would cast the scientist in an unfavorable light by her or his peers. Rarely, especially in geology, is there an absolutely clear conclusion, having 100% certainty. In science, conclusions are based on the "facts" available, always with the recognition that perceptions of "truth" change as more data are available on which to base a conclusion. Yet, in our court system a judgment must be made in a timely manner. The court cannot wait for scientific ideas to evolve toward some absolute certainty.

The expert witness's certainty and integrity are central to persuading the finder of fact, be it a judge or jury, of the legal and scientific positions being advanced by one side. Therefore, it is critical that the scientist understand what the lawyer means when she or he speaks of the absolute need for certainty. Likewise, the lawyer needs to understand what the scientist means when he or she says, "I'm not sure." These apparently opposing views of truth and certainty actually may not be at odds.

In this chapter we address these conflicting views of trial testimony in the context of our experience in the Love Canal case. In the Love Canal litigation, the State of New York and federal gov-

The opinions and analysis expressed in this article are those of the authors and do not reflect the opinions, position, or policies of Attorney General Dennis C. Vacco or of the New York State Department of Law.

Feld, J. A., Hernan, R. E., and Mickelson, D. M., 1998, Glacial geology, law, and the Love Canal trial, *in* Welby, C. W., and Gowan, M. E., eds., A Paradox of Power: Voices of Warning and Reason in the Geosciences: Boulder, Colorado, Geological Society of America Reviews in Engineering Geology, v. XII.

ernment were seeking to identify the pathways through which hazardous chemicals migrated from a chemical waste disposal site to the surrounding neighborhood. Geologic testimony was basic to proving the government's case. Dr. Mickelson served as a geologic expert for the State of New York, Ms. Feld was an in-house science expert on the staff of the New York State Attorney General's office, and Mr. Hernan was an assistant attorney general for the New York State Attorney General's office.

BACKGROUND

Love Canal was dug in the 1890s by William Love as part of a proposed electric power generating scheme in the Niagara Falls area (Fig. 1). The project failed and the 914-m (3,000-ft) portion of the canal that had been dug near the Niagara River remained water-filled and unused.

The Hooker Chemical Corporation first leased, then purchased the Love Canal site in the 1940s. Dumping of toxic chemicals occurred in the northern section from 1942 to 1946, and then in the southern section from 1946 to 1954, with some dumping in the central section in 1953–1954. Eventually, an estimated 22,000 tons of chemical waste were dumped in the canal (Table 1). The chemicals were dumped directly into the canal without containers, in metal drums that were often old and rusted, or in fiber drums commonly used for filter cake residues. The drums sometimes broke as they were being dumped into the canal. In places, dams were constructed across the canal; in other places, pits for disposal were dug outside the original boundaries of the canal. The pits were about 8 m (25 ft) deep and 8 m (25 ft) across. Pits were filled to within meters of the ground surface with drums and uncontainerized waste, and then covered with a thin layer of soil or fly ash.

During the dumping period, fires and explosions occurred in the canal, shooting flames as high as the homes that were built adjacent to the canal. In the postwar period, as the city of Niagara Falls grew, more residences were built in the area surrounding the canal. During the 1950s, houses were built immediately adjacent to the canal on nearly all available lots on 97th and 99th Streets (Fig. 1).

In 1952, Hooker was approached by the Niagara Falls School Board to buy a part of the Love Canal property (the central section where no dumping had occurred as yet) in order to build a new grade school. At first Hooker declined because it was concerned about liability from the wastes, but within a month it reconsidered and agreed to donate the property for $1 on the condition that the School Board take the entire property *and* indemnify Hooker for any claims. Hooker also retained the right to continue dumping until the school was built. By the time the 99th Street School was built in 1954, chemical wastes had been dumped in part of the central area of the canal next to where the school was built.

Contrary to some popular opinion, neither the school nor any homes were actually built on top of the waste disposal areas on the Love Canal property. Instead they were built directly adjacent to the disposal areas. However, the canal property itself was used

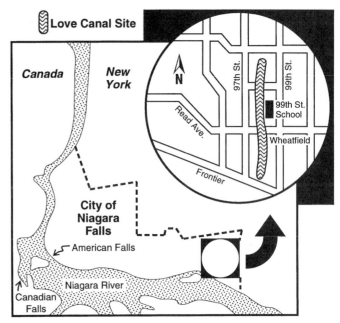

Figure 1. Location map of Love Canal showing detailed map of neighborhood.

extensively as a playground by the school children and the residents in the area. From 1954 through the mid-1970s, there were numerous incidents in which the ground subsided, or drums and toxic wastes rose to the surface, thereby endangering and burning children playing on the school grounds. For instance, children were burned as a result of playing with a chalk-like substance that was actually benzene hexachloride; in the outfield of a baseball field constructed on top of the backfilled canal, small "volcanoes" appeared, spewing out thionyl chloride; and a private inground swimming pool was lifted ~1 m out of the ground, likely the result of reactions occurring among chemicals underneath.

By the mid- to late 1970s, in addition to the surface exposures, the waste was entering the basements of homes adjacent to the canal. Contaminated water as well as darker, nonaqueous phase materials were found in basement sumps. Complaints to local health authorities intensified by 1976, and state and federal authorities became aware of the site and its problems. Studies were undertaken in 1977 and 1978 to determine the nature and extent of the hazards, and some possible ways to remedy the situation. Conditions deteriorated, and in August 1978, the State of New York and President Carter declared a state of emergency at Love Canal. The 99th Street School was closed and more than 200 families were relocated and their homes were purchased by the government. Based on further studies and uncertainties about the nature and extent of the risks at Love Canal, approximately 500 additional families were relocated in 1980, and their homes were bought by the state.

The governments instituted measures to remediate Love Canal beginning in late 1978. The remediation has been substantially completed, at a total cost to the governments of more than $200 million. Waste has not been removed but is being contained by collection trenches and treated. The entire area is monitored by a system of ground-water monitoring wells. Houses on 97th and 99th Streets were demolished, and the debris is being stored on site.

THE LITIGATION

In December 1980, Congress passed the Superfund law (*Comprehensive Environmental Response, Compensation, and Liability Act*, 42 U.S.C. Section 9601 et seq.) largely in response to Love Canal and several other environmental disasters. The Superfund law provided a fund to pay for remediation of contaminated sites such as Love Canal, and the ability to sue the responsible parties to recover these remediation costs. In 1979 and 1980, the state and federal governments instituted a lawsuit against the chemical company that had bought the Hooker Chemical Corporation and that was legally responsible for the actions of Hooker. In addition to the state and federal lawsuits, several thousand private lawsuits were filed separately against the chemical company by residents of the Love Canal area for personal injuries and property damage. Some of those have been settled, and some are still pending.

In response to the governments' lawsuit, the chemical company claimed that others were to blame for Love Canal. The company claimed that the use by the city of Niagara Falls of the canal for a brief period in 1953–1954 for garbage disposal, and the city's construction of sewers in the area of the canal contributed to the migration of chemicals from the canal. The company also had claims against the state based on the fact that in 1968 the state acquired, by eminent domain, a small piece of the southern portion of the Love Canal property as part of a highway construction project. The company alleged that the moving of a sewer as part of that project caused some migration of the chemicals away from the canal. In addition, the company argued that the federal government, in particular the U.S. Army, had dumped chemicals in the canal.

In addition to all of the legal disputes that needed to be addressed, many scientific questions arose during the course of the litigation. Where exactly were the boundaries of the landfill? Was it common practice to dispose of wastes in open pits, as Hooker had done? What was known about the toxicity of these chemicals in the 1940s and 1950s? Should Hooker have known that these chemicals would migrate to surrounding areas? What exactly were the migration pathways for the chemicals?

To answer these and many more questions that would arise during the litigation, the parties held at least eight years of pretrial discovery. During the course of this discovery more than 20 scientific experts were deposed and testified in areas such as photogrammetry, risk assessment, toxicology, solid waste engineering, and geology. As the pretrial discovery progressed, it became clear that the determination of the subsurface pathways through which the chemicals migrated from the canal to the surrounding neighborhood would become the critical issue in determining whether others besides the chemical company would be liable for the

TABLE 1. CHEMICALS DISPOSED OF IN LOVE CANAL BY HOOKER CHEMICAL CORPORATION, 1942–1954*

Type of Waste	Physical State	Total Estimated Quantity (tons)
Miscellaneous acid chlorides other than benzoyl - includes acetyl, caprylyl, butyryl, nitro benzoyls	Liquid and solid	400
Thionyl chloride and miscellaneous sulfur/chlorine compounds	Liquid and solid	500
Miscellaneous chlorination - includes waxes, oils, naphthenes, aniline	Liquid and solid	1,000
Dodecyl (Lauyl, Lorol) mercaptans (DDM), chlorides and miscellaneous organic sulfur compounds	Liquid and solid	2,400
Trichlorophenol (TCP)	Liquid and solid	200
Benzoyl chlorides and benzotrichlorides	Liquid and solid	800
Metal chlorides	Solid	400
Liquid disulfides (LDS/LDSN/-BDS) and chlorotoluenes	Liquid	700
Hexachlorocyclohexane (Lindane/BHC)	Solid	6,900
Chlorobenzenes	Liquid and solid	2,000
Benzylchlorides - includes benzyl chloride, benzyl alcohol, benzyl thiocyanate	Solid	2,400
Sodium sulfide/sulfhydrates	Solid	2,000
Miscellaneous 10% of above		2,000
Total		21,800

*From Interagency Task Force on Hazardous Wastes, Draft Report on Hazardous Waste Disposal in Erie and Niagra Counties, New York, March 1979, reproduced in Tarlton and Cassidy, 1981.

cleanup and damages. To address the issues related to contaminant migration, the parties relied on the testimony of experts in the fields of soil science, hydrogeology, contaminant fate and migration, clay mineralogy, and glacial geology.

SITE CONDITIONS: GEOLOGY AND HYDROGEOLOGY

The area of the Love Canal landfill is characterized by poor natural drainage due to several factors including (a) the relatively flat topography, (b) the presence of subsoils of low permeability, (c) the shallow depth of the nearby rivers and streams, (d) the high rate of precipitation, and (e) the absence of a well-developed natural drainage network. As a result, the Love Canal area historically has experienced a high water table and both subsurface and surface drainage problems.

The geologic setting of the Love Canal landfill is typical of many hazardous waste sites in the area surrounding the Great Lakes in the northern United States and southern Canada. Figure 2 illustrates the general stratigraphy at the Love Canal and surrounding area. In general, the following stratigraphic sequence is present. Above the Lockport dolomite, diamicton (presumably till) several meters thick is present. This is overlain by ~5 m of clayey lake sediment, presumably deposited in Lake Wayne or Lake Warren, early postglacial lakes in the Erie basin (Fig. 3a). This sediment generally contains less than 5% sand, 25 to 50% silt, and 50 to 75% clay. The lower part of the unit is soft, unfractured, and has a high natural moisture content. The upper part of the unit (stiff clay in Fig. 2) is saturated, but much stiffer with ~10% less natural moisture content (Mickelson et al., 1994), and it is fractured. The matrix between the fractures is oxidized compared to the soft gray clay beneath. The transition between stiff and soft clay takes place over less than 0.5 m.

Above, the clayey lake sediment is oxidized sand with some interbedded silt that is 1–2 m thick. This was deposited in Lake Tonawanda (Fig. 3b) between about 12.4 and 11 ka, before the Niagara Gorge had developed in its present location (Calkin and Feenstra, 1985).

While this general stratigraphy was undisputed, the mechanisms by which the contaminants migrated through the subsurface was very much disputed.

THEORIES OF CONTAMINANT MIGRATION

Early in the development of the technical case it became evident that issues relating to the subsurface migration of the contaminants from the landfill would be important to proving liability. As far as the governments were concerned, the issue of liability in this regard seemed clear: Chemicals, which had admittedly been dumped by the chemical company, had migrated, via the surface and subsurface, to the surrounding homes and properties, causing widespread contamination. It turned out that proving liability, however, was not this simple because of the necessity of disproving several alternate theories advanced by the chemical company.

Southern drain theory

During the first 10 years of pretrial discovery, migration of aqueous phase contaminants through the upper silt and sand (Fig. 2) was thought to be the primary issue of concern. One of the early theories of aqueous phase migration advanced by the chemical company was called the "southern drain theory." In essence, the company's theory was that the clayey material surrounding Love Canal prevented lateral migration of waste. They also claimed that inward ground-water gradients existed before, during, and after disposal and that water levels in the canal were controlled by a southern drain, which served as a ground-water discharge point from the canal to the Niagara River. The company further claimed that when the state built the LaSalle Expressway at the southern end of the canal in 1968, it blocked this discharge to the Niagara River, causing the water in the canal, which contained dissolved waste constituents, to rise and eventually overflow the top of the clay and migrate laterally through the upper silt and sand to the surrounding properties.

The state spent many years developing expert testimony to investigate and ultimately refute the southern drain theory. Geologists, hydrogeologists, and soil scientists conducted drilling and geophysical investigations, and reviewed historical maps and aerial photographs for evidence of a southern drain from the Love Canal area. The results of these investigations indicated that there was no evidence of a southern drain from the Love Canal area. These conclusions were developed by the state's experts and were documented in reports during the required pretrial discovery period. After extensive discovery, the state was able to effectively refute this theory of aqueous phase migration from the canal. The "southern drain theory," in effect, was abandoned by the chemical company several years prior to the beginning of the trial.

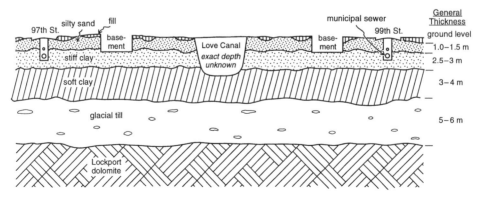

Figure 2. Generalized stratigraphic section of the Love Canal area. (Modified from Tarlton and Cassidy, 1981.)

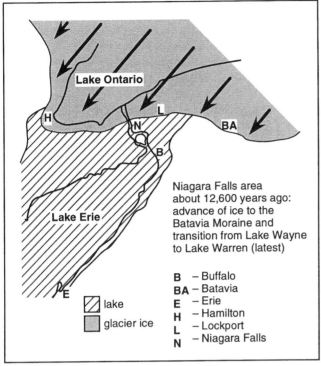

Figure 3a

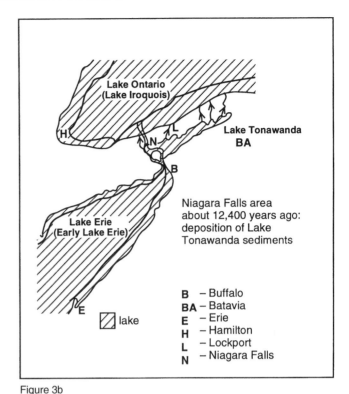

Figure 3b

Figure 3. Sketch map showing Love Canal region at time of deposition of clay (a) and silty sand (b) units.

Stress relief theory

In the late 1980s, the chemical company advanced an alternative theory to support its claim that the state was liable for the off-site migration of contaminants from the Love Canal landfill. Ongoing investigations by the governments had clearly indicated that, in addition to aqueous phase migration, dense nonaqueous phase liquids (DNAPLs) had also migrated through the subsurface to the surrounding properties. DNAPLs were found not only in basements and sumps, but also surrounding the landfill in some of the fractures in the stiff silty clay. The state's theory of migration was that waste, which had been placed at elevations above the base of the fractures, had freely migrated from the canal into the fractured subsurface and to surrounding properties. Furthermore, the state claimed that because the DNAPL elevations in the canal were above the base of the fractures in the silty clay (Fig. 2), the DNAPL, under the force of its own density, began to migrate from the canal soon after the chemical company began filling the canal.

The company claimed that at the time of waste disposal the fractures in the stiff silty clay were not open fractures and, therefore, could not have provided a pathway for the migration of the DNAPLs. It claimed that the fractures were opened only as a result of "stress relief" caused by the excavation of basements and by the governments' construction and relocation of storm sewers surrounding the Love Canal landfill in the 1970s. Thus, the company's position was that the state was responsible, in part, for the

release of contaminants from the landfill. It was at this point in the pretrial discovery that the state decided to hire a glacial geologist to provide expert testimony regarding the age and genesis of the fractures in the stiff silty clay surrounding the Love Canal landfill.

HOW TESTIMONY ON GLACIAL GEOLOGY WAS USED

The state needed to determine whether the fractures in the stiff silty clay predated sewer construction and in all likelihood predated construction of the canal itself. The expert was asked to answer two fundamental questions: (1) Could the fractures in the stiff silty clay provide an avenue for contaminant movement away from the canal? and (2) Did these fractures exist, in an open state, prior to the state's construction of the sewer lines?

When developing expert testimony, it is critical that the expert develop his or her opinions based on as much firsthand evidence as possible. Although it is legally proper for an expert to rely on evidence and testimony proffered by other experts, firsthand evidence is extremely important in establishing credibility with the trier of fact, who in this case was the judge. While access to the canal property was not possible (remedial activities, including the construction of a cover, had already been undertaken), the expert was able to make observations nearby and use extensive information previously collected. Fortunately, a large clay pit, located less than 3 km from the canal, was accessible to the trial team. The stratigraphy exposed in this pit is the same as that reported by investigations at the Love Canal site. In addition, extensive on-site and off-site investigations had been conducted during the late 1970s and early 1980s that provided information regarding the subsurface stratigraphy at the Love Canal landfill. Over 1,000 soil borings, soil probes, and test pit profiles were described by soil scientists and geologists, and field samples were collected and analyzed for grain size distribution and clay content.

The information collected, together with information observed at several smaller exposures in the Niagara Falls area, was used to develop opinions regarding the age and genesis of the fractures in the stiff silty clay in the Love Canal area.

The stiff clay in the Love Canal area contains numerous near-vertical fractures. Many of these display a polygonal pattern in plan view, with their spacing ranging from a few centimeters to more than 0.5 m. Coatings of gray, oriented clay 1–3 mm thick line the fracture faces (Fig. 4), and plant roots extend down to the base of the fractures, which are found ~3 m below ground level.

To determine whether these fractures formed as a result of stress relief from the excavation of the nearby clay pit or predated the excavation of the clay pit, backhoe trenches were excavated tens to hundreds of meters away from the clay pit. Walls of the backhoe trenches had similar polygonal fractures with oriented clay coatings and plant roots that clearly predated the excavation of the backhoe trenches. These older fractures could be distinguished easily from the fractures caused by stress relief that had formed perpendicular and parallel to walls of the backhoe trenches within several hours of excavating the trenches. These younger fractures had no oriented clay coatings. Substantial amounts of water drained from the older fractures, clearly indicating the potential for water flow.

Not only did the nature of the fractures help explain their age, but also their presence helped explain some of the seemingly anomalous sample results. In fractured clay deposits contaminant movement is usually restricted to the fractures themselves. Site

investigations that use borings to map the distribution of contaminants often produce puzzling results because borings that do not intersect fractures often do not show evidence of contamination. As an example, one soil investigation conducted at Love Canal in 1980 included 64 bore holes surrounding the canal (New York State Department of Health, 1980). Most of these extended 0.5–1 m into the soft clay, but four went to refusal at the top of the dolomite. Contaminants were found in the upper sandy sediments and in fractures in the hard clay in many, but not all, of the borings. Of the 64 borings, field records showed 38 had a chemical smell, 29 had oily liquid traces, and 35 intersected at least one fracture. Some of the borings showed no contamination even though they were surrounded by other borings that had oily films on fracture faces or strong chemical odors. Figure 5 illustrates this contamination pattern, which is typical of fractured media from part of that study. This spotty distribution of contaminants could lead one to conclude erroneously that the contamination is not widespread in the fractured clay.

In summary, the geological conclusion was that the stiff clay in the Love Canal area is fractured throughout and that these fractures provide a potential pathway for migration of contaminants away from the canal. This conclusion was supported by the testimony of a clay mineralogist whose research indicated that certain DNAPLs cause the clay minerals adjacent to the fractures to desiccate. The desiccation leads to a widening of the fractures and allows for an increase in the rate of contaminant migration. It was concluded further that these fractures very likely were older than the sewer excavations and likely were older than the original canal excavation. The level of confidence in the opinions regard-

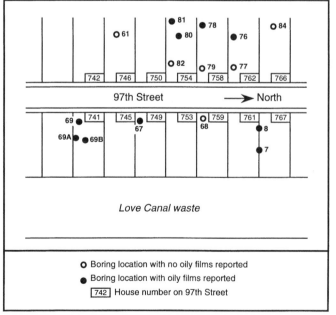

Figure 5. Sketch map of section of 97th Street properties and location of boreholes (New York State Department of Health, 1980) showing spotty distribution of described contaminant. Waste is contained in, but does not necessarily cover all of areas shown as Love Canal waste.

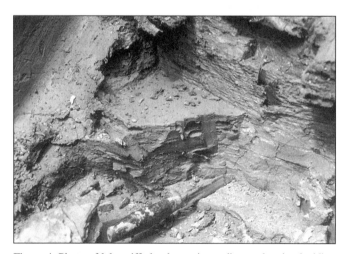

Figure 4. Photo of lake stiff clay lacustrine sediment showing bedding planes and fracture faces. Knife is pointed at intersection of two near-vertical fracture faces. Rootlets are present along fracture. Knife handle is 10 cm long.

ing the specific age of the formation of the fractures led to vigorous discussion of how geological conclusions can be presented fairly and clearly in the courtroom.

COLLIDING WORLDS OF LAW AND SCIENCE

As is often the case with expert testimony, the level of certainty and the scientific basis of the conclusions are both critical in countering alternate theories. There are two criteria to be met before expert testimony can be heard in federal court. State courts vary on this issue, but most often follow the federal rules or practice. First, the substance of the testimony must meet the requirements of the Supreme Court, established in the case of *Daubert v. Merrill Dow Pharmaceuticals, Inc.*, 113 S.Ct. 2786 (1993). Previous to this case, expert testimony had to rely on methodology that was generally accepted within the applicable scientific community. In *Daubert*, the Court replaced the older standard, with a flexible, five-factor test. Those five factors are (1) whether the technique or theory can be or has been tested, (2) whether the theory or technique has been subject to peer review and publication, (3) the known or potential rate of error, (4) the existence and maintenance of standards and controls, and (5) the degree to which the theory or technique has been generally accepted in the scientific community. At the same time, the Court in *Daubert* also held that the trial judge had the obligation to evaluate any proffered expert testimony, prior to the jury's hearing it, to ensure that the testimony met the five-part test.

In addition, and more relevant here, the witness must be prepared to say that her or his expert opinions are based on a reasonable degree of scientific certainty. Without such reasonable degree of scientific certainty, the so-called expert would be offering the trier of fact, be it judge or jury, only speculation, which is neither legally sufficient, nor particularly helpful. It is in meeting this second criterion that lawyers and scientists most often have conflicts.

In preparation of the geology testimony for the Love Canal litigation, it became clear that there were misunderstandings between lawyer and scientist. The lawyer wanted to know: Is that certain? Are you sure? Why can't you be certain? The scientist wanted to know: How can one be certain about that? What is "certainty"?

In discourse among scientists "certainty" suggests, indeed demands, quantification, most often as a statistical probability that something is true or not, usually with a 95% probability or confidence level. Even with such probability scientists are careful to qualify any conclusion by adding "based on the available data" or similar caveat.

In discourse among lawyers "certainty" demands only a 51% probability or confidence level. That is because "a reasonable degree of scientific certainty" in law means that the assertions by the expert must be more probably true than not true.[1] Thus, courts have adopted the 51% demarcation between what is admissible evidence and what is not. As the Court said in *Daubert*: "There are important differences between the quest for

truth in the courtroom and the quest for truth in the laboratory. Scientific conclusions are subject to perpetual revision. Law, on the other hand, must resolve disputes finally and quickly." (113 S. Ct. at 2798). Parties to lawsuits need, indeed demand, that their disputes be resolved—fairly, quickly, and finally. Fifty-one percent may be less certain than 95%, but courts cannot wait for such greater certainty to develop.

Most scientists are uncomfortable with giving testimony, under oath, that something is "true" without qualification, even though they have been assured that when the attorney says "true" he or she means "more likely than not." Once the expert can say that a certain fact is more probably true than not, then the lawyer is comfortable that the expert testimony will be heard by the court. But the lawyer now has to be persuasive, to convince the court, or jury, that this expert opinion is well-founded, authoritative, and should be believed. For this objective the lawyer needs the scientist expert to be, and to appear to be, absolute, certain, and unequivocal. But the objective can be accomplished not by stretching the substantive opinions, not by, in the world of the scientist, exaggerating the "truth." Rather, this objective can be accomplished by the authoritative tone, the manner and confidence exhibited by the expert in opining what is "more likely true than not."

CONCLUSIONS

An eight-month trial was held in 1990–1991 to determine the claims by the state for punitive damages against the chemical company, and the chemical company's claim that others were responsible. The U.S. District Court for the Western District of New York found, on the facts, that the chemical company's conduct was negligent and, indeed, inexcusable at times, especially with regard to incidents where children were exposed to chemicals at Love Canal (*United States v. Hooker Chemicals and Plastics Corp.*, 850 F.Supp. 993, W.D.N.Y. 1994). But, considering all the circumstances, the Court held that the company's conduct was not so outrageous as to warrant punitive damages. At that time the court did not rule on the chemical company's claims that the state or others were liable for the release of contaminants. In the summer of 1994, the company settled its liability with the State of New York for about $130 million; in 1995, it settled with the U.S. government for $129 million. Thus, the determination of the specific subsurface pathways and the impact on those pathways, if any, of actions by the city and state and others was never reached by the court. Nevertheless, the experience was most helpful in understanding how the disciplines of law and science interact, or collide. What started out as conflicting views of the legal process and conflicting views of what is meant by "certainty" and "truth" in science and law turned out to be reconcilable. The

---

[1]In other contexts, the law sometimes imposes a different standard. In certain cases a party has to prove its case by clear and convincing evidence (e.g., cases where fraud is alleged) and, of course, a prosecutor has to prove criminal charges beyond a reasonable doubt.

apparent conflict was resolved through a clear understanding of the separate role of expert and lawyer, and the meaning of certainty in each participant's world.

In the case of Love Canal, expert geological testimony, with regard to fractures, covered the following points and was given to a reasonable degree of scientific certainty: (1) the clay was deposited in an early stage of Lake Erie, (2) overlying silt and sand were deposited in Lake Tonawanda, (3) many fractures were present and open enough to allow passage of water and contaminants before the digging of sewer trenches in the 1970s, (4) many fractures likely were present before the Love Canal was excavated in the 1890s, and (5) the fractures likely formed during mid-Holocene when ground-water levels were lower.

Thus, even though the geologist could not state conclusively the age of the fractures, his opinion that the fractures were almost certainly older than the age of the sewer excavations, and likely older than the canal itself, met the required legal standard of "more likely than not." Therefore, this testimony was admitted at trial as evidence that the chemical company was liable for the off-site migration of the chemicals at Love Canal and was used further

to defend against the company's claim that the state's excavation of the surrounding sewers caused this off-site migration.

REFERENCES CITED

Calkin, P. E., and Feenstra, B. H., 1985, Evaluation of the Erie-basin Great Lakes, *in* Karrow, P. F., and Calkin, P. E., eds., Quaternary evolution of the Great Lakes: Geological Association of Canada Special Paper 30, p. 149–170.

Comprehensive Environmental Response, Compensation, and Liability Act, 42 U.S. Code Section 9601 et seq., 1980.

Daubert v. Merrill Dow Pharmaceuticals, Inc., 113 S.Ct. 2786 1993.

Mickelson, D. M., Edil, T. B., and Wang, X., 1994, Holocene groundwater levels and the development of fractures in till and lacustrine sediment of the Great Lakes region: Boulder, Colorado, Geological Society of America Abstracts with Programs, v. 26, no. 7, p. 300.

New York State Department of Health, Division of Environmental Health, 1980, Love Canal Litigation Soil Sampling: Available from the New York State Department of Law.

Tarlton, F., and Cassidy, J. J., 1981, Love Canal: A special report to the Governor and legislature: Albany, New York State Department of Health, 69 p.

United States v. Hooker Chemicals and Plastics Corp., 850 F.Supp. 993 (W.D.N.Y. 1994).

MANUSCRIPT ACCEPTED BY THE SOCIETY JUNE 5, 1997

Geological Society of America
Reviews in Engineering Geology, Volume XII
1998

Expectations of geological science:
Yucca Mountain site characterization, Nevada

Thomas W. Bjerstedt*
U.S. Department of Energy, Yucca Mountain Site Characterization Office, P.O. Box 30307, MS 523, North Las Vegas, Nevada 89036

ABSTRACT

The U.S. Department of Energy (DOE) has brought data, analyses, and conclusions on landscape stability and denudation rates from the Yucca Mountain site characterization program to the U.S. Nuclear Regulatory Commission (NRC) for evaluation. In the United States the NRC must license a geologic repository to dispose of spent nuclear reactor fuel and high-level radioactive wastes from military reprocessing through phases of construction, operation, and closure. The DOE reported rates of hillslope denudation at Yucca Mountain, valley incision in bedrock over the repository block, and alluvial stream incision on the major drainage system in the area. These data were presented in combination with a regulatory compliance argument that concluded extreme erosion had not occurred during the Quaternary Period and that erosion would not jeopardize performance of a geologic repository system over the next 10,000 years, if located there.

The NRC defined "extreme erosion" and the duration of the Quaternary Period in a qualitative regulatory context as one of 24 "potentially adverse conditions" (NRC, 1991) to be evaluated during site characterization. The DOE made a compliance argument using the NRC's regulatory requirement, supplemented by qualitative definitions from internal NRC guidance. The NRC was critical of the DOE's technical documentation and compliance argument because (1) the erosion assessment used time-averaged denudation rates, (2) erosion rates for the most recent 10,000 to 100,000 years of the Quaternary Period were not provided, and (3) multiple dating methods were not used to establish age of the surficial landforms examined.

The DOE encountered several difficulties interpreting the regulation and its administrative record, framing a compliance argument, and documenting the data, analyses, and conclusions from a field study program. Among these, (1) the DOE misinterpreted the regulation and its administrative record by primarily relying on extant written guidance to explain how the NRC staff interpreted their regulation; (2) the DOE had no knowledge of how the NRC would evaluate a limited and specific compliance argument against their regulation; (3) the DOE's technical documentation, in retrospect, was not robust enough to meet the NRC's expectations of high confidence in conclusions accompanied by low uncertainty; and (4) the NRC's comments implied expectations for geochronologic accuracy and degree of resolution that may be considered beyond the state of the practice.

*Present address: Texaco Exploration and Production Inc., P.O. Box 60252, 400 Poydras Street, New Orleans, Louisiana 70160.

Bjerstedt, T. W., 1998, Expectations of geological science: Yucca Mountain site characterization, Nevada, *in* Welby, C. W., and Gowan, M. E., eds., A Paradox of Power: Voices of Warning and Reason in the Geosciences: Boulder, Colorado, Geological Society of America Reviews in Engineering Geology, v. XII.

The DOE's documentation and the NRC's evaluation of it confronts the question of, how much information is enough?, in this case, to satisfy a limited and specific regulatory requirement from the United States' geologic disposal program. The dialog is also a calibration point gauging how well geology's epistemological limitations meet regulatory expectations for licensing a facility required to perform successfully for millennia. As the geologic repository program prepares for licensing just after the turn of the twenty-first century, this learning experience provides insight on the importance of the DOE's documentation, the effectiveness of communication between the DOE and NRC, and the flexibility that the NRC brings to bear in evaluating the DOE's compliance arguments.

INTRODUCTION

The Nuclear Waste Policy Act (NWPA) of 1982 established the United States' national policy of deep geologic disposal of commercial spent reactor fuel and vitrified glass waste from military reprocessing. The U.S. Department of Energy (DOE) is characterizing a site at Yucca Mountain, Nevada, for a potential geologic repository. The U.S. Nuclear Regulatory Commission (NRC) must license and regulate a repository over a period of about 100 years that includes phases of construction, operation, post-waste emplacement monitoring, and closure. A repository must contain and isolate the inventory of radionuclides over a 10,000-year period, or a different time period to be specified by the U.S. Environmental Protection Agency (EPA) in a new rule-making process that began in 1996.

The NRC's repository regulation, Title 10, Code of Federal Regulations (CFR), Part 60, "Disposal of High-Level Radioactive Wastes in Geologic Repositories" (NRC, 1991) was finalized in June 1983. It is a substantial regulation of 26,700 words that will require a great volume of documentation to present a case for compliance. In 10 CFR Part 60.122 there are 24 "potentially adverse conditions" (PAC). PACs are undesirable attributes of a repository site. For each PAC the DOE needs to show in a licensing proceeding either that it (1) is not present, (2) does not affect the ability of the site to isolate waste, (3) can be remediated, or (4) that favorable attributes of the site compensate for it. Extreme erosion during the Quaternary Period is one PAC. Yet, neither extreme erosion or a standard for comparison is defined in the regulation.

The DOE described field and laboratory studies in a site characterization plan (SCP) (DOE, 1988) to collect the information needed to prepare a case for compliance with the NRC's regulation. In March 1993, the DOE submitted documentation of technical data, analyses, conclusions, and a compliance argument to the NRC that the extreme erosion PAC is not present at the site. In August 1994 the NRC provided nine comments that explained their basis for not accepting the DOE's conclusions. In 1995 the DOE authorized collection of limited additional data to address the NRC's criticisms.

The NRC's evaluation of the DOE's data and compliance argument on erosion (denudation) rates at Yucca Mountain revealed high expectations for the accuracy and degree of resolution delivered by dating techniques, and that the specific dating technique used by the DOE did not meet these expectations. This chapter explores whether the expectation is well matched to (1) the limitations of the science, (2) scientific experience in framing a compliance argument for the time frame that is required, and (3) the precedent now being set with an unexercised regulation on this unprecedented human activity. To better understand the NRC's regulation, the DOE accessed written guidance that explained how the NRC staff interpreted it, but had no guidance or foresight into how NRC would evaluate compliance against it. As a result, the DOE's technical documentation was not robust enough to meet the NRC's expectation of high confidence in conclusions accompanied by low uncertainty.

How a geoscientist's work and conclusions are evaluated under a regulatory paradigm has not often been explored in the literature (Meehan, 1984). Geologists can be surprised by how their work is evaluated in a nuclear regulatory environment where there are different expectations for how one demonstrates the presence or magnitude of physical phenomena than in, for example, professional journals. The DOE's experiences with the extreme erosion PAC shows how different the regulatory paradigm is, and why it is different.

Reasonable assurance

The NRC's standard of proof, *reasonable assurance*, (McGarry and Echols, 1994, p. 1406) has evolved from power plant licensing and regulation of the engineered systems built to contain a nuclear chain reaction over an operating lifetime of about 40 years. In practice, reasonable assurance means high confidence in conclusions accompanied by low uncertainty. A geologic repository, in contrast to a reactor, is a passive system with no moving parts. It is a network of underground drifts in a chosen rock where specially designed large metal containers of spent fuel and high-level radioactive waste are emplaced. The goal of geologic disposal above the water table in the unsaturated zone, as at Yucca Mountain, is to keep waste as dry as possible for as long as possible to minimize the likelihood that radionuclides are carried by water away from the repository environment into the biosphere. In essence, a repository is designed to transfer long-lived radioactive waste from the time scale of human experience, to the scale of geologic time. Repository licensing will subject the geologic data and engineered design developed during site characterization to a legal process where findings of fact and conclusions of law are made on compliance to the requirements of the regulation (McGarry and Echols, 1994).

Can the *reasonable assurance* standard be applied as it has in the past to project the performance of what is primarily a geologic system over 10 millennia and more? Although the licensing proceeding will be unprecedented, the nation expects the DOE and the NRC to make the necessary judgements and decisions required by law (NWPA, 1983) at a sustainable cost and on a schedule compatible with those costs being borne by those who benefited from nuclear technologies. Although the case that the DOE brings forward for licensing will be evaluated within the parameters of administrative law, findings and conclusions will not be made in a state of complete knowledge or certainty in the knowledge that is brought forth (McGarry and Echols, 1994; 1995). Confidence in these conclusions also needs to take account of the limitations for what the geological sciences can demonstrate (Van Konynenburg, 1994a, b).

SITE CHARACTERIZATION AND A TOPICAL REPORT

In December 1982, the Nuclear Waste Policy Act (NWPA, 1983) authorized a program of parallel characterization of multiple sites in different geologic media. The statute was amended in 1987 to direct the DOE to characterize only the Yucca Mountain site in southern Nevada (Fig. 1). The DOE has been studying the Miocene rhyolitic volcanic tuffs underlying Yucca Mountain since the early 1980s to determine if the location is suitable for a repository. The DOE's site characterization plan (SCP) outlined substantial study programs to assess tectonism, seismicity, igneous activity, ground-water quantities and movement, and a comparatively modest program to study erosion (DOE, 1988, p. 8.3.1.6-1 to -31). Project scientists from the U.S. Geological Survey (USGS) and Los Alamos National Laboratory developed studies on landscape stability (e.g., surficial deposits mapping, study of hillslope evolution, and soil studies) from which denudation rates were calculated. Denudation rates were determined because erosion can be defined to exclude mass-wasting processes (Bates and Jackson, 1980, p. 210), for example, debris flows.

Although the DOE interchanges use of the terms denudation and erosion, the DOE's experimental design was to determine denudation rates as a means to assess erosion and long-term landscape stability. Bates and Jackson (1980, p. 167) regard denudation as the ". . . laying bare, uncovering, or exposure of bedrock . . . through the removal of overlying material by erosion." Denudation integrates the cumulative episodes of downcutting, deposition, and stasis that took place on the landscape around Yucca Mountain, and therefore takes into account process rate changes through time, such as short-duration changes in erosion rate that may correspond to different climatic regimes.

Through these studies, it was soon apparent that Quaternary erosion rates at Yucca Mountain were very low. The DOE's

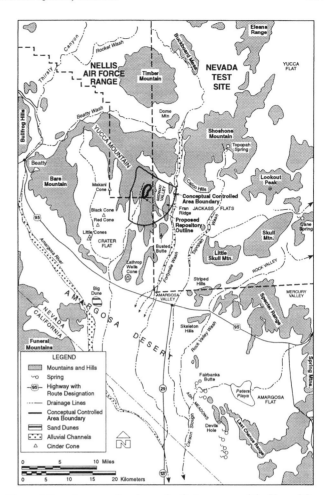

Figure 1. Location map showing major features around the Yucca Mountain site. The potential repository location lies within the conical outline marking the controlled area at the junction of federal land controlled by the Nevada Test Site, Nellis Air Force Base, and the Bureau of Land Management. Stippled areas represent highlands.

management was encouraged by these results, and in 1991 decided to prepare this work for presentation to the NRC in a topical report after the principal investigators published, or had papers accepted by, refereed journals. A topical report is a means to present methodologies proposed for characterizing the site or the results of applied methodologies to the NRC staff to seek informal agreement that the methodology or application is acceptable for citation in a future license application.

INTERPRETING THE REGULATION

It is the DOE's responsibility to (1) interpret the regulation and available administrative record, (2) develop the experimental approach, (3) gather data and draw conclusions, and (4) show regulatory compliance in a way that can be defended. Ideally these activities are sequential. In this case the first three steps proceeded in parallel, and an additional variable was introduced. While site characterization proceeded, the NRC sought to clarify parts of their regulation with supplementary internal guidance.

Potentially adverse condition

PAC 16 (NRC, 1991) is "Evidence for extreme erosion during the Quaternary Period." This PAC was developed because a repository site needs to avoid a geologic setting where, (1) erosional processes capable of unroofing a repository over a 10,000-year performance period are present, (2) degradation of the landscape over time could lead to a decrease in overburden that affects radionuclide releases from a repository, or (3) the magnitude and frequency of seismic activity or climatic change has been, or could be, such as to make the site susceptible to erosional modification in the future. The current preliminary repository design allows at least 200 m of overburden above the potential repository. Except near the eastern edge of the repository block, the thickness of stratiform welded and nonwelded tuff overburden is everywhere greater than 200 m (Fig. 2). In order to show that a PAC is not present or does not affect a repository's performance the DOE must show that assumptions were not used that underestimate the effect of the PAC on performance, and that the investigation considered the extent to which the PAC may be present but still undetected.

What is 'extreme erosion'?

In response to public comment 543 on draft 10 CFR Part 60 (NRC, 1983, p. 382) the NRC staff defined extreme erosion as ". . . the occurrence of substantial changes in land forms (as a result of erosion) over relatively short intervals of time." Thus, a qualitative definition superposes the qualitative statement of the PAC in the regulation. A new question emerges as a result of this response. How long are "relatively short intervals of time?"

How long is 'during the Quaternary Period'?

Another question of definition for the extreme erosion PAC centered on the meaning of "during the Quaternary Period." The DOE is required to, "demonstrate a sufficient understanding of the recent geologic past such that geologic changes can be projected over the intended period of performance with reasonably high confidence" (NRC, 1992, p. 4). In responding to comment 525 on their draft regulation, the NRC sought to avoid the problem of defining when the Quaternary Period began by stating that the DOE's investigations needed to look at the phenomenon during the Quaternary Period (NRC, 1983, p. 373). Is this a distinction without a difference? The DOE also was to assume that for "regulatory purposes" the Quaternary Period began 2 Ma unless a justification for another date is provided (NRC, 1992, p. 2: NRC, 1983, p. 373). The NRC staff also stated that ". . . recent history (i.e., the Quaternary Period) is a better indicator of possible future activity than is the distant geologic past" (NRC, 1992, p. 3). In order to "demonstrate a sufficient understanding," the DOE's studies needed to span the duration of the Quaternary with emphasis on the late Quaternary.

MAKING A COMPLIANCE ARGUMENT

While gathering the NRC's written interpretations and internal guidance about the extreme erosion PAC, the DOE's data collection program proceeded to conclusion. To calculate denudation rates, one needs a measure of material removed and the amount of time required to remove it. A dating technique capable of spanning the duration of the Quaternary Period was needed, one that could integrate unresolvable and undetectable short-term periods of erosion. If deposits that could be dated occurred on Yucca Mountain

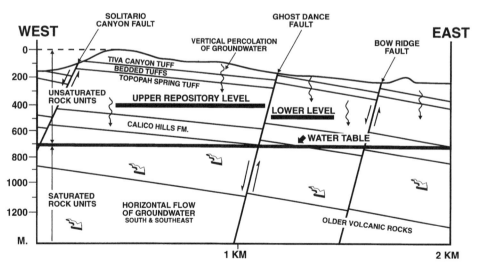

Figure 2. Schematic east-west cross section of Yucca Mountain showing potential repository horizon in the Topopah Spring Tuff, volcanic stratigraphy, the unsaturated zone, and water table. Ground-water flow in the saturated zone is primarily south-southeast.

hillslopes, if their age approached the duration of the Quaternary Period, and if a geologic context existed within which erosion could be measured, the stability of these hillslopes over time could be determined. The DOE reasoned that if extreme denudation rates on large-scale landforms are not present, then neither could erosion rates in any local area on the hillslopes be extreme.

The DOE prepared a topical report (DOE, 1993) that stated the regulatory motivation for the work and reported a site-specific analysis of the following items: hillslope evolution and hillslope denudation rates, valley-cutting rates over the potential repository block, and stream incision rates in alluvium including the base-level history of the major regional drainage and the first-order ephemeral streams over the repository block. The regulatory and technical assessments together concluded that the extreme erosion PAC was not present at Yucca Mountain.

How the DOE defined 'extreme erosion'

Because NRC's regulation and internal guidance contained only qualitative and subjective guidance to design a study program in the field, the DOE decided to use a practical definition for extreme erosion by presenting a contrast. This contrast was based first on a typical definition of the word extreme: something at the far end of a range, exceeding the ordinary, or of the greatest severity. Second, the DOE compiled a table from the literature that reported denudation rates calculated from various rock types in various climates throughout the United States and the world (DOE, 1993, Table 3). These rates were compared with the denudation rates calculated at Yucca Mountain (DOE, 1993, Table 5). Denudation rates over the entire United States, for example, range from 2–15 cm/k.y. and averages about 4 cm/k.y. Hillslope denudation rates determined for Yucca Mountain are about 0.2 cm/k.y., near the lowest rates determined in the United States. Not only has erosion not been extreme during the Quaternary at Yucca Mountain, but it has been significantly lower than average.

How the DOE defined 'during the Quaternary'

The DOE defined the beginning of the Quaternary Period at 1.6 Ma, and thereby its duration. This date has been endorsed by the Geological Society of America in the "Geologic Time Scale" (Palmer, 1983) and in the "Decade of North American Geology" series (Morrison, 1991). These literature sources are considered authoritative by the geologic community in this country, and certainly provide more basis than the NRC's seemingly arbitrary assignment of 2 Ma (NRC, 1992, p. 2: NRC, 1983, p. 373). The DOE's study, therefore, needed to characterize erosion rates and processes during the Quaternary, a period spanning the most recent 1.6 m.y. of earth history.

The DOE's technical and compliance argument

This paper discusses the interface between science and the regulatory environment. The USGS and Los Alamos National Laboratory geologists who performed the DOE's studies have published the data, analyses, and conclusions from much of this work in peer-reviewed journals (Harrington and Whitney, 1987; Whitney and Harrington, 1993), and in references cited in these works. The DOE's topical report recapitulated this work, included additional information for context, explained how site-specific erosion rate calculations were made, and discussed the assumptions underlying field sampling and the analytical technique used to date the boulder deposits.

Project geologists were drawn to the prominent colluvial boulder deposits on hillslopes in the area (Fig. 3) and the shallow incised channels adjacent to them (see also Whitney and Harrington, 1993, Fig. 1). Whitney and Harrington (1993) explained the climatic factors responsible for the formation and preservation of colluvial boulder deposits on hillslopes and why these geomorphic surfaces are key to understanding long-term stability of the landscape. The boulder deposits were a natural focal point to interpret the events and process that have acted on hillslopes over time. Establishing their age was the first step.

Calculating denudation rates

Project geologists used the varnish cation-ratio dating (VCR) technique to establish age estimates for a selection of boulder deposits on Yucca Mountain and nearby hillslopes (Fig. 4). The VCR technique yields an indirect estimate for age from a curve that must be calibrated with other dated deposits in the area intended for use (Harrington and Whitney, 1987; Whitney and Harrington, 1993, Fig. 8). The VCR dating method was a new

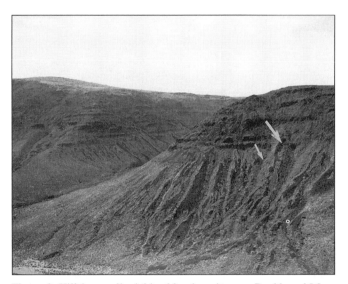

Figure 3. Hillslope colluvial boulder deposits near Buckboard Mesa (Fig. 1). See discussion in Whitney and Harrington (1993) on the origin of the boulder deposits. The large white arrow marks the dark, varnished surface of a boulder deposit. The smaller white arrow shows an adjacent channel from topographic inversion of the deposit in response to continued hillslope erosion after stabilization allowed varnish formation to begin. The channel depths furnish a measure for the amount of hillslope erosion that occurred since the deposit became stabilized.

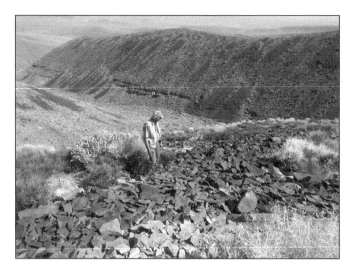

Figure 4. Varnished, boulder-sized clasts from the YME-1 colluvial boulder field (Whitney and Harrington, 1993, Fig. 2). Note the varnished deposits on hillslope in background. Boulder deposits on the upper slope of the bedrock ridge are in situ, and talus mantles at the slope toe are stabilized by varnished boulders that armour the surface.

and promising technique under development in the mid-1980s. The DOE's geologists concluded that VCR dating (1) was a suitable technique to use on the aphanitic tuffaceous and basaltic substrates on and around Yucca Mountain, and (2) was capable of spanning the 1.6 m.y. duration of the Quaternary Period (DOE, 1993, p. 32). The capability of acquiring ages directly from geomorphic surfaces with cosmogenic radionuclides was not widespread in the mid-1980s. Under this circumstance the DOE expected that VCR dating was a scientifically valid technique to estimate the age of the boulder deposits.

Whitney and Harrington (1993, Fig. 2) sampled and analyzed 11 boulder deposits for age estimates. The analysis of rock varnish chemistry showed that the boulders in these deposits were in place from 0.17 to 1.38 Ma, providing a data set that reaches substantially into the early Quaternary. The boulder deposits are stabilized not only by large clast size, but usually also by cementation to a pedogenic carbonate layer beneath them (Whitney and Harrington, 1993, Fig. 7). Once an age estimate for a boulder deposit was obtained, the depth of channel incision into adjacent colluvium and bedrock (ranging from 1 to 2.5 m deep) can be measured to calculate a denudation rate over the time since the boulder deposit became stable (DOE, 1993, p. 47). The average hillslope denudation rate calculated in this way was 0.19 cm/k.y. (DOE, 1993, Table 5).

Quaternary alluvium and valley fill in the basins around Yucca Mountain and colluvial deposits on hillslopes have been stable through the middle to late Quaternary due to low rates of tectonic activity and climatic fluctuations that have not been great (Whitney and Harrington, 1993). Climatic influences on erosion are minimal. Short-term climatic fluctuations during glacial and interglacial periods over the last 10 to 100 k.y. that are discernable with proxy data from the geologic record places bounds on future conditions. Wetter and cooler periods can be expected in addition to the hotter and dryer conditions of today. In the current climate, localized mobilization and transport of unconsolidated soil and rock typically occurs in debris flows on sparsely vegetated hillslopes after short but intense rain events (Whitney and Harrington, 1993, p. 1015–1016). Debris flows do not erode bedrock (DOE, 1993, p. 22), they merely transport loose material downslope. Hillslopes under wetter and cooler pluvial conditions, in contrast, are better stabilized by vegetation during runoff events and tend to be periods of relative stability or aggradation of unconsolidated materials (C. Harrington, personal communication, 1994).

Stream incision rates in alluvial deposits were derived from dated terrace surfaces near Fran Ridge that have been cut by Fortymile Wash, a short distance east of Yucca Mountain's bedrock ridges (Fig. 1). Based on two end-member scenarios then permitted by the data, a minimum stream incision rate is 42 cm/k.y. and a maximum rate is 222 cm/k.y. (DOE, 1993, p. 55). The latter estimate presumes a scenario of downcutting to bedrock, not a likely possibility given that approximately 130 m of alluvium underlies the wash. Mapping of surficial deposits along Fortymile Wash that was completed after the topical report was written does not support the latter scenario that downcutting could have proceeded to bedrock.

The Fortymile Wash drainage system has been aggrading during the Quaternary (DOE, 1993, p. 54). Local base level is the Amargosa Desert (Fig. 1). Southward, Fortymile Wash splays out into a series of shallow bifurcating channels that drain toward the ephemeral Amargosa River. There is no evidence of active or recent headward erosion from the main Fortymile Wash system into the first-order ephemeral streams over the Yucca Mountain block. Thin alluvial deposits and debris flows cover the floors of steep-sided valleys that have been cut into the Tiva Canyon Tuff of the Paintbrush Group, (Fig. 2) a 12.7-Ma welded-tuff caprock on Yucca Mountain. Trenching into the thin valley fill shows no downcutting into smooth, concave-upward bedrock valley floors (DOE, 1993, p. 54)

An eastward drainage from the crest of Yucca Mountain was established by tectonic activity soon after deposition of the Tiva Canyon Tuff. The volcanic layers dip gently to the east (Fig. 2) and caused downdip erosion of bedrock valleys. A downcutting rate of 0.8 cm/k.y. or less (DOE, 1993, p. 55) was calculated for these bedrock valleys, based on depth from adjacent ridge crests. This rate is truly a long-term average because it includes the late Miocene, a period of caldera formation and greater tectonic activity in the Great Basin when rates of downcutting were more rapid.

Repository performance period: 10,000 years

If hillslope denudation rates are projected over 10,000 years, degradation of hillslopes is expected to be less than 2 cm (DOE, 1993, p. 46). No downcutting of bedrock in the valley floors over the Yucca Mountain block would be expected over 10,000 years, only movement of alluvium and debris in the valleys. During the same period, between 4 and 20 m of incision in Fortymile Wash could occur (DOE, 1993, p. 55), with a good argument that the lower bound of this range is most realistic, because downcutting to bedrock is not a credible scenario.

NRC'S COMMENTS

The NRC staff forwarded nine comments on the topical report in August 1994 (NRC, 1994a) that expressed three basic criticisms on the DOE's approach to the study and the compliance argument. These criticisms can be traced to three root causes, (1) the NRC defined the PAC in a way that did not limit the period over which the DOE needed to "demonstrate a sufficient understanding" to the most recent 10–100 k.y., (2) the DOE did not have advance insight to understand how a compliance argument using time-averaged Quaternary denudation rates could be judged deficient by the NRC, and (3) the DOE did not know that the NRC would expect any dating technique used to establish a geochronology to be corroborated by other technique(s) to achieve an adequate level of confidence in the age estimates.

New performance measure for the PAC?

Comment 1 states, "By relying on long-term denudation rates to define the absence of the potentially adverse condition, the topical report does not address the regulatory requirement for the PAC, set forth in 10 CFR 60.122(c)(16), concerning evidence of extreme erosion during the Quaternary Period" (NRC, 1994a, p. 1). The DOE's compliance argument for extreme erosion did not cover a period of 10–100 k.y. before present. In comment 1 the NRC went on to recommend, "DOE should use a methodology that provides information on the 'extreme erosion rates'; those erosion rates which may have been experienced in the general Yucca Mountain area during relatively short periods of time, on the order of those periods of time equal to the regulatory period of performance (i.e. 10,000 to 100,000 years)." As part of the basis for comment 1 the NRC explained, "The purpose of the extreme erosion PAC is to assure a program of exploration and analysis which will ensure sufficient site characterization information to allow a projection of the erosion rates that could be expected during the period of intended repository performance—presently 10,000 years" (NRC, 1994a, p. 1).

Although 10 k.y. is the current period of regulated performance, the language of the PAC led the DOE to believe that the Quaternary Period was the time frame of interest. Furthermore, the DOE believed that if a relatively well preserved mid- to late Quaternary alluvial and hillslope record showed little modification of these deposits, and that interpretations for how the landscape had evolved during the Quaternary were consistent across multiple lines of evidence, then a firm basis existed to show that conditions that might occur over the next 10 k.y. were well bounded.

The NRC apparently expected most, or at least more, attention to be focused on the recent part of the Quaternary record, but

no quantification of this time frame was offered in the repository regulation beyond reference to "relatively short intervals of time" in the NRC's response to comments (NRC, 1983, p. 382) or ". . . recent history (i.e., the Quaternary Period) is a better indicator of possible future activity than is the distant geologic past" in internal guidance (NRC, 1992, p. 3). The only quantification of the PAC offered by the NRC occurred in comments on the topical report.

In their comment 1, the NRC superposed a quantitative definition onto a regulatory requirement that had previously been defined qualitatively; "substantial changes in land forms (as a result of erosion) over relatively short intervals of time" (NRC, 1983, p. 382). A new performance measure for the site, extreme erosion during the Holocene, is implied by expecting compliance to be based on time periods of 10–100 k.y. The DOE did not expect to establish a geochronology to calculate erosion rates within such a recent and narrow temporal window, or that not doing so would fail to "demonstrate a sufficient understanding" of the geologic processes during the Quaternary. Consider these two scenarios, (1) there are few deposits 10–100 k.y. old to date or few techniques appropriate to date them, and (2) the deposits that can be dated are much older than 10–100 k.y., as are all of the boulder deposits studied (range 0.76–1.38 Ma). In either case, is it obvious how a successful compliance argument can be made?

Time-averaged approach

The second criticism in the NRC's comments (NRC, 1994a, p. 1) is closely related to the first; that a time-averaged approach for determining erosion rates was inadequate. In another basis for comment 1 NRC stated, ". . . estimates of erosion rates based on net erosion over hundreds of thousands or even millions of years may be inappropriate. It is feasible that much of the incision of a surface which is 500,000 years old could have occurred over perhaps 10,000 years or less. If this is the case the shorter time interval could constitute a period of extreme erosion. However, averaged over a 500,000 year interval, estimated erosion rates would be 50 times less than the actual rates during the erosional episode (NRC, 1994a, p. 1)." The NRC states elsewhere, ". . . DOE's assessment relies on average denudation estimates over long intervals of time (i.e. in excess of 100,000 years) rather than on periods of extreme erosion that have occurred during the Quaternary, which if they recur, could have an adverse effect on repository performance" (NRC, 1994a, cover letter).

The NRC stated that a time-averaged approach did not take account of the potential to have higher erosion rates under different climates during the Quaternary. This criticism, and the one implying a performance measure of 10–100 k.y., strike at the heart of how geologists interpret earth history; time-averaging and the capability for any dating method to resolve a point in time from the geologic past. At the root of this criticism would seem to be an expectation for accurate dating of very young, inorganic terrestrial deposits. It is difficult enough under ideal conditions to expect dating techniques to resolve geologic events or deposits less than 100 k.y. old with high confidence and low uncertainty, but the same expectation for 10 k.y. simply pushes the science beyond its capabilities. All dating techniques have error bars on age assignments, and for deposits on the order of a few tens of thousands of years old the error can exceed the age of the deposit. Among techniques potentially available, applications also are limited by a specific geologic terrane and the need for a geologic context that can provide meaning for the dates acquired.

The DOE would be hard pressed to design a field study program to test the scenario the NRC offers above. Assume that one of the following hypothetical scenarios results in a 1-m-deep channel being cut adjacent to a 500-k.y. colluvial boulder deposit: (1) few low frequency/high magnitude events within a 10-k.y. period, (2) several low-frequency/high-magnitude events within a 100-k.y. period, or (3) many high-frequency/low-magnitude events over a 500-k.y. period. The geologic record is the same in all instances: 1 m of incision in 500 k.y., or an average of 2 cm over 10 k.y. regardless of which process scenario is most correct. Would additional data provide critical information about the Quaternary erosional history to justify the cost to acquire it? Given that there is over 200 m of bedrock overburden at the repository location, what insights might accrue by acquiring additional data trying to distinguish which process scenario is most correct?

The NRC raised the issue of time averaging in comment 43 on the DOE's SCP (NRC, 1989, p. 4–42). This comment stated that time-averaged values for geologic phenomena, including erosion, may not yield conservative estimates. The NRC's comment on the SCP came too late to influence the DOE's experimental design for erosion studies that were under way while the NRC commented on the DOE's SCP and drafted guidance to try to clarify parts of their repository regulation. Only in their 1994 comments on the topical report did the NRC explicitly state that examination of the most recent 10–100 k.y. of the Quaternary Period was the most important aspect of the DOE's argument.

The NRC's comment 43 warned the DOE about possible concerns over a time-averaged approach. Was that counsel ignored by the DOE, or perhaps not understood when faced with the need and practicality of designing a field study program? Project geologists approached their evaluation of landscape stability and erosional processes at Yucca Mountain as surface-process geomorphologists would intuitively approach such a problem. Examining the most temporally stable deposits in this terrane, aside from the bedrock itself, was key to understanding how stable the landscape has been through time and what modifying processes acted upon it. No experimental design presented itself to gather a data set to test NRC's observation in comment 43, "Failure to consider maximum conditions in predicting erosion over the next 10,000 years may result in an underestimation of the effect of potential erosion" (NRC, 1989, p. 4–42). If 1 to 2.5 m of channel cutting occurred in bedrock and unstable colluvium during the part of the Quaternary Period the VCR technique spanned (0.76–1.38 Ma), then DOE reasoned that "maximum conditions" over 10 k.y. had been taken into account.

The DOE concluded that the Yucca Mountain landscape has been stable through the mid- to late Quaternary as indicated by low denudation rates. If that conclusion is judged to be biased by having studied the oldest and most stable deposits in the area, how would geologists remedy such a criticism and design an approach to determine how *unstable* the landscape has been during the Quaternary? Would an experimental design to seek out and study the youngest deposits provide the same insights about long-term stability over millennia?

VCR dating technique inadequate

The third criticism in NRC's comments (NRC, 1994a, p. 7–13) focused on the DOE's use of the VCR technique. The NRC stated the technique was controversial (NRC, 1993), and the NRC was critical of the means by which the VCR technique was calibrated, was critical of the DOE for using it in absence of other techniques, and in the end judged that the results obtained from its application were inadequate to support a licensing action (NRC, 1994a). Through their comments it was clear that the DOE could not just apply the state of the practice for the technique in a suitable terrane, but was obligated to provide the geochemical justification for how the technique worked. Then, as now, the mechanism(s) for selective cation depletion in rock varnish over time requires additional basic research, though some relationship between cation depletion and age is certain enough.

A field trip held by the DOE for the NRC staff in February 1994 allowed interaction with DOE's principal investigators on the outcrop. Despite this two-day visit not a single concern out of 21 provided to the DOE before the visit (NRC, 1994b) were allayed, although specific attempts were made to do so in the field. The NRC believed that the DOE's field sampling program and analytical method for measuring varnish parameters was linked to assumptions about how varnish formed, and how the colluvial boulder deposits themselves formed, that tended to yield older ages than the true age of the deposits. If deposit ages were overestimated, the calculated process rates would be underestimated.

To resolve this criticism, DOE is corroborating the VCR technique by direct dating of bedrock and selected boulder deposit surfaces using a cosmogenic radionuclide, Beryllium[10].

As the data set continues to be developed, early results of Be^{10} dating of a boulder deposit sampled at Little Skull Mountain (LSM site 1; Whitney and Harrington, 1993, Fig. 2) shows that the Be^{10} results (405–675 ka; C. Harrington, unpublished data) overlap by 30% with the 500–930 ka age estimate determined at that location with the VCR technique. Will the Be^{10} application bypass similar questions on the theoretical basis for this technique, for example, atmospheric production rates for Be^{10}, or inherited exposure on the boulders sampled? Cosmogenic dating with Be^{10} is an application used by practicioners only over the last few years. There has not been much time to explore weaknesses in its theoretical basis and uncertainties in various applications in the literature. Will Be^{10} be able to resolve ages on the order of 10–100 k.y.?

Although the NRC considered the VCR technique to be

controversial, little controversy existed at the time it was adopted for the DOE's erosion studies. Much of the subsequent debate in the geologic literature over how or under what circumstances rock varnish can be used as a dating tool was generated by the scientists working on the DOE's program. They tested some assumptions used by others in early applications of the VCR dating technique and improved its theoretical basis to develop an application for Yucca Mountain.

IS EROSION A PERFORMANCE ISSUE?

In 1995 the DOE authorized the collection of additional data to address the NRC's August 1994 comments on the topical report. Cosmogenic Be[10] dating of selected boulder deposits and bedrock exposures is one part of that work. Another is examining the sensitivity of (1) calculated erosion rates to variation in the estimated VCR ages of boulder surfaces, and (2) estimated VCR ages to variation in the age of the alluvial surfaces (established with thermoluminescence, Uranium-trend, and Uranium-series techniques on buried caliches and soils) that were dated to construct the calibration curve in the Yucca Mountain area (Harrington and Whitney, 1987; Whitney and Harrington, 1993). These analyses show that sources of variation, or uncertainty, in estimated ages could sum to increase denudation rates by about 40% (C. Harrington, personal communication, 1996), increasing the calculated erosion rates on hillslopes from about 2 cm/10 k.y. (DOE, 1993), to about 2.6 cm/10 k.y. When these sources of uncertainty are taken into account, mid- to late Quaternary denudation rates at Yucca Mountain are still far below average for the United States, and for similar rocks in similar climates worldwide (DOE, 1993, Table 2).

Repository performance is not sensitive to the denudation rates that the DOE has determined at Yucca Mountain, or to rates 10 to 100 times higher (DOE, 1995, p. 2–39). If one assumes for the sake of argument that hillslope colluvial boulder deposits are much younger than the DOE's data indicates, that erosion rates are significantly greater as a consequence, and that the denudation rates on hillslopes are 100 times greater than the maximum rate calculated from the hillslopes examined at Yucca Mountain (0.57 cm/k.y.) (DOE, 1993, Table 5), it yields a denudation rate of 57 cm/k.y. Over a period of 10 ky the landscape degradation expected in this scenario would be 570 cm/10 k.y.—less than 6 m.

There exists wide latitude for uncertainty in understanding exactly what the true erosion rates at Yucca Mountain have been during the Quaternary. Even with erosion rates 10 to 100 times greater than the DOE calculated, (1) an unroofing scenario for a repository is incredible, and (2) exposing a potentially important hydrologic contact above the repository horizon between welded and nonwelded tuff layers is also exceedingly remote (Fig. 2). The bedded tuffs and its basal contact with the Topopah Spring Tuff of the Paintbrush Group (Fig. 2) is a hydraulic interface thought to be an important controlling element on water infiltration through the unsaturated tuff layers comprising the mountain.

CONCLUSIONS

Repository programs in other countries have not proceeded to a focused site-specific study as the United States has at Yucca Mountain. The human and institutional experience of projecting the geologic performance of a site in combination with an engineered repository system over millennia is nascent. The experience of gathering and presenting geologic evidence to demonstrate regulatory compliance over such a period is equally unprecedented. The DOE's first test of the repository program's regulatory structure with real data and a compliance argument was disappointing in retrospect. The lessons learned from trying to address the requirements imposed by an eight-word PAC can be applied in the period before entering a licensing phase with the NRC just after the turn of the twenty-first century. There are three areas for improvement.

The first is the importance of communication to help define expectations, especially subtleties in how the NRC interprets their regulation that could be lost to those who did not participate in writing it, and the DOE's intentions or plans for how to comply with it. The second is the importance of good documentation prepared in a manner that is most useful to the regulatory audience. The third is the need for flexibility and careful appraisal for what the geologic sciences can demonstrate. To be successful, the DOE needs flexibility in setting geologic and engineering specifications and requirements for the natural and man-made components of a repository system, and the NRC needs flexibility in evaluating the compliance arguments that are made.

The DOE proceeded to develop a topical report to test the regulation, and as a result, can make two conclusions about the experience with respect to documentation, and one more generic conclusion that bears upon all three areas mentioned above: (1) the topical report would have benefited from including additional information in the geotechnical basis for the compliance argument (e.g., such as a corroborating dating technique), and (2) the persuasiveness of the DOE's submittal was affected by targeting the specific and limited issue in the PAC, because corroborating data from other site characterization study programs were not brought in to show the internal consistency of the DOE's conclusions. As for the generic conclusion; debate about how well we understand site-specific attributes like PACs is diminished if it takes place outside a holistic context that includes the physical process models and numeric models developed from them to explain the performance of a site as a total system of natural and engineered barriers. Attention may not be focused on a site's most important attributes. In an era of limited resources, this is very important.

Communication

To successfully interpret the regulation and its administrative record, to develop a scientific approach, and to package data and conclusions demonstrating regulatory compliance in a way that can be defended requires communication with the regulator. It also requires a working relationship that permits ease in communicating to (1) detect differences in how the regulator interprets their regulation, (2) clarify expectations, and (3) indicate intentions so as to minimize surprises. The quality of more frequent opportunities for communication that technology now allows (for example, videoconferencing), is still dependent on a willingness to listen.

At their root the NRC's criticisms arose because effective communication of two things were lacking; the NRC's expectations and the DOE's intentions. Defining expectations in how the NRC interprets their regulation is important because the DOE may have a different interpretation when faced with the practical matter of designing a data collection program, framing a compliance argument with available capabilities and technology, and prudent management of resources. Resources are simply not available to the geologic disposal program so as to satisfy the expectations of all critics or sustain a scientific investigation into perpetuity.

In communicating expectations, the NRC is faced with two end members—overspecification and silence. Between these a balance must be struck. In the former, extensive written acceptance criteria for compliance may give satisfaction to the regulator that expectations have been communicated. Overspecification, especially too early in the investigation, risks overwhelming a project in detail and promotes tracking of comments and concerns that become moot given (1) time, (2) the insights provided by additional data, and (3) maturation of understanding. It constricts options that should be open during a period of exploration and site characterization, before the formality of licensing. Silence, on the other hand, risks that a project does not move toward completion.

In communicating intentions, the DOE needs to address the regulation's past administrative record and ensure that the chosen approach is sound by including the basis on which it should be considered adequate. Informal discussions can take place between the DOE and NRC staffs, and these opportunities can be used to explore ideas and approaches. Communication that is early enough allows feedback on how a compliance argument might be evaluated, or the acceptability of alternative approaches.

Documentation

The DOE's site characterization phase is now concluding and the project is now at the threshold of entering a compliance phase. The documentation of the DOE's scientific design and technical approaches, assumptions, alternative interpretations, sources of uncertainty, and conclusions need to be written for the correct audience. The data or information that allows the NRC to independently assess the DOE's conclusions must also be provided.

Writing regulatory documentation is an acquired skill that most universities do not prepare geologists to do well. Geologists working toward advanced degrees are focused toward independent research that can be quite narrow in scope: designing research programs, and reporting results in the professional journals of scientific societies. This research style of writing targets a specific audience and has a specific purpose. The research audience consists of similarly trained specialists: colleagues and generalists in the same discipline. This audience possesses a relatively homogeneous skill mix, where a common awareness of the technical lexicon is assumed and intuitive transitions in logic may go unexplained. The purpose is to advance the envelope of knowledge by using the scientific method to gather and report data and advocate interpretations or conclusions that readers may find persuasive or not. It is a style and purpose generally not useful to a regulatory agency.

The staff of regulatory agencies like the NRC evaluate geological work to make health and safety findings. The regulatory audience is likely to have a heterogeneous mixture of skills. Staff evaluating work may be geologic specialists in the work under review, but usually they are not. There typically will be a few specialists and generalists in earth science and other disciplines like engineering, and there are always legal specialists and managers (Fig. 5). Review teams may be composed of people having a mixture of these backgrounds and skills.

The purpose of regulatory documentation is to persuade. The preparer is an advocate of the data, interpretations, and conclusions it contains, and thorough documentation possesses the quality of being more persuasive. Documentation that provides the reasoning for choices, operative assumptions, and discussion of sampling or analytical uncertainty performs several important functions: (1) it is better able to persuade a primarily nonspecialist audience, (2) it allows work to be reconstructed without recourse to the original investigator, and (3) it is better able to withstand legal challenge. In regulatory documentation it is, therefore, important to explain basic physical principles for applied tech-

Who is the Target Audience?

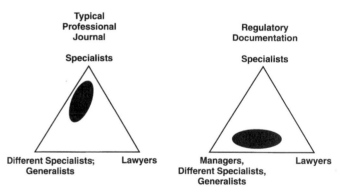

Figure 5. Ternary diagram showing the typical skill mixes for the readership of professional geological journals and that for regulatory documentation based on applications of geologic research. The writing in professional journals tends to be by specialists, for specialists, seeking to persuade each other rather than a broader audience. Documentation of geoscientific work for a regulatory audience needs to be written for a heterogeneous skill mix in order to increase the likelihood that the regulator will find interpretations persuasive and be convinced by the conclusions that are offered. Thoroughness in documentation is necessary to make data, interpretations and conclusions persuasive, independently reproducible, and legally defensible.

niques, decompose complex subject matter, and defend the rationale for choices in technique or approach that are made so that evaluators are better able to agree with the conclusions that are reached, even though this can result in a somewhat pedantic style of writing. Original data is required in tables or appendices and spatial reporting of field sampling programs needs to be precise enough to provide traceability and replication of sampling programs to allow an independent assessment to be performed.

Flexibility

Although the DOE has the burden of proof in a repository licensing action, the state of knowledge from site characterization will be far from complete (McGarry and Echols, 1995) and what we know will be uncertain (McGarry and Echols, 1994). A standard of proof based on the *preponderance of evidence* may be better suited for licensing a repository system for long performance periods than the NRC's traditional *reasonable assurance* when the limitations for what geological methods and tools can demonstrate are taken into account. An analogy is the difference between the standards of proof used in criminal (reasonable doubt) and civil proceedings (preponderance of evidence); however, the NWPA (NWPA, 1983, section 111[6][1] specifically cites the reasonable assurance standard for repository licensing. The challenge will be to make findings with reasonable assurance when in all likelihood the geoscience conclusions that underpin findings are based on a preponderance of evidence.

How the NRC views its administrative record (comment responses, internal guidance and positions, etc.) bears on the flexibility the NRC brings to evaluations of data, analyses, and compliance arguments. In studying any geologic system for isolating nuclear waste, flexibility, and the process of adaptation that is characteristic of the scientific method are important qualities to internalize.

Geologists can do a better job designing study programs and documenting their work to construct compliance arguments if (1) the regulation's expectations are understood in combination with all supplementary guidance, (2) guidance is placed in the context of a specific site, and (3) expectations do not require a degree of demonstration that is counterintuitive to what the science can demonstrate. With the example provided by the topical report, the DOE dealt with points 1 and 2 unilaterally, in a manner then judged to be reasonable but without prior NRC feedback. With respect to point 3, as this paper explains, the DOE viewed some of the NRC's comments as establishing problematic expectations for judging compliance.

The need for flexibility in setting requirements and specifications in the United States' geologic disposal program for high-level nuclear wastes was stressed by the National Academy of Sciences (NAS, 1990, p. 27–28). Flexibility in the evaluation of compliance documentation against a *reasonable assurance* standard is equally important (McGarry and Echols, 1994). Flexibility in evaluating data, interpretations, and conclusions in light of impacts on performance of the site as a total natural and engineered system is especially important. Arguments over interpretation of data, technical details, or importance of uncertainties can often be disposed when placed in a framework that weights their sensitivity to total system performance. The DOE needs to ensure that performance impacts and explanations for why performance is or is not sensitive to a parameter are documented so the NRC is not put into a position of being expected to draw these conclusions prima facie. In retrospect, the DOE's assessment of erosion and its sensitivity on system performance in the topical report was not as explicit as it could have been.

In the end, however, a wide variation in DOE's denudation rates for the Yucca Mountain site can be tolerated. If viewed from a performance perspective, the site is insensitive to the erosion parameter and the range of variation in the parameter can be adequately bounded to make a compliance case. DOE's hillslope denudation rates, valley cutting rates, and alluvial incision rates can be increased by 10 or even 100 times their calculated values over 10 k.y. and still have no likelihood of unroofing a repository, and very little likelihood of degrading the landscape to expose the hydrologically important bedded tuffs, locally incising the bedrock, or removing or redistributing enough alluvium to disturb the graded profile to base level in the Amargosa Desert.

Recent developments

A panel convened by the National Academy of Science in 1995 to look at the DOE's work on erosion, among other issues, offered technical comments on the VCR dating technique that touched on aspects of those made by the NRC (NAS, 1995). The DOE responded to the NRC's nine comments on the topical report (DOE, 1995) and in February 1996 a letter from the NRC (1) closed all nine open items related to their 1994 comments on the topical report, (2) stated that they would not rely on the VCR dating technique to support licensing conclusions without corroboration with another technique, (3) forward-referenced information they expected to see if DOE prepares a license application for Yucca Mountain (for example, Be^{10} dating results), and (4) stated that the NRC had no additional questions (NRC, 1996).

A new rulemaking by the EPA began in 1996 and is expected to revisit the 10,000-year performance requirement and establish a site-specific safety standard for Yucca Mountain. In response, the NRC will need to conform its existing regulation to the new EPA rule. The NRC may do this with a new site-specific regulation, or an amendment to 10 CFR Part 60.

Excavation of the underground access tunnels for the Exploratory Studies Facility were completed in April 1997. Two portals for the access tunnels enter the mountain from the east and ramps lead down westward to the potential repository layer about 330 m below the crest of Yucca Mountain. The volcanic stratigraphy overlying the potential repository layer is penetrated twice along an 8-km-long, U-shaped tunnel. Alcoves have been constructed and test programs are under way to provide insights that only in situ study allow, including the thermal impacts of simulated waste heat on the rock.

ACKNOWLEDGMENTS

This paper is based on an oral presentation at the "Geology, The Voice of Reason" session held during the 1994 G.S.A. Annual Meeting in Seattle, Washington, and the author's experience from 1990–1996 on the Licensing Team in the DOE's Yucca Mountain Site Characterization Office, Las Vegas, Nevada. Subjective judgements or recommendations are attributable to the author, but they are not made without considerable personal immersion in the regulatory environment that this paper describes. The comments of internal DOE and contractor reviewers and two anonymous G.S.A. peer reviewers assisted in sharpening the points made in this paper.

REFERENCES CITED

Bates, R. L. and Jackson, J. A., 1980, Glossary of geology: Falls Church, Virginia, American Geological Institute, 751 p.

Department of Energy (DOE), 1995, Response to NRC staff comments on the Topical report "Evaluation of the potentially adverse condition 'evidence of extreme erosion during the Quaternary Period' at Yucca Mountain, Nevada": Letter w/numbered enclosure, R. A. Milner to J. J. Holonich, dated April 13, 1995, 220 p.

Department of Energy (DOE), 1993, Topical report: Evaluation of the potentially adverse condition "Evidence of extreme erosion during the Quaternary Period" at Yucca Mountain, Nevada: Las Vegas, Nevada, U.S. Department of Energy, Yucca Mountain Site Characterization Project, YMP/92-41-TPR, 71 p.

Department of Energy (DOE), 1988, Site characterization plan, Yucca Mountain site, Nevada Research and Development Area, Nevada: Washington, D.C., U.S. Department of Energy, Office of Civilian Radioactive Waste Management, DOE/RW-0199, 5,385 p.

Harrington, C. D., and Whitney, J. W., 1987, Scanning electron microscope method for rock varnish dating: Geology, v. 15. p. 967–970.

McGarry, J. M., and Echols, F. S., 1994, Treatment of uncertainty in the NRC regulatory process, *in* Proceedings, Fifth International High-Level Radioactive Waste Management Conference, Las Vegas, Nevada: American Nuclear Society and American Society of Civil Engineers, p. 1404–1415.

McGarry, J. M., and Echols, F. S., 1995, Use of limited information in a license application to construct a repository, *in* Proceedings, Sixth International High-Level Radioactive Waste Management Conference, Las Vegas, Nevada: American Nuclear Society and American Society of Civil Engineers, p. 201–204.

Meehan, R. L., 1984, The atom and the fault: Experts, earthquakes, and nuclear power: Cambridge, Massachusetts, Massachusetts Institute of Technology Press, 160 p.

Morrison, R. B., 1991, Introduction, Quaternary nonglacial geology; Conterminous U.S., *in* Morrison, R. B., ed., The Geology of North America, Decade of North American Geology: Boulder, Colorado, Geological Society of America, v. K-2, p. 1–12.

National Academy of Sciences (NAS), 1990, Rethinking high-level radioactive waste disposal, A position statement of the Board on Radioactive Waste Management: Washington, D.C., National Academy of Sciences/National Research Council, National Academy Press, 34 p.

National Academy of Sciences (NAS), 1995, Review of U.S. Department of Energy technical basis report for surface characteristics, preclosure hydrology and erosion: Washington, D.C., National Academy of Sciences/National Research Council, National Academy Press, 131 p.

Nuclear Regulatory Commission (NRC), 1983, Staff analysis of public comments on Proposed Rule 10 CFR Part 60, Disposal of high-level radioactive wastes in geologic repositories: Washington, D.C., U.S. Nuclear Regulatory Commission, NUREG-0804.

Nuclear Regulatory Commission (NRC), 1989, NRC staff site characterization analysis of the Department of Energy's site characterization plan, Yucca Mountain site: Washington, D.C., U.S. Nuclear Regulatory Commission, NUREG-1347, 204 p.

Nuclear Regulatory Commission (NRC), 1991, Code of Federal Regulations; Title 10, Energy; Part 60, Disposal of high-level radioactive waste in geologic repositories: Washington, D.C., U.S. Nuclear Regulatory Commission, U.S. Government Printing Office, p. 85–118.

Nuclear Regulatory Commission (NRC), 1992, Meaning and use of the phrase "Quaternary Period" within 10 CFR Part 60: U.S. Nuclear Regulatory Commission, Draft Staff Position, Memorandum w/o numbered enclosure, R. Ballard to J. Holonich, dated August 17, 1992, 5 p.

Nuclear Regulatory Commission (NRC), 1993, Status of review of topical report on extreme erosion: Washington, D.C., U.S. Nuclear Regulatory Commission, Letter, B. Youngblood to D. Shelor, dated December 30, 1993, 4 p.

Nuclear Regulatory Commission (NRC), 1994a, NRC staff review of the U.S. Department of Energy topical report on extreme erosion: Letter w/numbered enclosure, J. J. Holonich to R. A. Milner, dated August 22, 1994, 20 p.

Nuclear Regulatory Commission (NRC), 1994b, Preliminary detailed concerns on the topical report "Evaluation of the potentially adverse condition of extreme erosion during the Quaternary Period at Yucca Mountain": Washington, D.C., U.S. Nuclear Regulatory Commission; Memorandum w/numbered enclosure, R. Ballard to J. Holonich, dated January 11, 1994, 5 p.

Nuclear Regulatory Commission (NRC), 1996, Issue resolution status report on the potentially adverse condition—Evidence of extreme erosion during the Quaternary Period at Yucca Mountain: Letter w/numbered enclosure, M. Bell to R. A. Milner, dated February 29, 1996, 17 p.

Nuclear Waste Policy Act (NWPA), 1983, Nuclear Waste Policy Act of 1982: Washington, D.C., Public Law 97-425, 42 U.S.C. 10101–10226.

Palmer, A. R., 1983, Compiler, The decade of North American geology, geologic time scale: Geology, v. 11, p. 503–504.

Van Konynenburg, R. A., 1994a, Science and licensing: Let's get off the collision course, *in* Proceedings, Materials Research Society Symposium on the Scientific Basis for Nuclear Waste Management, Boston, Massachusetts, December 1993: Materials Research Society, v. 333, p. 183–191.

Van Konynenburg, R. A., 1994b, Limitations on scientific prediction and how they could affect repository licensing, *in* Proceedings, Fifth International High-Level Radioactive Waste Management Conference, Las Vegas, Nevada: American Nuclear Society and American Society of Civil Engineers, p. 285–291.

Whitney, J. W., and Harrington, C. D., 1993, Relict colluvial boulder deposits as paleoclimatic indicators in the Yucca Mountain region, southern Nevada: Boulder, Colorado, Geological Society of America Bulletin, v. 105, p. 1008–1018.

Manuscript Accepted by the Society June 5, 1997

Geological Society of America
Reviews in Engineering Geology, Volume XII
1998

Providing valid long-term projections of geologic systems for policy decisions: Can we succeed? Should we try?

Jeremy M. Boak
Los Alamos National Laboratory, Los Alamos, New Mexico 87545
Holly A. Dockery
Sandia National Laboratories, Albuquerque, New Mexico 87185-1326

ABSTRACT

Many environmental problems require modeling of long-term interactions of man-made and geologic systems. By using the term "model," we acknowledge that we will never know whether our descriptions of geologic features, events, and processes are unique and represent absolute reality. "Validation" of a long-term predictive model means that, on the basis of tests of the assumptions, inputs, outputs, and sensitivities, the model adequately reflects the recognized behavior of the portion of the system it intends to represent. Adequacy is driven by the needs of the application for which the model is developed. Most environmental applications are overprinted with political, scientific, and social requirements that add subjective influences to the definitions and interpretations of measures of adequacy. Therefore no single measure can be developed for the adequacy of a model. The public, on the other hand, may expect "validation" to describe an unobtainable absolute demonstration of "truth."

Scientists assessing long-term risk use various mechanisms to establish the adequacy of their models such as: (1) expert judgment to assign appropriate ranges of parameters where data are sparse, controversial, or unobtainable; (2) conservatism in assigning parameter values and process descriptions, including ignoring some potentially mitigating processes; and (3) stochastic simulation to assess the effect of uncertainty in descriptions and the sensitivity of performance predictions to uncertainty, and to examine alternative scenarios and process models. Other measures are undertaken to demonstrate that the effort to ensure validity has been comprehensive, including: (1) documentation of the structure of models, including justification for assumptions and simplifications, as well as the examination of alternative conceptualizations for the system; and (2) review by the scientific community and those who have a stake in the decisions that these models support.

Legal precedent recognizes that decisions with large consequences often demand judgments of the validity of conflicting descriptions of reality. The stochastic nature of natural phenomena and the value of models as guides to judgment (not final answers) are both acknowledged. The problem of compounding conservatisms, which leads to an inherently unreal and thus invalid, model, may also be understood. The scientific community can usefully project the range of future behavior of systems and must do so if well-reasoned choices are to be made about how humans should affect those systems. Unfortunately, the consequences (costs and risks) of abandoning or overburdening efforts to make long-term projections are rarely examined as critically as are the efforts to project interactions of man-made systems with the geologic environment.

Boak, J. M., and Dockery, H. A., 1998, Providing valid long-term projections of geologic systems for policy decisions: Can we succeed? Should we try?, *in* Welby, C. W., and Gowan, M. E., eds., A Paradox of Power: Voices of Warning and Reason in the Geosciences: Boulder, Colorado, Geological Society of America Reviews in Engineering Geology, v. XII.

INTRODUCTION

In recent years there has been an increased emphasis on the need to validate ground-water models, driven largely by those engaged in radioactive waste disposal. . . . It is our intent to approach the question of validation on two levels: (1) the philosophical level, and (2) the practical level of validating a site-specific model. We will argue that, at both levels, validation has no place in hydrology.
                                   —Konikow and Bredehoeft, 1992, p. 75

Many environmental problems require modeling of long-term interactions of man-made and geologic systems. Examination of such long-term interactions has mainly been confined to investigations for disposal of radioactive wastes, generally high-level and transuranic wastes and spent nuclear fuel, because of the long half-lives of radionuclides and their continued hazard potential, even at low activities. However, the significance of such questions may be equally important for nonradioactive wastes, because some elements are also potentially hazardous at low concentrations and do not decay. Over periods shorter than the thousands to millions of years that are relevant to high-level radioactive waste disposal, geologic processes may still be complex enough to call the results of hydrologic, geochemical, and tectonic models into question.

It is not enough simply to project the consequences of geologic processes acting on human systems; it is necessary to show that we have adequate understanding of the processes acting in these systems. Such a demonstration is needed to assert that our understanding is sufficient to project the full range of reasonably likely consequences, given the variability and heterogeneity of the natural world (in both space and time).

The title of an international collective opinion of the Organization for Economic Cooperation and Development's Nuclear Energy Agency—*Disposal of Radioactive Waste: Can Long-Term Safety Be Evaluated?* (OECD/NEA, 1991a)—embodies the concern over such long-term projections. The validity of model projections arises as a problem primarily where modeling results are applied to legal and regulatory judgments regarding potential risks to populations and the environment. It is interesting that this reexamination of what constitutes scientific proof is driven by institutions that scientists commonly consider far less rigorous than the scientific community.

Certain premises that we take to be central to the scientific enterprise underlie our discussion of model validation. The first centers around the term "model." Konikow and Bredehoeft (1992, p. 75) define a model as "a representation of a real system or process." As they point out, different types of models exist, such as numerical or analytic, stochastic or deterministic. Their definition contains a crucial distinction that clarifies the scientific meaning of model validation. Because a model "represents" a system or process, it is not the original. By using the term "model," we already acknowledge that absolute validity or uniqueness does not exist, perhaps especially for descriptions of geologic features, events, and processes. The problem of nonuniqueness has been illustrated clearly for geochemical systems by Bethke (1992).

This lack of absoluteness does not mean that a validation exercise cannot be useful when properly constrained by the objectives of an application. Indeed, the programs for validation of hydrogeological models cited by Konikow and Bredehoeft (Swedish Nuclear Power Inspectorate, SKI, 1990, 1992) all concluded that validation was a continuing process that seeks adequate, not absolute, validation of models.

We also separate our use of the terms "validation" and "model validation" from the terms "verification," or "code verification," which have also been brought into the discussion about the application of models to long-term projections. Verification is appropriately applied to the process of determining whether a computer program has accurately embodied the equations set out as the basis for the program, and whether the numerical implementation of the equations converges appropriately. The questions asked are "Does the program calculate the formulas it says it does?" and "Will the model converge, given credible input parameters?" These questions can be answered with reasonable certainty, and therefore the implication of "truth" is limited and repeatedly testable. Validation, the assertion that a model describes the operation of a real system, is a thornier question.

MODEL VALIDATION: AN EXAMPLE

An example taken from a source (Science News; Peterson, 1992b) readily available to the average lay reader will illustrate the difficulty we have accepting the assertion of Bredehoeft and Konikow (1993) that the public has a clear and absolute perception of what constitutes validation. It also shows why we feel that relative validity can be understood and accepted by the public for models that describe long-term processes and that this relative validity actually represents what scientists have long acknowledged about scientific "proof." If, as Bredehoeft and Konikow point out, science is distinguished by its perpetual falsifiability, validation has always been a relative term when applied to scientific results. The example relates to Newton's model for the attractive force between two masses, a relationship commonly incorporated in models of complex geologic systems, including models of flow and transport in ground water.

Three hundred years of validating Newton's Law

More than 300 years ago, Isaac Newton devised a remarkably simple mathematical relationship to encapsulate how the force of gravity depends on the separation of two objects and their masses. Since then, researchers have sought possible deviations from Newton's gravitational law, but have generally failed to produce any compelling experimental evidence of such discrepancies. *Instead these efforts—especially over the last decade—have substantially increased the precision with which experiment agrees with theory.* (emphasis added)

The final results confirmed that Newton's law of gravity holds to within two parts in 10,000 for masses a few meters apart. 'We have plans to improve this further,' Paik says. (emphasis added) (Peterson, 1992b, p. 215)

The article (Peterson, 1992b) describes experiments testing validity of the Newtonian formulation for gravity using very precise measurements with what the experimenters call a "gravity gradiometer." Such experiments are commonly directed at determining whether some additional fundamental force might be identified, beyond gravity, electromagnetic, and nuclear forces (strong and weak).We note that any deviation that did appear would probably result in the formulation of such a fifth force, rather than an invalidation of Newton's "Law of Gravity." Thus, the way we construct models influences how we think about validity. These investigators, the article indicates, are interested in searching for gravitational waves, and are mainly concerned about extraneous effects. The article demonstrates that validation is, indeed, never absolute. However, one must ask, how many calculations including gravitational effects in hydrologic or geophysical models need incorporate the degree of precision required for these calculations? Is the Newtonian formulation conditionally valid for hydrologic and geophysical models?

Chaos and gravity on geologic time scales

The second article describes computations of the Earth's orbital motions for geologically significant periods. The complexity of such calculations is beyond the reach of analytical methods, but recent advances in computing have enabled calculation using "averaged" differential equations. These smooth out higher frequency variations in planetary motions, but incorporate long-term trends for the eight main planets. However, not all the chaos is removed:

Strikingly different methods of computing and tracking the evolution of planetary orbits now strongly suggest that chaos lurks in the planetary clockwork. . . . The presence of chaos would mean that although the solar system has apparently survived for more than 4.5 billion years in some semblance of its present form, nothing guarantees that its future holds no surprises. . . . Numerically solving, or integrating, the resulting set of equations—which include about 150,000 algebraic terms—shows that *the ability to predict the orbits of the inner planets, including Earth, declines sharply within a few tens of millions of years.* (emphasis added) (Peterson, 1992a, p. 120)

Thus, the geologic record extends for perhaps one hundred times the range over which our knowledge of gravity (including the relativistic effects) gives us the ability to project the orbital motion of Earth.

This result doesn't necessarily mean that Earth is likely to wander from its usual path in the next 10 million years or so, perhaps ending up on a collision course with Mars or Venus. It does suggest, however, that the traditional mathematical tools of celestial mechanics would fail to predict such an event far in the future. *In a chaotic system, there is no way to prove that something can't ever happen.* (emphasis added) (Peterson, 1992a, p. 121)

Does this, then, invalidate the use of the Newtonian formulation of gravity for geologic systems operating over geologic time scales? If so, what then, is the period or the scale over which Newton's model is valid, if any?

Relativistic gravity on geologic time scales

Finally, we examine the geological significance of the relativistic description of gravity. If Newton's formulation of gravity is valid, it should be valid over the long periods of time of interest to geologists, as suggested above. Kuhn (1970) has argued that Newton's formulation is not just an approximation of the actual behavior of the universe as described by Einstein. He asserts that Einstein's theory redefines how the universe works, invalidating Newton's Law. Recent calculations for the obliquity of Mars provide an interesting insight into the significance of that invalidation.

Wisdom and Touma's calculations show that orbital variations alone can cause such drastic changes. Their model suggests that the resulting tilt angles can range from about 11 degrees to 49 degrees. . . . Moreover, these irregular variations in the tilt of Mars over intervals longer than 10 million years appear inherently unpredictable. . . . *Indeed, different orbital models now qualitatively agree that the average obliquity of Mars abruptly increased about 4 million years ago.* . . . Curiously, Wisdom and Touma found *no such tilt transition when they excluded the effects of general relativity from their equations of motion for the planets.* (emphasis added) (Peterson, 1993, p. 132–133)

The question of interest remains whether invalidation of Newton's model for long-term projections of planetary motions means that we must abandon the term "valid" when discussing the influence of gravity gradients on the motion of water through porous media beneath the surface of the Earth.

Model validation: example results

The results of these examinations of Newton's model for gravitational attraction suggest that the model is reasonably valid for many of the uses geologists commonly require. These include defining gravity anomalies as exploration targets, launching satellites, and modeling flow and transport in ground water.

However, the Newtonian model is not adequately valid for a variety of applications of interest to the scientific community in general, and to geologists and planetary geologists in specific. Applications for which the Newtonian model is inadequately valid include ruling out the existence of a fifth force, modeling relativistic systems, and black holes, and long-term projections of orbits and obliquity, and their climatic effects.

MODEL VALIDATION: COMMON DEFINITIONS, A DEFINITION FOR LONG-TERM PREDICTIVE MODELS, AND SOME CAVEATS

Bredehoeft and Konikow(1993, p. 178) assert that "The word validation has a clear meaning to both the scientific community and the general public." We suggest this is not clear. One dictionary (Gove, 1965, p. 980) defines *valid* as:

1: having legal efficacy or force; esp.: executed with the proper legal authority and formalities 2a: well grounded: SOUND b(1): having a conclusion correctly derived from premises [~ argument] (2) correctly derived from premises [~ inference] 3: EFFECTIVE, EFFICACIOUS

The accompanying note on synonyms suggests that:

VALID, SOUND, COGENT, CONVINCING, TELLING mean having such force as to compel acceptance. VALID implies being supported by objective truth or generally accepted authority; SOUND implies being based on flawless reasoning and on solid grounds. . . .

This definition clearly admits a range of meaning to validity, from the judgmental (legal or other authority) to the logical (derived from premises or objective truth). Acceptability is as much a part of the common meaning of the word as is absoluteness.

Bredehoeft and Konikow (1993) state in the next sentence that "Within the scientific community the validation of scientific theory has been the subject of philosophical debate." If there is a philosophical debate, does it not likely arise from an issue about meaning? The debate arises largely because most scientists accept a working definition of validation without keeping constantly in mind the perpetual falsifiability of any of their conclusions. Few of our publications acknowledge that our models did not explicitly account for relativistic effects.

We present the following working definition of validation for models that project the long-term consequences of geologic processes:

Validation – the determination, based on tests of the model assumptions, inputs, outputs, and sensitivities that the model adequately reflects the recognized behavior of the portion of the system it intends to represent.

This definition is consistent with the definitions of Rechard (1995, p. Glos -20) for "validation" and "validation of an (applied) model," which stress that "few objections can be fairly brought" against something valid, and that "sufficient testing" and "sufficient accuracy" require subjective judgments made in the continuing process of validation of a model. Zuidema (1991, p. 22) makes it clear that validation is not absolute in discussing models when he uses phrases like, ". . . proving that the predictions are sufficiently 'close to the truth' (i.e., are valid) . . ." and, "in a strict sense, rigorous proof of matching 'the truth' is not possible because . . . models can only be disproven (invalidated) . . ."

In the collective opinion mentioned in the introduction (OECD/NEA, 1991a), the Organization for Economic Cooperation and Development's Nuclear Energy Agency (OECD/NEA) also stresses that validation is a process:

Model validation is the process of assuring that the models used adequately represent the real system behavior. . . . Validation of long-term predictions must focus on the adequacy of modeling processes that may define system performance under a reasonable variety of possible futures. There is no way to validate system performance predictions over long times, but the adequacy of specific aspects of the modeling may be

supported through a variety of laboratory, field and natural analogue studies.(OECD/NEA, 1991a, p. 18)

The International Atomic Energy Agency (IAEA) states that:

A model cannot be considered validated until sufficient testing has been performed to ensure an acceptable level of predictive accuracy (note that the acceptable level of accuracy is judgmental and will vary depending on the specific problem to be addressed by the model). (IAEA, 1982, p. 43)

The Radioactive Waste Management Committee of the OECD/NEA further notes that:

Validation efforts are a necessary part of the process to achieve confidence in predictive capabilities, and it is necessary to develop a strategy for establishing priorities with respect to validation (OECD/NEA, 1991b, p. 72).

It might well be that a repository built so that its performance can be assessed with high confidence is more acceptable than a repository aimed at maximum safety. (OECD/NEA, 1991b, p. 73)

The concept that further testing brings increased confidence, but not absolute confirmation, in projections of the long-term safety of geologic repositories for radioactive wastes is well recognized by the organizations whose representatives have sponsored the most intensive investigations of validation for hydrologic and geochemical models. The citations indicate that validation includes the identification of the parts of the system in which uncertainties have the greatest significance to the projection of performance. System processes or features that have little effect on the significant measures of performance may be adequately validated with little effort.

The OECD/NEA collective opinion points out that "the ultimate objective of safety assessments is to provide a basis for well-founded decisions about radioactive waste disposal systems" (OECD/NEA, 1991a, p. 18). This use of the term "validation" then refers to a process governed by evaluation of where a model might fail, a process terminated by some consensus that the remaining uncertainties are acceptable.

This usage *may* be misleading to the public; they may expect a model to present an unobtainable absolute validation —"the truth." Konikow and Bredehoeft do not provide evidence for their assertion that the operational definitions discussed above "are certainly contrary to the prevailing scientific and layman's view of validation" (Konikow and Bredehoeft, 1992, p. 78). One of us has participated in dozens of public tours to Yucca Mountain (the U. S. candidate site for geologic disposal of high-level radioactive waste and spent nuclear fuel), involving dialogue with hundreds of average citizens concerned enough to spend a day learning about these unprecedented activities. In those tours, such an expectation of absoluteness was not encountered.

Average citizens do not commonly discuss model validity, but they do recognize, in general, that absolute certainty with respect to long-term projections is not available. Perhaps it is the scientific community that considers what they provide to be "truth." Such an assertion has been made by a U.S. Geological Survey geologist responding to another scientist's plea for compromise in interpreting apparently conflicting age determinations of recent volcanism near Yucca Mountain. Apart from any definition of "valid," this erroneous view of science is dangerous both to the scientific community and to the public.

The *potential* for such misunderstanding, however, should not necessarily be grounds for rejecting the use of the term "validation." All earth scientists have been disturbed by the ability of elements of the public to misconstrue the meaning of "evolution" and "natural selection," but none has suggested that the terms should be abandoned because of this demonstrated, sometimes willful, misinterpretation. There are interesting parallels between the evolution/creation debate and the debate over disposal of radioactive wastes.

However, a conditional definition of validation places a substantial burden on the modeler to define and demonstrate adequacy. Decision-makers must also be responsible for understanding and defending the determination that models are adequately validated for the purpose for which they were developed. The opportunity exists for extended disputes about those definitions and demonstrations. These disputes can be conducted in the scientific literature, in the legal arena, or in the political realm.

RECOGNIZED MEANS OF VALIDATION

A variety of methods have been developed to evaluate the adequacy of models and to demonstrate that reasonable efforts have been made to examine significant potential failure modes for both the model and the derived estimates of long-term performance. We will discuss three mechanisms to establish the adequacy of models for long-term risk assessments: (1) elicitation of expert judgment, (2) conservatism, and (3) stochastic simulation.

Elicitation of expert judgment

Formal elicitation of expert judgment is used to assign appropriate ranges to parameters where data are sparse, controversial, or unobtainable. Keeney and von Winterfeldt (1989) provide a useful perspective on the use of expert judgment. Their approach stresses the appropriate uses of explicit and implicit judgment and the value of quantifying experts' judgments. Such elicitation has been used in a variety of cases (EPRI, 1986, 1993; Trauth et al., 1992; Hora et al., 1991; Barnard et al., 1992). In some instances, one of the major benefits of such elicitation is that different perspectives on a given parameter are uncovered, and the resolution of these differences refines the model at the same time that values for a model parameter are elicited.

Expert judgment, especially when formally elicited and documented, may increase confidence that relevant features of the system have not been overlooked. Additional viewpoints external to a working group can remind the group of features it may have ignored at early stages and failed to reincorporate. External viewpoints may also identify processes or scenarios that are significant in other fields and whose importance to the problem at hand may not have been recognized.

Conservatism

Conservatism consists of assigning values to parameters, or forms, to model structures that are likely to overestimate the likelihood of failure of a system. For a waste disposal system, one may purposely assign higher values of percolation flux to the system than are reasonably expected to occur. This approach increases the likelihood that the modeled containment will be breached and that releases will occur in the modeling exercise. In some cases, conservatism is attained by ignoring the benefit of subsystems that would not be expected to fail completely. Taking no credit for the performance of the subsystem assures that the estimate of total performance bounds the likely behavior. The Yucca Mountain performance assessments have commonly assumed, for example, that once a waste package fails through corrosion, it no longer exists (Barnard et al., 1992). The model ignored the substantial potential for the waste package and its corrosion products to retard the release of radionuclides. This approach was taken in part because the expected benefit of waste-package retardation was difficult to quantify. Conservatism in assigning parameter values and process descriptions, including ignoring some potentially mitigating processes, adds confidence that errors in projections overestimate the likelihood of failure. Interestingly enough, the use of conservatism causes one to simulate unrealistic values to increase confidence in the result, thereby invalidating the model in order to validate the result.

Conservatism has its pitfalls as a means of validating results. In complex systems, presumably conservative assumption may not turn out to be truly conservative with respect to performance. A model developed for the Yucca Mountain site that presumed that all flow through the rock occurred in fractures (Wilson, 1992) was thought to be conservative, because fracture flow provided a much faster pathway for contaminated ground water to reach the accessible environment. However, a logical consequence of the model was that very little of the fast-moving water contacted the waste packages, and the releases calculated were lower than those in the standard composite porosity model (Barnard et al., 1992). It may also be possible for an assumption to be conservative for one performance measure, but not for another. Finally, application of conservatism can lead one to stop investigating phenomena that lie outside the range of the "conservative" estimates used. Where complex nonlinear processes interact, the potential for ignoring significant possible future states (both favorable and unfavorable to performance) exists when realistic ranges are not investigated for the sake of conservatism.

Stochastic simulation

Stochastic simulation involves repeated running of a computer code using different sets of parameter values in each run, to evaluate the effects of heterogeneity in the system, or uncertainty in the future state, on the performance of the system. It is also possible to perform multiple runs with fundamentally different model structures to examine the effects of uncertainties about the system description. The development of increasingly sophisticated algorithms for sampling the multidimensional space of model parameters has enabled investigators to test the structure of their models as well as the potential performance of systems for which we cannot run the real-world experiment.

The effect of uncertainty in system descriptions. Any model intended to project the range of future behaviors of a natural system must account for the spatial and temporal variability of the parameters of the model. Stochastic simulation allows the modeler to look at many potential future states. Estimates of the uncertainty about a parameter value must incorporate the known variability of a given parameter (heterogeneity) and some estimate of the degree to which that known variability represents the true variability of the population of values for a parameter (uncertainty). Such estimates were vital to the studies of validation that Bredehoeft and Konikow (1993; Konikow and Bredenhoeft, 1992) criticize in their papers and a critical feature of most efforts to assess the long-term performance of human systems (Barnard et al., 1992; Wilson et al., 1994). Most studies proposed for the Yucca Mountain site are intended to provide adequate estimates of the ranges of parameters for models of the hydrologic behavior of the site. The regulations originally proposed for geologic disposal called for evaluation of the geologic record for 20 times the regulatory period, to increase assurance that uncertainties have been adequately addressed (Nuclear Regulatory Commission, 1983).

In their discussion of the failure of models to project future states adequately, Konikow and Bredehoeft (1992) give an excellent example of the failure to account for both elements of uncertainty. The failure of Swain's (1978) projection of the behavior of the Coachella valley aquifer resulted from the use of a deterministic model for the likely recharge. Based on the historic values, the model underestimated stream flow in tributary streams in the region during the performance period for which the model was constructed. The use of stochastic simulation would readily enable the expansion of the range of recharge values to indicate ranges of values for the head changes (which were the major performance measure for this study). Capturing the uncertainty about the historic record as well as its heterogeneity should have constituted a central part of any discussion of the validity of the model. The lack of this analysis seems a readily apparent flaw even without the demonstrable failure of the model to predict the head values.

The sensitivity of performance predictions to uncertainty. From the description in Konikow and Bredehoeft (1992), it seems likely that a stochastic simulation of the Coachella Aquifer model would have identified the recharge value as a sensitive parameter of the model, perhaps even for the historic range of values. Thus, this method might have identified in advance those parameters for which the residual uncertainty might be most important. It can also identify parameters for which no realistic value drives the sys-

tem projections outside the acceptable range. Stochastic simulation cannot, of course, address unidentified uncertainties.

Alternative scenarios and process models. Stochastic simulation also permits one to identify critical differences among various states for the future condition of a system (scenarios) and alternative descriptions of the processes acting on that system (conceptual and numerical models). As Konikow and Bredehoeft (1992) point out in their example for the Dakota Aquifer, not all measures of the validity of a model are equally significant. Alternatively, one may state this observation as the following: several models for a given system may be equally valid for some measures of system performance. Rather than invalidating the use of the term validation, these statements indicate that judgments of validity are application-specific.

OTHER MEANS OF VALIDATION

Other measures are undertaken to demonstrate that the effort to ensure validity has been comprehensively considered. These include documentation of the model structure and results and review by scientific and stakeholder communities.

Documentation of model structure and results

Documentation of the model structure should list assumptions and inputs to the model, and justify the assumptions, simplifications, and parameter ranges used. It should also discuss alternative conceptual approaches to modeling the system, and potential implications for performance of these differences. All of this information is intended to allow others to duplicate the model results, to evaluate for themselves the significance of alternative conceptual models, and to identify potential gaps in the model structure.

External review

Review by the scientific community and those who have a stake in the decisions that these models support decreases the probability of omissions in the model description. Such review may occur at many stages. Tsang (1991) has suggested that standard peer review may be limited in its value because peer reviewers commonly do not have time to form independent, site-specific perspectives of a given model. He recommends use of multiple assessment groups, which provide a potentially more continuous review of the model development. Keeney and von Winterfeldt (1991) suggest that external technical and stakeholder involvement is critical to defensible elicitation of expert judgments. Thus, many steps of review beyond the typical review of a finished product offer the potential to avoid mistakes in modeling complex processes.

REGULATION AND VALIDATION

The question of validity of models has greatest significance where scientific data and conclusions are brought to bear on difficult legal and regulatory decisions. It is here that the confusion that Konikow and Bredehoeft (1992) are concerned with is most likely to present a problem. The debate about the validity of conclusions with little immediate impact on society is largely a matter for the technical community, which is reasonably aware of the dangers of overgeneralization. Although it would be preferable if popular accounts of scientific advances and speculations adequately identified the caveats common in most scientists' writing, it is only when such caveats have bearing on important social choices that this lack can take on critical importance. Legal and regulatory precedent recognizes that decisions with large consequences often demand judgments of the validity of conflicting descriptions of reality. We will discuss three aspects of the problem of uncertainties about models applied to regulatory questions: (1) the role of models as guides to understanding, (2) the stochastic nature of real-world phenomena, and (3) the danger of compounding conservatisms.

Models and nonuniqueness

At least for the high-level radioactive waste disposal arena, where the issue of validation of long-term projections of man-made and natural systems has received extensive study and discussion, the problem of residual uncertainty has been recognized by the appropriate regulatory authority, the Nuclear Regulatory Commission.

The degree of certainty implied by statistical definition has never characterized the administrative process. It is particularly inappropriate where evidence is 'difficult to come by, uncertain or conflicting because it is on the frontiers of scientific knowledge.'
—Nuclear Regulatory Commission, as cited in McGarry and Echols (1994)

Stochastic phenomena

The NRC has also dealt with the difficulties of making reasonable decisions on technical questions where some issues remain unresolved due to residual uncertainties. In its implementing regulations for high-level radioactive waste disposal (NRC, 1983), it acknowledges both the inherent uncertainties of long-term performance and the lack of firm proof for any assertion about the performance:

The projected performance of a high-level waste (HLW) repository is inherently uncertain, reflecting the long time period of concern during which relatively rare geologic, climatic, and human-initiated disruptions might occur.

and

Because of the long time period involved and the nature of the events and processes of interest, there will inevitably be substantial uncertainties in projecting disposal system performance. Proof of the future performance of a disposal system is not to be had in the ordinary sense of

the word in situations that deal with much shorter time frames [i. e., nuclear reactor licensing]. Instead, what is required is a reasonable expectation, on the basis of the record before the implementing agency [NRC] that compliance will be achieved.
—Nuclear Regulatory Commission Staff, as cited in McGarry and Echols (1994, p. 1408)

Although clear differences may arise between the applicant and the regulatory agency about when adequacy has been achieved, the language of the regulator clearly indicates that certainty is not what is expected. It may be added that proof "in the ordinary sense of the word" is likewise much debated for many of the shorter periods mentioned, as should be the case if scientific laws remain indefinitely falsifiable.

Compounding of conservatism

A major risk of the insistence on assigning conservative ranges to parameters and to choosing always the most conservative model of a given system is the danger that the compounding of conservatisms will result in a model that poorly represents reality. It may represent only the most extreme of behavior and offer no insight about the likely performance of the system. A special danger of this problem is that it may lead to extensive investigation of fringe phenomena, to the exclusion of study of true sensitivities. This difficulty has been recognized by the NRC in ruling on nuclear power plant issues:

Conservatisms and margins for error in . . . calculations are necessary and desirable, but must be footed to some extent in reasonable, scientific ground. Conservatism upon conservatism can distort technical data to the point where it no longer meaningfully describes the mechanism at issue.
—Nuclear Regulatory Commission, as cited in McGarry and Echols (1994, p. 1409)

CONCLUSIONS

The scientific community can usefully project the long-range future behavior of systems. It must do so if well-reasoned choices are to be made about how humans should affect those systems. To do so, it must present models of geologic behavior and defend at least their relative validity. Validation has reasonable meanings to the scientific and regulatory communities, which commonly recognize the lack of absoluteness. Perhaps scientists must learn to qualify their use of the term "validate" to remind both themselves and the public of the perpetual tentativeness of their conclusions, but it is unclear that such qualification will retain its value through such repetition. Abandoning the term will not resolve the problems of: (1) misapplication of models, (2) the need for demonstrations of adequacy, and (3) the debate over the adequacy of such demonstrations.

There are consequences (costs and risks) of abandoning or overburdening efforts to make long-term projections. These consequences are rarely examined as critically as are the efforts to project interactions of man-made systems with the geologic environment.

It has been fashionable, at least momentarily, in political circles to raise concerns about the impossibility of providing absolute guarantees of safety and the cost of abdicating the difficult decisions about what is an adequate evaluation of risk. Opponents of such risk-based cost/benefit analyses have emphasized the impossibility of determining the value of intangible resources in order to judge adequacy. Some of the same people have been willing to impose restrictions on industry that challenge them to develop better scientific and technological solutions (for example, more fuel-efficient automobiles). Perhaps the demand for risk-based cost/benefit analyses for various federal actions will provide a similar technological drive to the scientists and engineers and others developing methods to characterize hazards, evaluate risks, and support legislative and executive decisions.

The greatest difficulties encountered in making the long-term safety assessments that we have been involved in came in the attempt to capture the wealth of scientific information in a way that is internally consistent and to interpret the results so that they made decision-making easier not harder. The need for earth scientists to become involved in this sort of integrative task of demonstrating the adequacy of current models, and the value of further refinement is more important to us than the terminology applied.

REFERENCES CITED

Barnard, R. W., Wilson, M. L., Dockery, H. A., Gauthier, J. H., Kaplan, P. G., Eaton, R. R., Bingham, F. W., and Robey, T. H., 1992, TSPA 1991: An initial total-system performance assessment for Yucca Mountain: Albuquerque, Sandia National Laboratories Report SAND91-2795, 376 p.

Bethke, C. M., 1992, The question of uniqueness in geochemical modeling: Geochimica et Cosmochimica Acta, v. 56. p. 4315–4320.

Bredehoeft, J. D., and Konikow, L. F., 1993, Ground-water models: validate or invalidate?: Ground Water, v. 31, p. 178–179.

Electric Power Research Institute, 1986, Seismic hazard methodology for the central and eastern United States: Palo Alto, California, Electric Power Research Institute Report EPRI NP-4726, Project 101-21, v. 1: Methodology, 216 p.

Electric Power Research Institute, 1993, Earthquakes and tectonics expert judgment elicitation project: Palo Alto, California, Electric Power Research Institute Report EPRI TR-1020000, Project 3055-13, 194 p.

Gove, P. B., editor-in-chief, 1965, Webster's seventh new collegiate dictionary: Springfield, Massachusetts, G. C. Merriam Company, 1221 p.

Hora, S. C., von Winterfeldt, D., and Trauth, K. M., 1991, Expert judgment on inadvertent human intrusion into the Waste Isolation Pilot Plant: Albuquerque, Sandia National Laboratories Report, SAND90-3063, 363 p.

International Atomic Energy Agency, 1982, Radioactive waste management glossary: Vienna, Austria, International Atomic Energy Agency TEC-DOC-264, 44 p.

Keeney, R. L., and von Winterfeldt, D., 1989, On the uses of expert judgment on complex technical problems: Institute of Electrical and Electronics Engineers Transactions on Engineering Management, v. 36, p. 83–86.

Keeney, R. L., and von Winterfeldt, D., 1991, Eliciting probabilities from experts in complex technical problems: Institute of Electrical and Electronics Engineers Transactions on Engineering Management, v. 38, p. 191–201.

Konikow, L. F., and Bredehoeft, J. D., 1992, Ground-water models cannot be validated: Advances in Water Resources, v. 15, pp. 75–83.

Kuhn, T. S., 1970, The structure of scientific revolutions (second edition, enlarged): Chicago, University of Chicago Press, 210 p.

McGarry, J. M., III, and Echols, F. S., 1994, Treatment of uncertainty in the NRC regulatory process, in High Level Radioactive Waste Management: Proceedings, Fifth Annual International Conference: La Grange Park, Illinois, American Nuclear Society, p. 1404–1416.

Nuclear Regulatory Commission (NRC), 1983, Disposal of high-level radioactive wastes in geologic repositories: Washington, D.C., Code of Federal Regulations, Title 10, Part 60, p. 597–628 [1986 Edition of Title 10].

Organization for Economic Cooperation and Development/Nuclear Energy Agency, 1991a, Disposal of radioactive waste: Can long-term safety be evaluated?: Paris, Organization for Economic Cooperation and Development Publications, 45 p.

Organization for Economic Cooperation and Development/Nuclear Energy Agency, 1991b, Disposal of radioactive waste: Review of safety assessment methods: Paris, Organization for Economic Cooperation and Development Publications, 77 p.

Peterson, I., 1992a, Chaos in the clockwork: Science News, v. 141, p. 120–121.

Peterson, I., 1992b, Taking the measure of Newton's gravity law: Science News, v. 142, p. 215.

Peterson, I., 1993, Tilted: Stable Earth, Chaotic Mars: Science News, v. 143, p. 132–133.

Rechard, R. P., 1995, An introduction to the mechanics of performance assessment using examples of calculations done for the Waste Isolation Pilot Plant between 1990 and 1992: Albuquerque, Sandia National Laboratories Report SAND93-1378, 301 p.

Swain, L., 1978, Predicted water-level and water-quality effects of artificial recharge in the upper Coachella Valley, California, using a finite-element digital model: U. S. Geological Survey Water-Resources Investigation 77–29, 61 p.

Swedish Nuclear Power Inspectorate, 1990, The International INTRAVAL Project—Background and results: Paris, France, Organization for Economic Cooperation and Development, 45 p.

Swedish Nuclear Power Inspectorate, 1992, The International HYDROCOIN Project—Groundwater hydrology modeling strategies for performance assessment of nuclear waste disposal—Summary Report: Paris, France, Nuclear Energy Agency, Organization for Economic Cooperation and Development, 182 p.

Tsang, C. F., 1991, The modeling process and model validation: Ground Water, v. 29, p. 825–831.

Wilson, M. L., 1992, Comparison of two conceptual models of flow using the TSA, in High Level Radioactive Waste Management: Proceedings, Third Annual International Conference: La Grange Park, Illinois, American Nuclear Society, p. 882–890.

Wilson, M. L. and 24 others, 1994, Total-system performance assessment for Yucca Mountain—SNL second iteration (TSPA-1993): Albuquerque, Sandia National Laboratories Report SAND92-0479, 815 p., 2 vol.

Zuidema, P., 1991, Predicting and judging long-term safety of high-level waste disposal: main approaches and key issues, in Disposal of high-level radioactive wastes: radiation protection and safety criteria: Paris, France, Organization for Economic Cooperation and Development, Nuclear Energy Agency, p. 17–27

MANUSCRIPT ACCEPTED BY THE SOCIETY JUNE 5, 1997

Printed in U.S.A.

Afterword

No better modern example of the growing shift in defining enlightenment by the mystical instead of the scientific might exist than "the environment." A greater emphasis on intuition and emotions, rather than intellect, has gained popularity in many influential institutions and cultures. Relativists argue that viewpoints other than scientific are equally valid and deserve respect. The scientific community can probably expect this trend to continue.

As several of the authors have shown, conflict arises as one principle pulls one way and another pulls the other way. Wars are fought—personal and political, petty and important—over which principle takes precedence. The process of truth-seeking is made difficult by sorting through what is known, what is not known, and what is believed.

These statements are not meant to espouse one viewpoint but to stimulate the reader to investigate the source of a stakeholder's position. Without passing judgment, we might consider working out a theory of the meaning and justification for belief systems and actions in the dilemmas encountered. What belief system is guiding a stakeholder's principles? Is it rationalism, empiricism, expertism, monotheism, pantheism, polytheism, or something else altogether? Are the stakeholder's actions those of tactical deceptions, intellectual dishonesty, willful ignorance, or good will? From these beliefs and actions, what are the results? Are they misconceptions, fallacies, media hype, or heightened understanding? By asking ourselves these questions, we can confront our own "paradox of power." Ultimately, perhaps we can find the most effective and meaningful passage to serving society and our profession well.

MG

Printed in U.S.A.